D0479337

EVERYWOMAN

by the same author

EVERYWOMAN

A Gynaecological Guide for Life

Derek Llewellyn-Jones, M.D.

With Illustrations by Audrey Besterman

Faber and Faber
London and Boston

First published in 1971
by Faber and Faber Limited
3 Queen Square London WC1
First published in this edition 1972
Reprinted 1973 (three times), 1974, 1976 and 1977
Second edition 1978
Set by Filmtype Services Limited, Scarborough
Printed by
The Riverside Press Ltd, Whitstable, Kent
All rights reserved

© 1971, 1972, 1978 by Derek Llewellyn-Jones

British Cataloguing in Publication Data

Llewellyn-Jones, Derek
    Everywoman. – 2nd ed.
    1. Gynecology 2. Obstetrics
    I. Title
    618   RG101

    Library of Congress Catalog Card Number
    77–30546

    ISBN 0–571–04961–3
    ISBN 0–571–04960–5 Pbk

Contents

Illustrations

Tables

Preface

When *Everywoman* was published seven years ago, I hoped that it would provide a helpful source of information for women who were interested in their bodies and in the changes which occur during each period of their lives. Judging from the gratifying sales of the book, my hope has been realized!

But because of changes in attitude to woman's role in society, and to her sexuality, and because medical science has made considerable advances, in all fields of study, including obstetrics and gynaecology, a revised edition is needed so that the information is as up to date as possible.

None of this alters my belief that modern woman is interested in her femininity and wants information, which all too often, she is not given when she consults a doctor. Too many doctors still behave in an authoritarian way (I'll tell the little woman as much as is good for her to know), rather than involving the woman in her own health care, as an active participant.

I wrote in the first edition that several women had been asked for their critical comment on certain chapters and I thanked them. I have extended this process in preparing this edition, especially in the rewritten Chapters. These are Chapter 5, About sexuality; Chapter 7, Birth control and family planning; Chapter 12, The three stages of labour; and Chapter 18, Breasts and breast-feeding. The manuscript of Chapters 5 and 7 has been critically reviewed by Mrs Delys Sargeant, the staff and the course participants of the Social Biology Resources Centre, the University of Melbourne. Chapter 12 has been discussed with members of the Childbirth Education Association and matters in Chapter 18 were discussed with members of the Nursing Mothers Association of Australia. I have also received information from members of both Associations which drew to my attention the problems of adjusting to parenthood (in Chapter 15). I had not realized the extent of the problems before I received their comments, and am currently investigating it further. These changes, and the others which I have made to most chapters, will, I hope, make *Everywoman* a helpful gynaecological guide for life.

Fig. 7/1, The growth of the world's population, has been redrawn from *Population Bulletin*, **18**, 1, 1962 with their kind permission. I should also like to thank the Ortho Pharmaceutical Corporation, Raritan, N.J., for their permission to reproduce the illustrations of the vaginal diaphragm, Fig. 7/5A, B, C and E. Figs. 9/2 to 9/11 have been redrawn from a series published in *Pregnancy in Anatomical Transparencies* by the Carnation Co., and I am grateful to them for their permission.

I would like to thank my secretaries, Mrs Jenny Smith, Mrs Barbara Hodgson and Mrs Carole Kirkland for their help in typing and retyping alterations, and for keeping me up to my revision schedule.

Finally, I am happy that I can change the dedication I made in the first edition to two very special women. I dedicate this edition of *Everywoman* to three very special women. The first two I have known and loved for longer, and more closely than any others. They are my wife Elisabeth and our daughter, Deborah. The third has only recently joined us. She is Deborah's daughter, Gemma.

DEREK LLEWELLYN-JONES
Sydney, 1978.

Chapter 1

A Woman is Different

Even in these days of unisex fashions, the distinction between a man and a woman is relatively easy! Not only does a woman's psychological make-up differ from that of a man – although exactly how much of this is due to the prevailing cultural attitudes is not clear – but quite obviously she is anatomically different. Amongst Western communities, the breast has a unique sexual symbolism, and even if fashion diminishes its rotundity, the hemispherical mammary glands are a potent attraction for the male eye. In more primitive communities, where breasts are habitually exposed, they have little sexual connotation, being considered for what they are – a source of nourishment for the infant.

The more specific anatomical differences are of the genital organs. The proud male external genitals – the penis and the testicles – are absent in woman, a fact which suggested to Freud that many of woman's sexual problems related to an envy for the absent penis and a complex that the testicles had been castrated. Woman was therefore a mutilated male, and inferior to man. Freud was in fact more than unfair to women, and considerably confused about women, possibly because of his own upbringing in a traditional Jewish middle-class family. He held that woman had a smaller intellectual capacity, a far greater vanity, a constitutional passivity, a weaker sexuality, and a greater disposition to neurosis. At the same time, he considered her enigmatic, her femininity a complicated process, her psychology involved. Studies over the past half-century have shown that Freud's view of woman as an inferior, mutilated male is incorrect, and his assessment of her inferiority and her instability is more an indictment of the cultural environment in which she is brought up, than of her inherited make-up. In other words, a woman behaves in a certain way because she is brought up to believe that society expects her to behave in that way. This does not imply that she is weaker or inferior to a man, even if both are brought up by society to believe this. Indeed, longevity studies show that the female is stronger than the male, less likely to be aborted when in her mother's womb, more likely to be born alive, less likely to succumb to infection in the first years of life, and more likely to live beyond the age of 65.

Given the opportunity, a woman can succeed in most activities as well as a man, but in one activity she is unique. The human female is a mammal. She carries her infant in the womb until it is sufficiently well developed to survive, or at least to suck, she suckles it and cares for it. This process of internal development of the infant is only possible because the womb – or uterus – is in a protected position, enclosed by the strong bones of the female pelvis.

Although the uterus is central to the anatomical difference between male and female, the most obvious differences are those of the external genitalia, which will be described first. After that, the internal genital organs, the vagina, the uterus, the oviducts and the ovaries will be described, for unless a woman has some idea of her anatomy, much of what follows in this book will be less easily understood.

THE EXTERNAL GENITALIA IN THE FEMALE

The anatomical name for the area of the external genitalia in the female is the *vulva*. It is made up of several structures which surround the entrance to the vagina, and each of which has its own separate function (Fig. 1/1). The *labia majora* (or the large lips of the vagina) are two large folds of skin which contain sweat glands and hair follicles embedded in fat. The size of the labia majora varies considerably. In infancy and in old age they are small, and the fat is not present; in the reproductive years, between puberty and the menopause, they are well filled with fatty tissue. In front (looked at from between the legs), they join together in the pad of fat which surmounts the pelvic bone, and which was called the *'mount of Venus' (mons veneris)* by the ancient anatomists, when they noted that it was most developed in the reproductive years. Both of the labia, and more particularly the mons veneris, are covered with hair, the quantity of which varies from woman to woman. The pubic hair on the abdominal side of the mons veneris terminates in a straight line, whilst in the male the hair stretches upwards in an inverted 'V' to reach the umbilicus (Fig. 1/2). The inner surfaces of the labia majora

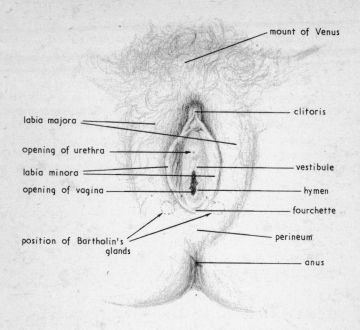

FIG. 1/1 The external genitals in a virgin

are free from hair, and are separated by a small groove from the thin labia minora, which guard the entrance to the vagina.

The *labia minora* (the small lips) are delicate folds of skin which contain little fatty tissue. They vary in size, and it was once believed that large labia minora were due to masturbation, which at that time was considered evil. It is now known that this is nonsense. In front, the labia minora split into two folds, one of which passes over and the other under the *clitoris*, and at the back they join to form the *fourchette*, which is always torn during childbirth. In the reproductive years, the labia minora are hidden by the enlarged labia majora, but in childhood and old age the labia minora appear more prominent because the labia majora are relatively small.

The *clitoris* is the exact female equivalent of the male penis. The fold of the labia minora which passes over it is equivalent to the male foreskin (prepuce). It is called the 'hood' and it covers and protects the sensitive end (or glans) of the clitoris. Some sexologists believe

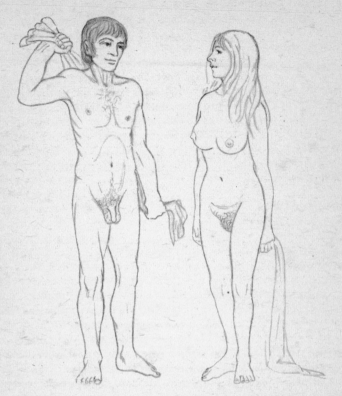

FIG. 1/2 The male and female from the front

that an 'adherent' hood reduces a woman's ability to achieve full
sexual pleasure, and have devised operations to 'free' the clitoris
from the hood – a sort of circumcision of the clitoris. It is unlikely that
the operation has anything more than a psychological effect and
should be avoided. The fold of skin which passes under the clitoris is
the equivalent of the small band of tissue which joins the pink glans of
the penis to the skin which covers it. It is called the *frenulum*.

   The clitoris is made up of tissue which fills with blood during sexual
excitement. The end of the clitoris is often very sensitive to touch, but
the area along the shaft of the clitoris, if stimulated, produces sexual
arousal in the same way that a man is sexually aroused when the shaft

of his penis is stimulated. In sexual intercourse, the movement of the man's penis in the vagina indirectly stimulates the clitoris and can lead to the woman having an orgasm. Many women do not get an orgasm during sexual intercourse but have deeply satisfying orgasms if they masturbate their clitoral area with their own finger or hand, or if their sexual partner caresses the area with finger or tongue (see page 76). The clitoris varies considerably in size, but is usually that of a green pea; as sexual excitement mounts, the clitoris increases in size. Once again this varies considerably between individuals.

The cleft below the clitoris and between the labia minora is called the *vestibule* (or entrance). Just below the clitoris is the external opening of that part of the urinary tract (the *urethra*) which connects the bladder to the outside world. In old women the urethral orifice may stretch, and the lining of the lower part of the urethra may be exposed.

Below the external urethral orifice is the hymen, which surrounds the vaginal orifice. The hymen is a thin incomplete fold of membrane, which has one or more apertures in it. It varies considerably in shape and in elasticity, but is generally stretched or torn during the first attempt at sexual intercourse. The tearing is usually followed by a minute amount of bleeding. In many cultures the rupture of the hymen (also called the maidenhead), and the consequent bleed, was considered a sign that the girl was a virgin at the time of marriage, and the bed was inspected on the morning after the first night of the honeymoon for evidence of blood. Although an 'intact' hymen is considered a sign of virginity, it is not a reliable sign, as in some cases coitus fails to cause a tear, and in others the hymen may have been torn previously by exploring fingers, either of the girl herself or of a consort. The stretching and tearing of the hymen at a first copulation may be painful, particularly if the partners are apprehensive or ignorant of sexual matters. If the couple are well adjusted, the discomfort is minimal. Childbirth causes a much greater tearing of the hymen, and after delivery only a few tags remain. They are called *carunculae myrtiformes* (Fig. 1/3). Just outside the hymen, still within the vestibule but deep beneath the skin, are two collections of erectile tissues which fill with blood during sexual arousal. Deep in the backward part of the vestibule are two pea-sized glands which also secrete fluid during sexual arousal and moisten the entrance to the vagina, so that the penis may more readily enter it without discomfort. These glands occasionally become infected. They are known as *Bartholin's glands*.

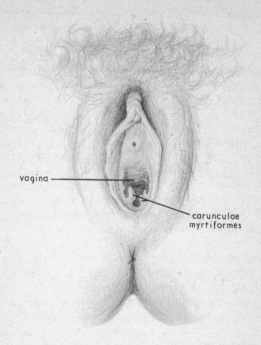

vagina

carunculae
myrtiformes

FIG. 1/3 The external genitals in a woman who has had a
child

The area of the vulva between the posterior fourchette and the
anus, and the muscles which lie under the skin, form a pyramid-
shaped wedge of tissue separating the vagina and the rectum. It is
called the *perineum*, and is of considerable importance in childbirth.

It is a matter of constant surprise to me that a large number of
women have never looked at their own, or any other woman's external genitals, and consequently are concerned that they may be
abnormal. I should say, first, that the diagram on page 17 is idealized
to some extent and that a considerable range of shapes and sizes of
the labia minora, the hymen and the hood of the clitoris are usual; so
that if a woman looks at her external genitals with a mirror (and
women should do this!) and finds that what she sees is not exactly like
the diagram she should not be worried, as biological variations are
very wide, particularly in the length and shapes of the labia minora.

This reluctance to look at one's own genitals is a feminine trait (after all, men constantly look at and touch their external genitals) and has its origin in the attitudes that many mothers give their daughters about their genitals. These attitudes are that the external genitals are 'private', ugly, should never be touched or 'played with', have a smell, and are 'dirty'. Such indoctrination in childhood can have sad consequences in a woman's image of her own body and in her sexual response. Even the medical word for the external genitals of a woman is negatively loaded: it is the *pudendum* – which derives from the Latin word *pudere* 'to be ashamed'. A woman should not be ashamed of or disgusted by her external genitals and should look at them to become familiar with their unique shape.

THE INTERNAL GENITAL ORGANS

The *vagina* is a muscular tube which stretches upwards and backwards from the vestibule to reach the uterus. As well as being muscular, it contains a well-developed network of veins which become distended in sexual arousal. Normally the walls of the vagina lie close together, the vagina being a potential cavity which is distended by intravaginal tampons used during menstruation, by the penis at copulation, and during childbirth, when it can stretch very considerably to permit the baby to be born. The vagina is about 9 cm (3¾ in) long, and at the upper end the *cervix* (or neck) of the uterus projects into it (Fig. 1/4). The vagina lies between the bladder in front and the rectum (or back-passage) behind. At the sides it is surrounded and protected by the strong muscles of the floor of the pelvis. Unless the vagina has been damaged, injured or tightened at operation, or has not developed due to an absence of sex hormones, its size is quite adequate for sexual intercourse. The woman who menstruates has a normal-sized vagina, and 'difficulty' at intercourse is not due to her being 'small made'. This is a myth. The cause lies not in the vagina, but in a mental fear of sexual intercourse which leads the woman to tighten the muscles which support the vagina to such an extent that coitus is painful.

The vagina is a remarkable organ. Not only is it capable of great distension, but it keeps itself clean. The cells which form its walls are 30 cells deep, lying on each other like the bricks of a house wall. In the reproductive years, the top layer of cells is constantly being shed

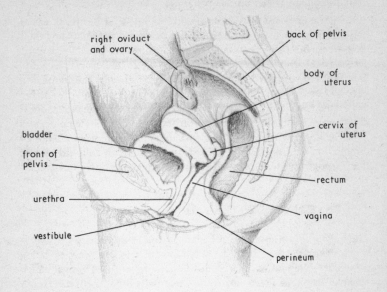

right oviduct
and ovary

back of pelvis

body of
uterus

cervix of
uterus

bladder

front of
pelvis

rectum

urethra

vestibule

vagina

perineum

FIG. 1/4 The internal genital organs of the female

into the vagina, where the cells are acted upon by a small bacillus which normally lives there, to produce lactic acid. The lactic acid then kills any contaminating germs which may happen to get into the vagina. Because of this, 'cleansing' vaginal douches, so popular at one time in the U.S.A., are unnecessary. In childhood, the wall of the vagina is thin, and the production of lactic acid does not take place. However this is of little importance, because the vagina is not usually contaminated at this age. In old age, the lining becomes thin once again, and few cells are shed. Because of this, little or no lactic acid is formed, and contaminating germs may grow. This sometimes results in inflammation of the vagina.

The *uterus* is an even more remarkable organ than the vagina. Before pregnancy it is pear-shaped, averages 9 cm (3¾ in) in length, 6 cm (2½ in) in width at its widest point, and weighs 60 g (2 oz). In pregnancy, it enlarges to weigh 1,000 g (2¼ lb), and is able to contain a baby measuring 40 cm (17 in) in length. It is able to undergo these changes because of the complex structure of its muscle and its exceptional response to the female sex hormones. The uterus is a hollow, muscular organ, which is located in the middle of the bony pelvis, lying between the bladder in front and the bowel behind (Fig. 1/4). It is pear-shaped, and its muscular front and back walls bulge into the cavity which is normally narrow and slit-like, until pregnancy occurs. Viewed from in front, the cavity is triangular, and is lined with a special tissue made up of glands in a network of cells. This tissue is called the endometrium, and it undergoes changes during each menstrual cycle. For descriptive purposes, the uterus is divided into an upper part, or *body*, and a lower portion, or *cervix uteri*. The word cervix means neck, so that the 'cervix uteri' means the neck of the womb. The cavity is narrow in the cervix, where it is called the cervical canal; widest in the body of the uterus; and then narrows again towards the cornu (or horn), where the cavity is continuous with the hollow of the Fallopian tube (Fig. 1/5). The cervix projects into the upper part of the vagina, and is a particular place where cancer sometimes develops. As it is readily accessible for examination, early changes in the cells indicating that cancer may be about to occur can be sought by special methods. This is discussed in more detail in Chapter 20. The lower part of the uterus and the upper part of the cervix are supported by a sling of special tissues, which stretch to the muscles of the pelvic wall in a fan-like manner. These supports may be stretched in childbirth, leading to a 'prolapse' later in life. With better obstetrics, this complication is today much less likely to occur.

Normally the uterus lies bent forward at an angle of 90° to the vagina, resting on the bladder. As the bladder fills, it rotates backwards; as it empties, the uterus falls forward. In about 10 per cent of women the uterus lies bent backwards. This is called *retroversion*. In the past it was considered a serious condition, causing backache, sterility and many other complaints. There were many operations for its cure. Today it is known that unless the retroversion is due to infection or to a peculiar condition called endometriosis, it is unimportant and is not the cause of the symptoms which were attributed to it. Surgery is not needed, and the patient can be reassured that the position of the uterus is normal for her.

The *oviducts* (or Fallopian tubes) are two small, hollow tubes, one on each side, which stretch for about 10 cm (4 in) from the upper part of the uterus to lie in contact with the ovary on each side. The outer end of each oviduct is divided into long finger-like processes, and it is

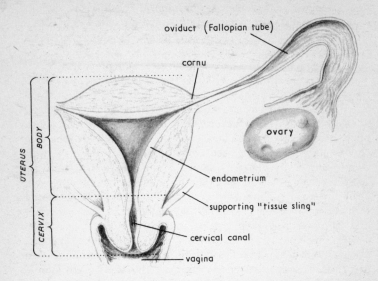

FIG. 1/5 The cavity of the uterus, and tubes

thought that these sweep up the egg when it is expelled from the ovary. The oviduct is lined with cells shaped like goblets, which lie between cells with frond-like borders. The oviduct is of great importance, as it is within it that fertilization of the egg takes place, and it is likely that its secretions help to nourish the fertilized egg as it is moved by the cells with long fronds towards the uterus.

The two *ovaries* are ovoid-shaped organs, averaging 3.5 cm (1½ in) in length and 2 cm (¾ in) in breadth. In the infant they are small, delicate, thin structures, but after puberty they enlarge to reach the adult proportions mentioned. After the menopause, they become small and wrinkled, and in old age are less than half their adult size. Each ovary has a centre made up of small cells and a mesh of vessels. Surrounding this is the ovary proper – the cortex – which contains about 200,000 egg cells lying in a cellular bed (the stroma), and outside again, protecting the egg cells and the ovarian stroma, is a thickened layer of tissue. The ovaries are the equivalent of the male testes, and in addition to containing the egg cells on which all human life depends, are a hormone factory producing the female sex hormones, which are so important.

As can be appreciated, the passage within the genital tract extends from the vestibule, along the vagina, through the cervix and uterus, and along the tubes to the ovaries. It is because of this that the male spermatozoa can reach the female egg for fertilization to take place within the body.

Chapter 2

How Human Life Begins

The human being, so complex in his behaviour, so different from his fellows, develops from a single fertilized cell. This cell – the fertilized ovum – divides almost at once into two identical cells. These two cells divide to make four identical cells, which then divide again, and so on. As they divide again and again, certain groups of cells become different, or differentiate, and form particular tissues or organs. For example, some cells form the bony skeleton, some the muscles, others the heart and blood vessels. Still others form the red blood cells which carry oxygen in the blood to the tissues, and others form the white blood cells which protect us against infections. Yet another group of cells multiplies to form the nerve cells of the brain and the nerves.

All these groups of cells with different functions have come from the single fertilized egg cell, and each and every cell has in its substance the information needed to perform the functions of any other cell, although once it has differentiated, it never does. Half of this information comes from the father's side of the family, and is transmitted in the spermatozoon which fertilized the egg. The other half comes from the mother's side, and is transmitted in the substance of the egg itself.

The information needed for the cell to perform its particular function is contained in the twisted strands of a substance found in the centre (or nucleus) of every cell. These strands are called chromosomes, and themselves are formed of long strings of several million beads, which are more properly called genes. The gene is the smallest unit of information, and is itself composed of twisted strands of a chemical called DNA (deoxyribonucleic acid). If you can imagine an ultra-sophisticated computer, which responds to requests fed in by giving out information, you have a pretty good idea of how the genes work in the cell. In any cell only a few genes operate to control the functions of that cell, the rest being covered over and inactive.

Each cell in the human body, with the exception of the egg cells in the woman and the spermatozoa in the man, contains 46 chromosomes. Forty-four of these chromosomes control all our physical characteristics and our body functions. These are called autosomes. The other two determine our sex. Recently it has been possible to take photographs of the chromosomes in the human body cells. In this way they can be displayed and measured. The two sex chromosomes can be identified easily. The smallest one has the shape of a Y, and is called the Y sex chromosome; the other has the shape of an X, and is called the X sex chromosome. Each of the millions of cells which make up a woman's body has 44 autosomes and two X chromosomes. A man's body cells have 44 autosomes, an X and a Y chromosome. You can see that even in the smallest body cell, a man is different from a woman because his cells alone have the Y chromosome.

As I have noted, the only cells in the body which do not have 46 chromosomes are the egg cells in the woman and the spermatozoa in the man. These two kinds of cells have only 23 chromosomes, and develop in special ways.

THE DEVELOPMENT OF THE EGG CELLS

Very early in life (about 20 days after fertilization) certain cells develop in the wall of the gut cavity of the embryo. These cells then migrate through the tissues to reach a thickened area lying in a ridge at each side of the midline of the gut cavity. This is the tissue from which the ovary will develop. By the 30th day after fertilization, the cells have settled in the tissue (which is now called a gonad), and have begun to multiply. By 140 days after fertilization (the 22nd week of pregnancy), a total of 7 million cells are found in the ovary, and many of them have acquired a coating of cells derived from the gonad. They develop within this protective coat and fluid appears in many of the cells. These are the egg cells (or *oocytes*), and the cells which contain fluid are called *follicles*. The cells which do not have the coating are destroyed, and by birth only 2 million oocytes remain. In the childhood years, many of the oocytes are destroyed and by puberty only 200,000 remain. Each month from puberty to the menopause between 12 and 30 of the oocytes develop further, and one which outstrips all the rest in growth is expelled from the ovary. This is the ovum which may be fertilized. Occasionally more than one ovum escapes from the ovary. If the additional ova are fertilized, twins, triplets or quadruplets will result, although twins may occur through another mechanism.

During its development in the ovary, the ovum divides into two daughter egg cells. This division is unequal, a large cell and a small cell being formed. Each of these cells has 23 chromosomes – 22 autosomes and an X chromosome. The large cell is the one which will accept the head of the spermatozoon into its substance at the time of fertilization, and will form the new individual. The small cell is pushed to lie just inside the zona pellucida, and has no further function. It is called a *polar body*.

THE DEVELOPMENT OF THE SPERMATOZOA

It can be seen that all the egg cells in the ovary of the female are formed before birth, and none can be formed later. The male is different, spermatozoa are continually being formed in his testicles from puberty onwards, and into old age.

The spermatozoa are formed from parent cells found in the testicles. They undergo several changes before becoming mature, and during the changes the number of chromosomes in each spermatozoon is reduced by half. The mature spermatozoon therefore has 23 chromosomes. Twenty-two of these are autosomes and one is a sex chromosome. Since the parent sperm cell had 44 autosomes, an X and a Y chromosome, it follows that when it divides to form the spermatozoa, each will have 22 autosomes and an X or a Y chromosome (Fig. 2/1). In this way two equal populations of spermatozoa form, and when you remember that each time a man has an orgasm he ejaculates between 100 and 400 *million* spermatozoa, they are large populations of cells. One population of spermatozoa has 22 autosomes and an X chromosome, the other 22 autosomes and a Y chromosome. If a spermatozoon carrying the Y chromosome fertilizes the egg, the new cell will have 44 autosomes, an X chromosome and a Y chromosome. The baby resulting from this will be a boy. If the spermatozoon which fertilizes the egg is one with 22 autosomes and an X chromosome, the resulting cell will have 44

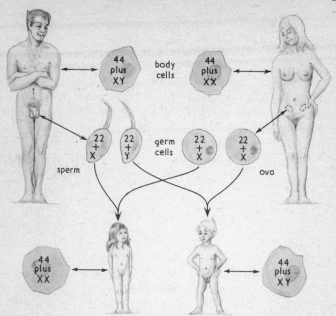

FIG. 2/1 The chromosomes of the ovum and
spermatozoon

autosomes and two X chromosomes. The baby resulting from this
will be a girl (Fig. **2/1**). This means that the father determines the sex
of the child.

THE FERTILIZATION OF THE EGG

A new life begins when a single spermatozoon, out of the millions
which were deposited in the upper part of the vagina during intercourse, fertilizes the egg (or ovum). Of the millions of spermatozoa
deposited in the vicinity of the cervix, only a few thousand manage to
negotiate the twisting mucus tunnels of its canal to reach the cavity of
the uterus. Of these only a few hundred get through the narrow cornu
of the uterus to enter the oviduct, and only a few dozen swim up along
the oviduct, against the current made by the moving fronds of its
lining, to reach the ovum. Only one penetrates through the cells and
tough, glistening, transparent 'shell' (the zona pellucida) which

surrounds the egg. Once the spermatozoon has penetrated the 'shell' of the egg, it alters the zona pellucida in some way, so that no other spermatozoa are able to penetrate it. In this way only one spermatozoon fertilizes the ovum. The new life actually begins when the chromosomes of the ovum and those of the spermatozoon fuse together. Under the control of the genes, the cell then divides again and again until a human being is formed, as was described in the opening paragraph of this chapter.

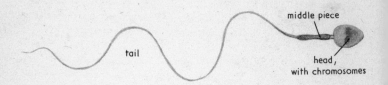

FIG. 2/2 The spermatozoon. The length is 0.05 mm and the thickness of the tail is about half that of a fine hair. It is only visible under a microscope

The spermatozoon has a head, a middle piece and a tail (Fig. 2/2). The head contains the chromosomes, the middle piece supplies the energy, and the tail propels it on its journey through the woman's genital tract (Fig. 2/3). When the spermatozoon reaches the ovum, its head penetrates the outer shell, and enters the substance of the egg. The head then separates from the middle piece and tail, which remain stuck in the shell and are destroyed.

When the head of the spermatozoon enters the ovum, its nucleus (which is the part containing the chromosomes) loses its wall and the chromosomes are exposed. Simultaneously, the wall surrounding the nucleus of the ovum is shed. The two sets of 23 chromosomes move together and fuse, so the number of chromosomes in the cell is 46 once again (Fig. 2/4). In this way the number of chromosomes in the human body cell is kept constant at 46.

A woman is a woman because each cell in her body (with the exception of the egg cells) has 44 non-sex chromosomes and two X sex chromosomes. Her femininity is further confirmed by the fact that none of her body cells contains a Y chromosome. In the absence of a Y chromosome, her internal and external genitalia will develop in a feminine way. There is also some evidence that the absence of a Y

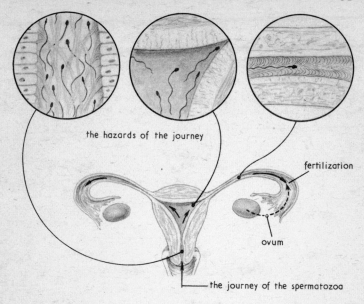

the hazards of the journey

fertilization

ovum

the journey of the spermatozoa

FIG. 2/3 The journey of the spermatazoa through the genital tract

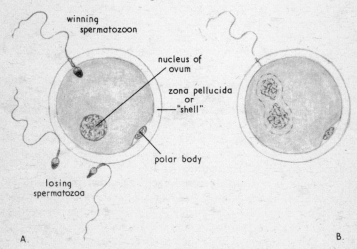

winning spermatozoon

nucleus of ovum

zona pellucida or "shell"

polar body

losing spermatozoa

A.

B.

FIG. 2/4 Conception. The sperm head is seen in the substance of the egg in A, and the two exposed masses of genetic material are seen in B. Almost immediately they fuse and a new individual is formed chromosome tends to make her 'psychologically' feminine. The effect of this is small, however, compared with the very considerable psychological pressures during childhood which confirm her in her feminine role. From the time she can notice anything she is treated as a girl; she is shown to be different from boys; she performs different tasks; is expected to behave differently, and so rapidly realizes that she is female.

Chapter 3

The Start of Femininity

The moment that the newborn baby is breathing properly, the doctor examines it to make sure it is normal in every way, and hands it to the mother to fondle and cuddle. She has done something no man can do – she has matured a new life in her uterus for 40 weeks and her baby has been born.

The newborn baby is totally dependent on others for all its needs, and forms its first physical contact with its mother. If she is going to breast-feed the baby, its first real tactile contact is the soft, warm breast, which provides a pleasant food. Even if she does not breast-feed her baby, it is she who cuddles the infant, lavishes affection on it, and performs the many tasks needed to sustain its life. The emotional links between infant and mother are strong, and a bond can also develop between infant and father if he plays a proper role, sharing with his wife the care of the child. But the bond between the infant and mother is so strong that the development of the growing child is influenced considerably by its character. If the mother is a warm, friendly person, the chances are that the child will develop in a similar way. If the mother is hard and unyielding, the child may reflect these characteristics, and find it difficult to adjust to a more normal human relationship in adult life. The sexual implications of this are no less important for the female than for the male.

The first sense an infant develops is touch, and although the warmth it obtains from cuddling is pleasurable, the infant soon begins to explore. The first explorations are necessarily confined to his own body, and the infant finds that touching the genital area produces pleasurable sensations. Similar pleasurable sensations are produced when the baby is bathed or the nappies (diapers) are changed. These explorations are completely normal. It is now known that most small children masturbate. This is easier to see if the child is a boy, but girls masturbate by 'rocking', which stimulates the area around their clitoris.

As the infant becomes a small child, its curiosity about the body increases. Most children explore each other's bodies and interact with each other (including sexually) in play. We do not know when this body exploration is interpreted by the child as erotic. By the age of 3, genital comparison is normal, as is body exploration. This sex play is valuable for it helps the child become familiar with its own body and that of others. If parents treat sex as 'dirty', and threaten to punish a child found engaged in sexual play, the child may develop attitudes to sex which will mar his or her adult life.

THE FEMALE ROLE

Children of both sexes if left alone will occupy themselves in the same way, will play the same games and will see no difference (other than an anatomical one) between each other. However, few children are left in this natural state. From the moment the baby becomes a child, the parents reinforce the sexual difference between boys and girls, and emphasize their different roles. This sexual differentiation is also emphasized by the manufacturers of children's goods, finding its most ridiculous and extreme expression in the U.S.A. in the manufacture of 'bras' and cosmetics for children of 10 and 11. By all these influences, a gender role is established for each child, a role which is necessary for the survival of the nomadic tribe when man must hunt for meat and woman must cook, care for the children and occasionally grow vegetables. Moreover, the organizational pattern of tribal life demands that each sex knows its own duties and has its own responsibilities. Despite the television set, the car, the electric cooker, the water-heater and the suburban 'dream-home', we are in many ways as tribal as the natives of New Guinea or Equador. This tribalism may well be necessary – it certainly exists – and in its cultural atmosphere a girl is to a certain extent indoctrinated that her role is that of housewife and mother; one of her main objectives to get married and have children; her future to be encompassed by the walls of her 'dream-home'; her thoughts bounded by the family.

GYNAECOLOGICAL CONDITIONS IN CHILDHOOD

Since the genital organs are immature and have not been stimulated by the sex hormones which will be produced by the ovary at puberty, gynaecological problems in infancy are uncommon. However, two require mention, as they may cause distress.

The 'genital crisis'

A few female infants either bleed slightly from the vagina, or develop enlargement of the breasts which secrete a watery solution in the first weeks of life. These conditions are called the 'genital crisis', and are due to the passage from the mother to her baby of certain hormones. Following birth, the hormones no longer pass, and in a few infants the symptoms mentioned may occur. They are without significance; no treatment is required as they settle down and disappear within a few days.

Inflammation of the vulva and vagina

In small children the vulva and the vagina may become inflamed and sore. The inflammation may be due to irritation from soaps used for washing, to lack of washing and poor hygiene, which permit bacteria to grow, or to the introduction into the vagina of some object.

The condition is very painful, and medical help should be sought. Meanwhile, certain general principles of treatment can be adopted. These are: (1) general cleanliness, using only a mild soap, or none at all, for washing the child's vulva, (2) careful drying and powdering after vulval washing, and (3) the wearing of light, cotton panties day and night to prevent the child from scratching the area.

Chapter 4

Adolescence

The period of life between childhood and maturity is adolescence, which biologically extends from the age of 10 to the age of 19. The most important event in adolescence, as far as the girl and her mother are concerned, is the onset of menstruation, which may occur at any time between the ages of 10 and 16. The time of onset of menstruation is called the menarche. In rural societies the menarche was a mark that the girl was now a woman, and could take up the duties and obligations of womanhood. This cultural attitude is retained in many societies today. For some reason, which may be connected with better nutrition, the age of the onset of menstruation has become earlier. In Britain the average age of the onset of menstruation is now 13 years, compared with 15 years a century ago. It seems that the daughters of better-off parents tend to start menstruating a little earlier than those whose parents are poor, but the average difference is no more than 6 to 9 months. The old belief that the menarche occurred earlier in girls living in the hot tropics does not appear to be true, and the average age of onset of menstruation depends more on the socio-economic status of the parents than on the climate.

The menarche, however, is only the culminating change in a sequence which has altered the girl into a young woman. These changes are due to a series of interactions between several glands in the body. The controlling gland is a special part of the brain called the *hypothalamus*, which, working with the pituitary gland, controls the subsequent events. For reasons which are not yet clear, the hypothalamus begins to secrete substances called releasing factors about four years before the menarche. The releasing factors pass down the blood vessels connecting the hypothalamus to the pituitary, where they cause the release of several chemical substances, called hormones. One of these hormones is the growth hormone which causes the spurt of growth that precedes the menarche. The girl begins to grow about four years before the menarche, and the rate of growth is greatest in the first two years, slowing down as the menarche approaches.

Two other hormones secreted by the pituitary gland are of particular importance to women as they act on the egg cells in the ovaries. In Chapter 2 it was noted that by the time of birth, fluid had appeared in many of the egg cells, which were then called egg follicles. The first of the hormones which affects the egg cells is called the follicle-stimulating hormone (or FSH), because it stimulates the growth of some of the follicles. At first only a very few follicles grow, and as they do so their surrounding mantle of cells manufactures a hormone called oestrogen. This hormone is the one which makes a female child become a woman. The stimulated follicles produce oestrogen for about a month, and then die. But by this time other egg follicles have been stimulated, and these secrete oestrogen in their turn. As time passes, more follicles are stimulated each month (eventually between 12 and 20 being stimulated), so that there is a gradual rise in the amount of oestrogen produced by the ovaries. Oestrogen has many effects. It stimulates the growth of the ducts of the breasts and the area under the nipples, so that this becomes enlarged. It stimulates the growth of the oviducts, the uterus and the vagina. In the vagina it thickens the vaginal wall, and causes increased vaginal moisture. It causes fat to be laid down on the hips. It slows down the growth spurt which was started earlier by the pituitary growth hormone, so that the mature girl is generally not as tall as the mature boy.

As time passes, the amount of oestrogen in the circulation rises more rapidly, and the menarche is near. The rising levels of oestrogen stimulate the growth of the lining of the uterus, the *endometrium*, but at the same time 'feed-back' reduces the quantity of follicle-stimulating hormone secreted by the pituitary. Once the level of follicle-stimulating hormone begins to fall, the growth of the follicles in the ovaries and the secretion of oestrogen are reduced. The blood vessels supplying the lining of the uterus become kinked and break, so that bleeding occurs in the uterus. The endometrium crumbles. Blood and endometrial cells collect in the uterus, and then escape through the cervix into the vagina. Menstruation has started – the menarche has arrived.

The average age at which various changes occur is as follows:

Age 9–10	The bony pelvis begins to grow and to attain a female shape.
	Fat begins to be deposited, commencing the changes in shape to that of a woman.
	The nipples bud.
Age 10–11	The nipples increase in size.
	Hair begins to appear over the pubis.
Age 11–13	The area beneath the nipples develops.
	The internal and external genitals grow and develop.
	The vaginal wall thickens, and vaginal secretions may appear.
Age 12–14	The breasts develop further, and the nipples become darker in colour.
Age 13–15	Hair increases over the pubis, and appears in the arm-pits.
	Spots appear on the face of about half the girls.
	The menarche occurs, but the first few periods occur at irregular intervals.
Age 15–17	Increased fatty deposition occurs on the hips and the breasts.
	The periods become more regular.
Age 16–18	Growth of the skeleton ceases. The girl has now reached her maximum height.

MENSTRUATION

At intervals from the menarche – irregularly at first but with increasing regularity as time goes by – the girl 'has her periods', or menstruates. Within 4 to 6 years of the menarche (by the age of 17 to 19), her menstrual pattern will have become established. Each individual has her own pattern, but in most women menstruation occurs each month (unless pregnancy intervenes) until about the age of 45, when it becomes increasingly irregular once again. For convenience, the menstrual cycle is considered to start on the first day of menstruation (day 1), and to end the day before the next menstruation starts. The menstrual cycle therefore includes the days when bleeding occurs and the interval between each menstrual period. In most women the cycle varies in length from 24 to 34 days, averaging 29 days. But even the woman who says she knows exactly on what day menstruation will start is often a few days out either side. In adolescence, until the pattern has been established, menstruation tends to occur at irregular intervals, usually of longer duration than normal, but occasionally more frequently. In the first year or two after the menarche, the periods may only recur twice or three times a year, and when they do occur may be heavy. Sooner or later, however, a regular rhythmic pattern is established.

The menstrual cycle

It has been said that menstruation is 'the uterus weeping because pregnancy did not happen'. Bleeding from the crumbling of the lining of the uterus is the culmination of a series of interlocked events which prepare the uterus to accept a fertilized egg. If pregnancy does not occur, this prepared lining is shed from the uterus, and the whole cycle of events begins again.

The ultimate 'controller' of these events is the hypothalamus, and even this part of the brain is affected by emotions and upsets. This is demonstrated by the fact that menstruation may cease after a particularly strong emotional upset, or if a girl leaves home and changes her occupation. The duration of time during which menstruation ceases is variable and the periods usually return after two or three months; but in some patients the absence of the periods, which is called amenorrhoea, may last for more than a year. Such patients require careful investigation to exclude an underlying disease which may cause amenorrhoea. Luckily the cause is not usually a disease, and menstruation can be restored with certain drugs if this is considered desirable. It should be stressed that if there is no underlying disease, the absence of menstruation is of no importance. Contrary to a popular myth, menstruation does not clean the body, and the absence of menstruation does not mean that 'dangerous substances' are dammed up within the uterus.

As the sequence of events leading to each menstrual period is complicated, it is perhaps best to start at the time of menstruation and trace what happens up to the time of the next menstruation.

During menstruation the hypothalamus sends quantities of the FSH-releasing factor to stimulate the cells in the pituitary gland which manufactures FSH. The amount of FSH in the blood rises and stimulates a number of egg follicles in the ovary, usually 12 to 20. These follicles grow, and as they do so they manufacture oestrogen, so that the amount of this special female sex hormone increases in the blood. As has been noted earlier, oestrogen has several effects upon the tissues which make up the genital tract, but the one in which we are particularly interested is its action on the lining of the uterus. Oestrogen stimulates the lining to grow. At the end of menstruation most of the lining has crumbled away and, mixed with blood, has been shed as the menstrual flow. The lining is made up of narrow tubes, called endometrial glands, set in several layers of cells, called endometrial stromal cells. Oestrogen makes the glands grow, and the layers of stromal cells increase, or proliferate. Because of this, the changes in the uterus are called proliferative, and this part of the cycle is called the proliferative phase of the cycle.

As the follicles grow, the amount of oestrogen in the blood continues to rise, and by 13 days after the onset of menstruation, it has increased six-fold above the level found at its onset. The rising blood levels have an effect called a 'feed-back' on the hypothalamus, causing a reduction in FSH-releasing factor, but making the hypothalamus release another substance called the LH-releasing factor. This factor is carried down the blood vessels which connect the hypothalamus to the pituitary gland, where certain specialized cells produce a substance called luteinising hormone, or LH (Fig. 4/1). This hormone is so-called because it induces one of the egg follicles to burst and expel its contained egg, and it then changes the cells which make up the follicle to a bright yellow colour. The Latin word for yellow is 'luteus' – hence the luteinising, or yellow-making hormone. At about the 14th day after the onset of menstruation (in a girl with a normal cycle, or later if the cycle is prolonged unduly) a sudden surge of luteinising hormone sweeps through the blood stream. It reaches the ovary, where it induces 'bursting' of the egg follicle which has grown the most, and which is blown-up and tight like a tiny balloon. During growth, this particular follicle has swollen and moved through the ovary to reach its surface, where it makes a tiny bulge that can be seen by the naked eye. Suddenly, under the influence of the luteinising hormone, the follicle bursts and the egg is pushed out, together with the fluid in which it lay. The egg is caught in the finger-like ends of the oviduct which caress the ovary at this time, and is moved slowly but gently into the cavity of the oviduct tube,

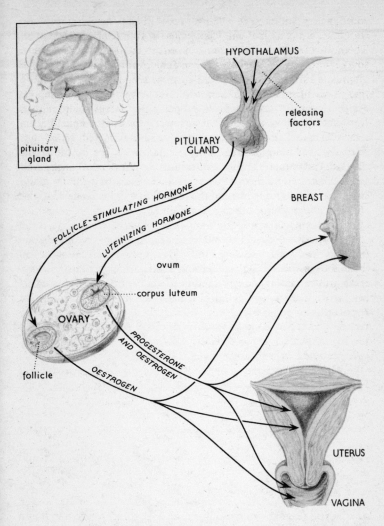

FIG.4/1 The control of menstruation

where fertilization takes place, if this is to happen (Fig. 4/2).

Once the egg (or ovum) has been expelled, the now empty follicle collapses, and the luteinising hormone acts on the cells of its wall, turning them yellow. The collapsed follicle is called a yellow body, or, in Latin, a *corpus luteum*. The change in colour of the cells of the corpus luteum is due to a change in their activity. Now not only do they continue to secrete oestrogen (along with the other 11 to 19 stimulated follicles which failed to grow so quickly), but uniquely they also manufacture a new hormone called progesterone. The name is apt, for the hormone prepares the uterus for pregnancy (*progestos*) – hence pro-gest-erone (-one indicates the kind of chemical substance). Progesterone is the second main female sex hormone. It has many actions, but the main ones are that it relaxes smooth (involuntary) muscle; increases the production of the waxy secretions of the skin; and raises the temperature of the body. This is why it is normal for women in the second half of the menstrual cycle to have a temperature up to 37.4° Centigrade, or 99.5° Fahrenheit. The most important progestational effect of progesterone is its action on the uterus. Progesterone thickens the lining of the uterus, and induces the glands to secrete a nutritious fluid and become succulent, so that the fertilized egg may be nourished during the time it needs to take root or implant in the lining of the womb. The part of the menstrual cycle after ovulation is called the luteal or the progestational phase.

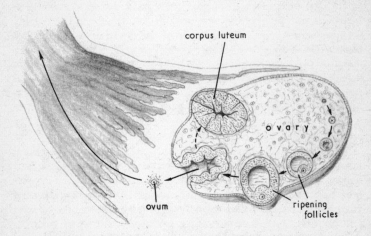

FIG. 4/2 The growth of stimulated follicles in the ovary during a menstrual cycle

Unless the egg is fertilized and implants onto the endometrium, the yellow body in the ovary dies (as do the other stimulated follicles). If this happens, the level of oestrogen and progesterone in the blood falls. This has two effects: firstly, the restraint on FSH-releasing factors by the hypothalamus is removed, and FSH production by the pituitary gland increases. Secondly, without the stimulation of oestrogen and progesterone, the now thick, juicy lining of the uterus begins to shrink, and in doing so kinks the tiny blood vessels which supply it. The kinked blood vessels (really blood capillaries) break, and patchy bleeding occurs in the deeper layers of the lining. This separates the lining above the blood; it crumbles and is shed into the uterine cavity, together with blood. Within a few hours, the amount of blood in the uterine cavity is such that the uterus contracts, expelling the blood through the cervix into the vagina. Menstruation has begun.

'Protection' during menstruation

No woman wants to discolour her clothes with menstrual blood. In the past a rag was used which was placed over the vulva, and which is the origin of an English name for menstruation, 'the rags'. Today clean, absorbent, easily disposable materials are used to make sanitary pads and intravaginal tampons, the two usual ways of dealing with menstrual loss. The sanitary pad has the disadvantage that it may chafe the upper thighs as it lies applied to the vulva, and may be apparent, particularly in sports clothes. The latter objection is more often in the mind of the wearer than of the observer, and if menstruation is considered a normal function (which it is), it is surely unimportant if others know that a menstrual period is in progress. It is only in communities which consider menstruation something of which to be ashamed and to be hidden that these attitudes apply.

The intravaginal tampon has the advantage that it is convenient, inconspicuous and effective. There is no truth in the belief that it is dangerous to collect menstrual blood in the vagina. Since the tampon must be introduced into the vagina, it should not be used in the early years of puberty, but by the age of 16 or 17 it may replace the sanitary pad, provided the girl can introduce it without discomfort. A disadvantage is that occasionally a tampon may be forgotten and left in the vagina. This can lead to a most offensive vaginal discharge. Women who have profuse periods also find that the tampon is inadequate to mop up the blood loss, and may find a sanitary pad more satisfactory. The choice is that of the girl – neither method is superior to the other, both being satisfactory.

Myths about menstruation

In primitive cultures, menstruating women were regarded not as dirty, but as evil and dangerous. The loss of blood to primitive races was a loss of life. As menstrual blood emerged from the same passage as did the baby, but seemed in some way to prevent pregnancy, it was felt to be a danger to growing things. A menstruating woman therefore could damage crops, cause animals to abort, turn wine into vinegar and turn milk sour by her presence. These primitive beliefs are still accepted in parts of Europe today, and it is believed that if a menstruating woman makes jam it will not keep; if she touches wine, beer or milk it will go bad; if she touches buds they will wither; and if she rides a pregnant mare it will miscarry. In most societies it was therefore felt imperative that a woman, at the time of the menstrual period, withdrew from the life of the community, and remained secluded and hidden from view in the house. Whilst menstruating, she could not touch food or cook, nor should her shadow fall on another woman, particularly if she was pregnant. These strange prohibitions are found in Australian Aboriginal tribes, and amongst the highly intelligent but superstitious Hindu cultures. Almost all societies have surrounded menstruation with myth and ritual. Both the Jews and the Muslims have elaborate rituals for purification following menstruation, and even in modern Western society strange traditional beliefs persist. Certain foods, especially pineapple and raspberries, are thought to be 'bad' if eaten during menstruation. Washing the hair is believed to lead to an increased menstrual loss, and to the development of a cold or pneumonia.

Of course, there is no basis of truth in any of these beliefs. Provided the menstrual flow is not too heavy and the girl wishes, she can take part in any activity. She can ride, swim, work or walk, wash her head or her feet, eat what she likes, bathe or shower, dance or drive. It is also a myth that menstruation is necessary for a woman's health. The basis of this myth is that the menstrual blood, in some obscure way, washes 'bad substances' from a woman's body. This is quite untrue. Menstruation has two psychological functions. It indicates to a woman that she is still in the period of life when she can conceive children and it indicates to her that she has not conceived. If she has no desire to have children, or has completed her family, there are no physical or psychological reasons why she should menstruate. But unless she takes drugs (such as the injectable hormonal contraceptives) or has had her uterus removed surgically, her biological rhythm will ensure that menstruation will continue.

Menstrual irregularities in adolescence

The menstrual cycle is repeated throughout the reproductive years, unless pregnancy occurs. At each extreme – that is in adolescence and near the menopause – the cycles are less regular, and ovulation may not occur. In these cycles the endometrium is only stimulated by oestrogen, and only FSH is secreted (in any quantity) by the pituitary gland. The menstrual cycles tend to be irregular in duration: they may be as short as 12 days, or as long as 3 or 4 months. The duration and amount of menstrual bleeding is also variable: it may be scanty and of short duration, or heavy and long. If the bleeding times are too heavy or too prolonged, the girl should consult a doctor who can give hormonal treatment for a few months to regulate the periods. During this time, the girl's own rhythm is established. In most cases, the irregularity is not too inconvenient, and the knowledge that normal cycles will eventually appear is sufficient reassurance. But if there is any doubt, the girl should consult a doctor.

DELAYED ONSET OF MENSTRUATION

Of even more concern to the girl, and more particularly to her mother, is when the periods fail to start. If menstruation has not started by the age of 16, and particularly if the girl is of short stature, a doctor should be consulted. He will take a very careful history, will require to make a full physical examination, and finally will need to make a pelvic examination (although in some cases an examination by inserting a finger into the rectum will give sufficient information). If at the end of this time the doctor has not been able to find out why the periods have not started, the girl should be referred to a gynaecologist so that special investigations can be started. The investigations are fairly simple and include the examination under a microscope of cells taken by a swab from the inside of the cheek. A sample of the girl's blood is taken and the levels of FSH, oestrogen, progesterone and a hormone, called prolactin, are measured. Some of the blood is treated in a special way so that the chromosome pattern of the body cells can be determined.

DYSMENORRHOEA

Many girls suffer from painful periods. This is called dysmenorrhoea. Dysmenorrhoea does not usually start until two or three years after the menarche, and usually only occurs if the menstrual period follows a cycle in which ovulation occurred. Occasionally dysmenorrhoea occurs in a period in which ovulation did not occur (called an 'anovulatory cycle'), particularly if the menstrual blood clots in the uterus, and the small clots are then expelled.

The pain is cramp-like in character, felt in the lower abdomen, and usually starts 24 hours before the menstrual period and lasts for the first 12 hours of bleeding, when all the discomfort goes.

The cause of dysmenorrhoea is unknown, but the most acceptable theory is that the pain is caused by spasm of the uterine muscle, due in turn to an immature blood supply. The cause of the pain is therefore similar to that which occurs in your arm if you tie a tight band around the upper part. Cultural beliefs, and the concept that menstruation is the discharge of waste products, have the effect of increasing the pain sensation. Thus adolescents in 'primitive races' are said to suffer less dysmenorrhoea than girls in more sophisticated Western societies. It is by no means certain that this is true, but Western society in calling menstruation 'the curse', the 'poorly time' and the 'unclean time' (as in the Bible) only intensifies the erroneous belief that menstruation is something of which to be ashamed, and not the naturally occurring shedding of the uterine lining prepared for a pregnancy which failed to occur.

Probably 50 per cent of women complain of dysmenorrhoea at some stage of their life. Usually the peak years are between 17 and 25, and the condition is relieved or cured by pregnancy. Because of this high incidence, a bewildering variety of treatments have been prescribed in the past, and continue to appear today. Some of the more bizarre methods, such as exotic spinal and pelvic exercises, Sitz baths, cold showers, and surgical operations for removing the nerves of the pelvis, are now of only historical interest, but others which are equally wild appear from time to time.

The great majority of girls need no more than an explanation of what dysmenorrhoea is, a sympathetic attitude from parents which is neither too hard nor too pitying, and the use of aspirin or other pain-relieving drugs. If the pain is so incapacitating that the girl has to go to bed, or has associated vomiting, the use of oral contraceptives ('the Pill') will usually prevent dysmenorrhoea. Another hormonal treatment, which prevents dysmenorrhoea apparently without stopping ovulation, has been introduced recently. Although effective, neither of these treatments should be used until the girl has been examined by a doctor.

EMOTIONAL CHANGES IN ADOLESCENCE

With the hormonal tides which ebb and flow before and after the menarche, with increasing knowledge and with increasing information (and misinformation) received from her peer-group, the adolescent has to adjust to a new identity – that of a young woman. In the adolescent period of transition, she has to emerge from the family orientated dependent tranquillity of childhood and enter the frustrations, competitiveness and trauma of adult life. Successful adaptation demands that she matures not only biologically but emotionally and socially as well. In the initial period of biological development she begins to become much closer to other teenagers than to her family. From them, she learns of different attitudes to morality and to sexuality. She now has to resolve a conflict. She has to decide which set of values she should adopt, or more accurately, how many of her parents' values she will reject. And at this time she begins to feel the force of new, ill-understood heterosexual attractions.

The great majority of adolescents adjust with little trouble, but during the period of adjustment are moody, irritable, apparently irrational and 'difficult'. These are outward expressions of inward conflicts, of frustrations, of doubts, even of despair. The adolescent resents adult criticism, particularly when she is told to behave one way by parents who are quite clearly behaving in an entirely different way.

Adults complain about the irresponsibility of teenagers, about their lack of respect, about their morals and about their promiscuity.

Yet it is difficult to ask teenagers to develop responsibility when adults seem to be rejecting it, and when society seems to be fragmenting. It is particularly difficult to ask young people to maintain sexual responsibility, when the mass media constantly emphasize that all wants can be instantly gratified. The adolescent needs understanding and love. And she needs to be able to talk to someone close to her, not to have to talk to her parents as strangers. If parents are unable to answer her questions regarding social, moral and sexual attitudes, they have failed as parents, and should not blame their child if she appears to have failed them.

As I shall mention in the next chapter, sexual problems arise in nearly 50 per cent of marriages and, although many are apparently only minor, they can and do much to cause marital discord. It is now clear that many of the problems occur because sex is thought of as 'dirty' or 'indecent' or something to be hidden by one or other partner. The importance of a healthy attitude towards human sexuality in childhood and adolescence is crucial, and this is mainly the responsibility of the child's parents. Parents should be aware of their important function in educating their children to a healthy sexuality by their words and their 'non-verbal cues', that is, by the way they behave themselves in sexual matters. Both are important.

In childhood, a boy or a girl should be able to say with conviction by the age of 2 'I am a boy' or 'I am a girl'. As the child grows older its interest in sex increases. Young children, for example, explore their own and their playmates' bodies in games such as 'playing doctors' or 'mothers and fathers'. Young children find that stimulation of their genitalia is pleasurable: boys fondle their penis, girls 'rock', indirectly stimulating their clitoris. These preliminary explorations should be treated by parents with respect and acceptance and neither condemned nor punished. When children ask questions about sexual matters, their questions should be answered factually and the child should be given access to accurate printed information, including pictures. Parents should always stress that sex is a natural function but that it carries responsibilities to another person.

In adolescence, the needs for privacy, for intimacy and for erotic expression should be recognised by the child's parents; and parents should try to stress that there are satisfying, non-exploiting ways of meeting these needs. They should also accept that much information (and misinformation) comes from other children in the child's group. To put it in a sentence: an adolescent should have been helped to be aware of her own body, to be able to touch it joyfully, and to see it as a uniquely personal possession, so that later she will be able to respond when in close joyous touch with another person's body. If she can achieve this contact she will also be able to communicate her needs to the other person, as you will see in Chapter 5.

Edward Brecher, in *The Sex Researchers* has put the matter very clearly:

'The moral for parents of the next generation of little girls seems to me crystal clear. The repression of masturbation and other forms of childhood sexuality is not going to lead your daughter to maintain her chastity until marriage, or to remain faithful and monogamous thereafter. But if your intention is to spoil your son's and your daughter's *enjoyment* of their future sexual experiences, including marital coitus, then the castigation of childhood masturbation and other forms of sexuality as shameful and filthy is almost guaranteed beyond your expectations'.

Chapter 5

About Sexuality

In these days of change – social, educational and sexual – the differences between men and women have been reduced considerably. Although a woman tends to have less well-developed muscles than a man, she can equal him in physical and mental stamina, and is able increasingly to perform jobs which have been reserved for men in the past. The degree to which this change has occurred varies between countries but, more and more, the two sexes are performing the same work and are sharing responsibilities previously reserved for one or the other. Political power, industrial power and military power – the three props which support Western society at present – are still predominantly male preserves, but even here increasing numbers of women are playing a significant part and sharing power with men.

In the earliest tribal societies, the culture was predominantly feminine, centring around childrearing, food-getting and home-making. The women tilled such fields as there were, and cultivated the edible vegetables. The men had far less responsibility; they brought in food from hunting, they took part in certain rituals necessary to bring rain or deflect the anger of the gods, and they occasionally helped with certain limited duties. Once nomadic tribes settled, cultivated fixed fields and domesticated animals, man began to dominate society. Man's status in his tribe could be measured by the number of his cattle or goats, and women became debased to be possessions of man, ranking only a little above his cows. In the West, by the Middle Ages, women of the peasant class had lost all of their traditionally dominant duties and now worked in the fields and in the house under the guidance and dominance of the man, who considered woman his chattel. If a woman was born into the upper classes, she did little except grace the house, organize the servants and act chiefly as a toy or pet for her husband. Even so, her position was not without merit. The organization of a great establishment, many of which were self-contained communities, took skill and knowledge. Educated women of the seventeenth and eighteenth centuries took the same pride in the way they managed their households as they did in learning to play musical instruments, or embroider intricate pieces of needlework and to paint.

In India, Hindu society had strict rules for the conduct of the sexes, which hardly changed over 1,000 years. The woman entered her husband's family at marriage and the primary object of marriage was the birth of a son so that the family line might continue. The woman was therefore totally subordinate to her husband, who believed that she was inferior to man, less able to resist temptation and therefore weaker. Because of this, it was his duty to protect his wife with 'the respect due to his mother' but also to regulate her behaviour to his desires.

The Christian cultures of the West also held that woman was inferior to man and, following St Augustine, believed that sexual intercourse was permissible only for the purpose of producing children, a belief similar to that of the older Hindu religion. The pronouncements of the early Christian theologians were further codified during the turbulence of the Reformation, when male dominance and female subjugation were confirmed. In such an environment men were able to insist on their exclusive right to the women they owned. The woman was to be a virgin at marriage and monogamous after marriage, so that the man could be certain that any child she conceived was his. This encouraged the belief that only heterosexual intercourse was normal, and that only orgasm achieved during heterosexual intercourse was proper. Other forms of sexual pleasure, such as masturbation, clitoral or penile manipulation, or homosexual relationships were evil. A 'double standard' of sexual behaviour was established, in which the male was permitted to seek sexual satisfaction with women and even encouraged to do so, whilst the female was expected to avoid sexual relations until marriage and then submit to the dominance of her husband.

This rigid pattern of male dominance and female submission was changed to some extent by the influence of Sigmund Freud towards the end of the nineteenth century. He insisted that sex was a basic instinct which should be enjoyed by both men and women. Other psychologists amplified Freud's original work by confirming that sex should extend beyond the mere physical act of copulation to involve the emotional responses of both partners. In other words, both partners needed to have a knowledge of, and involvement in sex for the further development of their personalities.

Despite this evidence, the double standard remains remarkably strong in much of Western society. People, both men and women, are conditioned by their upbringing, and by the prevailing cultural attitudes, to believe that men, by virtue of being men, are sexually knowledgeable, aggressive and have an urgent, highly demanding, sexual drive. Many people are taught that sex is a man's 'reponsibility'; he should always take the initiative for sex, and in sexual encounters he is the master, the woman the passive servant. Many people think that women should be sexually innocent, relatively inert, rarely initiating sex and never obviously pursuing the man. It is also thought that a woman should value her sexuality as a necessary precursor to reproduction, rather than something deeply pleasurable in itself, and that a woman is expected to suppress her sexual feelings or to perceive them as something not 'quite nice'. Many women brought up to expect that their sexual arousal will be slow, will depend on their partner to be aroused and believe that they do not need to be aroused as often and as much as a man. Because of all this, in many relationships, a woman is treated as, and accepts the role of, a sexual puppet, available for a man when he requires release of sexual tension. She may be regarded by him lovingly, valued for her qualities as a housewife and mother, accorded respect when she adds to the family income by working, but he never treats her as a human being who has equal sexual needs.

Unfortunately, if a man believes that a woman has a reduced sexuality, compared with his, and if he treats her as his sexual possession, he will 'use' her sexually. He may condescend to stimulate her sexually in a perfunctory way, but his real objective is to reach his orgasm at his speed without really considering her sexual needs. If 'his' woman manages to reach an orgasm during sexual intercourse that is great. If she does not, he need not worry unduly, as women are 'known' to be less sexually responsive than men. But, paradoxically, a man may expect a woman to reach an orgasm during sexual intercourse, preferably simultaneously with his orgasm. If a woman fails to reach an orgasm, the man may feel sexually inadequate, his masculinity suspect, as he has learnt that a man 'gives a woman her orgasm'. So that he will not feel disappointed, or to protect his masculine self-image, many women attempt to 'fake' orgasms.

This attitude is beginning to change as women obtain emancipation politically, socially and sexually. But the majority of women are still confused about their sexuality, because parents, by their behaviour to each other and within the family, reinforce the 'double standard' of sexuality. This behaviour may convince the girl that human sexuality is something which cannot be discussed and which is a taboo subject. Such conditioning can cause a woman to suppress her sexuality; not necessarily her desire for sex but certainly her full enjoyment of sex.

A woman will only obtain full sexual pleasure when she and her partner have equality in sexual matters, and when the sexual pleasure is mutually shared, something that is done together, rather than to the other person; something with each other, rather than for the other. Women will only be sexually equal when men accept that a woman is not merely a sexual receptacle, and when women accept that a man is not merely a sexual instrument.

Many groups within our society resist the idea of a woman having sexual equality. Some people fear that the change will diminish the status of those women who prefer to remain 'mere housewives'. Some men fear it will place heavy burdens on them to prove their masculinity. As long as a man has only to express to the woman, by word or gesture, that he wants sex, so long as he only has to obtain an erection and reach an orgasm at his desired pace, he is in control of the situation. But if he has to consider the woman's sexual needs, he has to be more perceptive and more receptive. He may even feel that a woman's sexual equality is a threat to his sexuality. Some men and women resist the change to sexual equality because of inhibitions towards sex which they acquired during their early upbringing. One such inhibition is that sex is dirty and should be 'indulged' in secretly rather than enjoyed mutually. Some men and women also fear that woman's sexual equality will diminish her 'femininity'. These fears are all groundless. All have the effect of reducing the right of women to equality with men in all spheres of life and particularly in the sexual sphere.

Sexual and socio-economic emancipation do place additional burdens on a woman, particularly if she is sharing her life, whether married or not, with a man who rejects her views. Because of cultural attitudes, rather than biology, a woman is expected to manage her home and rear her children without necessarily receiving help. Biologically, it is true that only a woman can breast-feed a baby, but there is no reason why a man should not share in all the other home-making and child-rearing functions. As more women prove themselves the equal of men in practically every field of human endeavour, it is extremely galling to discover that many men expect their women to give up their careers on marriage, or, if the woman has to work to supplement the family income, refuse to help in the house. This can place an intolerable strain on a woman and, so far, Western society has done little to help women solve this problem. A new approach to the partnership between a man and a woman is needed and this should start in childhood. Children should be brought up to accept that domestic chores should be shared, that the kitchen and the nursery are as much the joint responsibility of the father and mother as is the bedroom.

It is equally important to women's dignity that society accepts the idea that not all women believe that the 'be-all and end-all' of their life is marriage. Only a woman can conceive and bear a child, but this in itself does not mean her life can only be fulfilled if she carries out this biological function. To bring up a girl to believe that she is unfeminine unless she marries and becomes a mother, is probably one of the most dangerous heresies of this century. Some women may never have the opportunity to marry, others have no desire to do so. They can still live full, active and stimulating lives as single women, as personalities in their own right. Once this fact is accepted, many outmoded conventions will disappear from our society.

Meanwhile, convention still requires that a woman must display a willingness to be a housewife, a mother and have the capacity to be sexually attractive to a man. A woman is also taught to be sexually available to a man, particularly if she is married to him. Some women who do not enjoy sexual intercourse, make themselves 'available' for their man to have sex with because they are afraid that they will lose the man's love if they challenge his sexual expertise by suggesting ways in which they might enjoy sex more. Some women 'trade sex for love' and believe their man gives love for sex. Other women trade sexual intercourse for body contact and the close touch of another human, rather than for the emotional and physical sensations of intercourse, and especially of orgasm, which because of the man's insensitivity, may be minimal. It is becoming accepted, at last, that women have no less enthusiasm for sexual intercourse and no less enjoyment of sexuality than men. It is true however, that some women take longer than men to reach their full sexual response; but a woman's total sexual response exceeds that of a man and, once aroused, women can often have orgasms more frequently than men.

In our society, a woman will only achieve her full potential for sexual pleasure if she is able to let her partner know her sexual needs and desires, confident that he will respond understandingly and lovingly. Equally, she must be just as responsive to his sexual needs and desires.

Unfortunately, because of the way children are reared in our society and our 'hang-ups' about expressing emotions, many couples are unable to let each other know how they feel and what their emotional needs are. One of these emotional needs is the need to be sexually fulfilled. What stimulates a person sexually, what 'turns them on' is an individual matter. It is based on the person's memories and experiences. If you are unable to express your special needs to your partner and he, or she, is unable to guess them, your sexuality will be less enjoyable than it should be. Your partner may 'know' what you want, but often this 'knowledge' is based on myths, not on the reality of your sexuality.

THE SEXUAL DRIVE

At puberty, the sex hormones, oestrogen in girls and testosterone in boys, increase in quantity and 'stimulate' the person's sexual drive, which has been developing slowly since infancy, so that his or her desire for sexual pleasure increases.

Your sexual drive is not your capacity to have sexual relations but your desire or urge for sex. It is determined largely by the attitudes towards sexuality you have acquired during your up-bringing. Your sexual beliefs and attitudes are formed by what you have learnt from your parents and other adults, which in turn depends on their attitudes and beliefs. In late childhood and in adolescence these attitudes may be influenced by the sexual values of your peer-group from whom you 'learn' a good deal about sex. Some of this information is inaccurate, some is not, but you form your sexual values from these examples and from your own experience.

In our kind of society, girls are thought to be more inhibited about sex than boys, because girls are given different values about sex. This has led to the belief that in adolescence and when adult, women are less sexual; they 'demand' and 'need' sex less often than men; they respond sexually more slowly, and they reach orgasm less rapidly and less often than men. Because of this, many women still believe that they have a lower sex drive than men, which is not true. Biologically, a woman's sex drive is no different from that of a man, but if a mother has taught her daughter, by example or by words, that sex is 'dirty', that sex outside marriage is 'sinful' and that it is a wife's 'duty' to submit passively to her husband's sexual 'demands', rather than enjoying sex, her sexuality may be impaired. As I mentioned in the last chapter when I quoted Edward Brecher, the importance of sensitive sexual upbringing by informed parents and teachers is obvious, if a person is to achieve his or her full potential for sexual pleasure.

The intensity of a person's sexual drive is not only influenced by their upbringing but also varies at different times during their life. It is believed that it decreases in intensity as people grow older. This is untrue and many people have a high sexual drive well into old age. A person's sexual drive is influenced by many factors. For example, pressure of work, fatigue, chronic pain, anxiety about a job, excessive alcohol or a defective relationship with one's sexual partner can reduce the drive of men and women, whilst the demands of child-rearing (see p. 259) can reduce it in women.

There are many ways in which you may solve the problem of having a different sexual drive compared with that of your partner, if this occurs, as it may, from time to time. One of these ways (and you may have found others) is for you to share your feelings, so that your partner understands the kinds of feelings you have about your sexual desires. If you can do this, your sexual relationship is likely to be enhanced, as each of you will understand and accept that sex is not something done to the other, but a pleasurable activity enjoyed together.

Unfortunately, because of the inhibitions about sex we acquire from our parents and others during our up-bringing, and because of our own 'hang-ups', many of us do not have a sexual relationship in which each partner is considered to have equal needs. Many people find it difficult to talk openly about their sexual desires and needs, so that they do not find out what is right, sexually, for each person in the relationship. Your unwillingness, or inability, to talk openly with your partner about your sexual needs, may be one facet of an inability to relate to each other emotionally in other matters. If you have emotional barriers, sexual or other, your relationship may be unequal and perhaps fragile, and frustrations can mount.

Women in our society seem to be especially affected by the inability to express sexual and other emotional needs, and the resulting frustrations can be damaging to health. The frustrations may be pushed deep into the woman's unconscious mind to emerge as depression, fatigue or irritability, or they may be expressed in a bewildering variety of gynaecological disorders, such as pain in the lower abdomen, backache, increased vaginal discharge or changes in the quantity and duration of menstruation. In all of these conditions, the problem originates in the mind, not in the pelvis; they are psychosomatic in origin, but that makes them no less real.

It is interesting to speculate on the extent to which sexual problems are present because of the 'work-ethic' of Western society. A man will spend long hours attending to his business, or working at his job. He may come home tired and frustrated, and expect his wife to console him; but to him sex, like work, has its special place and special time. It may be subordinate to work, and the time spent on establishing a warm, mutually pleasurable relationship is thought to be less important than the time spent at work, at sport or in the pub. The man may be insufficiently sensitive to realize that his wife has also had a tiring, frustrating day. He needs sex for consolation; but because of the double standard of sexuality he can only envisage sex as something to be 'indulged' in, rather than something to be shared. In this type of situation the resolution of the couple's sexual problems will depend on their ability to give time to the pleasure of their sexual relationship, and to know that both of them have sexual and other emotional needs which they want to share with the other.

SEXUAL AROUSAL AND EXCITEMENT

What is it that attracts one person to another, whilst both ignore a third person? The answer is not yet known, but it seems likely that each person begins developing his or her own pattern, or scenario, in childhood. In the scenario, the person, who is the 'writer' of his or her own sexual arousal script, builds it up from childhood memories and fantasies, adolescent fantasies and experiences, and a selection of the information obtained from parents and peers. The scenario is added to, modified, expanded and re-written again and again as the person grows up, until he or she creates a unique, individual pattern of sexual arousal. In the scenario, the 'writer' has created and identified the type of person by whom he or she is sexually excited. When he or she meets such a person, sexual arousal occurs, and if this is reciprocated by the other person, who has his or her own scenario, the couple make closer contact. The contact may be emotional, or physical, but is usually both. With the contact, the couple explore each other's personality and become closer, or separate, as they learn more about each other.

If the contact becomes closer, their sexual arousal and excitement increases. All the senses – sight, sound, taste, smell and touch, may be involved in increasing your sexual arousal. Sight appears to be a potent stimulus for men, and both advertizers and publishers of erotica play on this by using women's bodies as sexual symbols. In Western nations, a woman's breasts, suggested through clothing, or naked, and her buttocks are considered to be sexually arousing to men.

The smell of a clean body is stimulating to both sexes, and in many cultures including our own, perfume, usually sold under a sexually provocative name, is used by women for their own pleasure and is sexually exciting to men. Unpleasant odours can be sexually repellent. Women have a more precise sense of smell than men, so that an unpleasant smell from a man can depress them sexually. Sound, of voice or of music, can be sexually arousing, as can the taste of a partner's hair, lips or body.

For many people, the touch of body contact is the most sexually exciting of all the senses. Most men and women become sexually excited when they kiss or hug each other, particularly when those parts of the body which they find most erotically arousing are caressed. Each person has his or her own erotically arousing parts of the body. Most men are aroused by the sight and feel of a woman's breasts, buttocks and vulva, and most women are aroused by the buttocks and genitals of a man. Other people are aroused by different areas of their body. Only you can find out what part of your body, and your partner's body, arouses you the most.

Sexual excitement, which is an emotion, leads to a physical sexual response, which can be observed and described. Some of what follows has been known for centuries, but some was only discovered by Dr Masters and Dr Johnson in 1966.

Since human sexuality is a shared experience and each partner obtains, or should obtain, pleasure and fulfilment, I think it appropriate to describe what happens to each sex if sexual excitement continues and is not suppressed.

The Sexual Response of Men

The most obvious sign of sexual excitement in a man is the erection of his penis, which enlarges both in length and in diameter. With further excitement, a clear secretion, which may be scanty or profuse, emerges from the 'eye' of his penis and lubricates the glans, whether he has a foreskin or not. Once the man's penis is erect, he is in a stage when additional sexual excitement will make him want to have sexual intercourse, or to have his penis stroked so that he can reach orgasm and ejaculate. In erection, the penis approximately doubles its length and measures 9.5 cm (4 ins). There are several fallacies connected with the penis. The first is that the larger the penis, the better is the man as a lover; this is not true, as the size of the penis is not related to its function. A man with a small penis is as sexually adequate as a man with a large penis, and can provide as much sexual satisfaction. A second fallacy is that the circumcised male takes longer to reach orgasm, and so may more readily help a woman to reach an orgasm. The evidence is that there is no difference in time to reach an orgasm between circumcised and uncircumcised men. There is, of course, a considerable difference between men in the time they take to reach an orgasm, but circumcision or its absence is not a factor.

Once penile erection has occurred and the arousal stimulus continues, the man either seeks to have sexual intercourse or masturbates. In essence, there is little difference as far as the penis is concerned. During coitus he thrusts his penis in and out of his partner's vagina; during masturbation he stimulates his penis by grasping it lightly and stroking the length of the entire organ.

As orgasm approaches, a time is reached when the man knows that within a few moments ejaculation will occur; the phase lasts about 3 or 4 seconds, and even if he ceased all movements of his penis, he knows that ejaculation is inevitable. There is nothing he can do to stop it. This time of 'suspended animation' is followed by a warm feeling along the shaft of his penis as the seminal fluid moves from the seminal vesicles, or collecting area, to the top of the penis. Then, spasmodically, three to six expulsive contractions of the muscles at the base of his penis lead to spurting of seminal fluid, and simultaneously the muscles of his thighs and lower abdomen jerk and thrust convulsively. During his explosive, expulsive period, he may clasp the woman tightly to his body. The 'crisis' or 'climax' passes with smaller contractions fading away. Immediately after ejaculation, the glans of the penis becomes momentarily exquisitely tender, and a feeling of warm, well-being envelops the man. It is usual for complete relaxation and short sleep to occur, the 'little death' of the French, during which time the penis becomes limp.

As a man grows older, certain changes in his sexual response may occur. He may take longer to get an erection, during foreplay his erection may disappear and return several times; he may take longer to ejaculate, and the period after ejaculation before he desires sexual intercourse again may increase, often to 24 hours. These changes vary in degree: some men experience no alteration in sexual response whilst in others the changes are considerable. It is important for a woman to know about these changes as she may feel that because her partner is slower to respond sexually, he no longer loves her, or that he finds her ageing, less firm body no longer sexually stimulating. Of course, this is possible; but it is equally possible that the changes are only due to increasing age, and that if she makes allowance for this, their relationship will be enhanced. This is more likely to occur if the partners are able to communicate with each other.

The Sexual Response in Women

The sexual response of a woman can be divided into four phases, which Masters and Johnson have called (1) the excitement or arousal phase, (2) the plateau phase, (3) the phase of orgasm, and (4) the phase of resolution.

Excitement Phase: This is initiated more by bodily contact with the male than by visual stimuli, although the sight of an attractive male may play some part. Sexual arousal varies in women depending on the time of the month. Many women have a heightened sexual interest at certain times, often at the midcycle or just before and during menstruation, but no consistent pattern can be determined. Tradition has held that sexual intercourse during menstruation is dangerous because the tissues are more fragile and liable to infection, but probably really because of the old Jewish law which held a woman to be 'unclean' during menstruation. This is unfortunate because some women are particularly aroused sexually at this time. There is no medical reason why a woman who desires sexual intercourse during menstruation should not have it. The tissues are not more fragile, nor is infection more likely to occur. There is no danger and the woman is not unclean.

The excitement phase of a woman tends to be slower to reach its peak, and to last for longer, than that of a man. During it her nipples become erect, and the areola around them becomes swollen and dusky. Her clitoris increases in size, mainly in width, and the 'lips' around the vaginal entrance become softer and thicker as they become congested with blood, forming soft swellings. These changes vary in degree from woman to woman.

At the same time as these events are occurring, fluid is entering her pelvic tissues, her vagina is becoming softer and some of the fluid seeps through the layers of tiny cells which make up the vaginal wall, so that it becomes lubricated. Two small glands which lie near the opening of the vagina also secrete fluid, so that both the vagina and its entrance become moist and slippery. If the man attempts to introduce his penis before the fluid has been secreted and the area has become lubricated, coitus may be painful. This is one reason, but not the only one, for a woman's partner to stimulate her by kissing and caressing her, until she is sexually excited. Simultaneously the tissues surrounding the lower one-third of the woman's vagina become swollen with blood, so that soft, warm, 'cushions' form which will caress the man's penis as it enters the vagina.

Plateau Phase: The woman is now in the plateau phase and if she has a sensitive, relating partner will want to feel his erect penis in her lubricated vagina. Even if he is not sensitive to her sexual needs, she is physically able to accept his penis without pain, although she may be resentful, or trade her vagina for the favours he gives her.

In a recent survey, many women said that the most pleasurable part, of sexual intercourse, apart from the orgasm itself, was the feeling of the man's penis entering the vagina. Also, the closer contact of the couple's bodies may stimulate her clitoral area directly, whilst the movement of the man's penis, by moving the lips around the vagina, stimulates it indirectly. This stimulation may bring her to orgasm. About one woman in three reaches an orgasm whilst the man is thrusting in her vagina, either before he ejaculates, simultaneously with his orgasm, or very soon after. But if a woman does not have an orgasm at this time, she may wish the man to help her have an orgasm by gently manipulating her clitoral area at her direction, or by caressing it with his tongue and lips, which is called cunnilingus. She may prefer to have an orgasm before they begin coitus, or after the man has ejaculated, depending on her mood and that of her partner.

Whatever the timing, she is in control and should let the man know what movements of his fingers or tongue stimulate her most and what movements distract her. Most women prefer to have the shaft of the clitoris stimulated rather than the tip (or glans), and finger stimulation is more comfortable if the area is moist. The man can obtain lubrication from her vaginal secretions or from his saliva. The woman should let her partner know what she wants, and he should accept that she knows what is most pleasurable to her, instead of doing what he assumes will give her most pleasure.

Orgasm: It is difficult to describe an orgasm as it is something each person feels and perceives in a unique way. Descriptions given by women suggest that an orgasm is a feeling of intense pleasure which is the peak of sexual arousal. Initially, the feeling is usually located deep in the pelvis, but later it spreads over the whole body. During the orgasm the person's feelings are concentrated on the sensations, largely to the exclusion of anything else. It begins with moments of stillness which are followed by uncontrollable muscle movements, a general tingling, a floating feeling, warmth, well-being, a release of mental tension, and exhilaration.

An orgasm is due to a reflex. Stimulation of the clitoral area, either directly when a woman masturbates or is caressed, or indirectly by the movement of the man's penis as he thrusts in her vagina, sends a message to her spinal cord. In the spinal cord, the reflex occurs and the message is relayed to the nerves which control the muscles of her pelvis. But whether the message is relayed at all, is increased in its intensity, or is inhibited, depends on the degree of control by her brain over the reflex. A woman who has no inhibitions about sex will probably enhance the strength of the message and will have an orgasm. If she has inhibitions or does not like the feeling that the man is 'using' her, she may fail to have an orgasm during coitus, although she can reach an orgasm by fantasizing when she masturbates.

A woman's orgasm is usually associated with the same jerking thrusting movements of the thigh and pelvic muscles, as those of a man, but some women remain still and rigid during the orgasm. A woman's orgasm only differs from a man's orgasm by the absence of ejaculation. Contrary to popular belief a woman does not have to arch her back or 'writhe' in ecstasy during her orgasm. The muscles of her womb and her vagina contract, and some women have a more intense orgasm if the erect penis is deeply inside the vagina at the time, so that it can be rhythmically gripped and released by the contracting vaginal muscles. It was believed until recently that women had two types of orgasm: the 'clitoral orgasm', and the 'vaginal orgasm'. An error of observation and of deduction by Freud is responsible for this. He maintained that the clitoral orgasm was an immature form, which was obtained by masturbation, and that vaginal orgasm only developed with sexual and psychological maturity, when the centre of sexual sensitivity was transferred from the clitoral area to the vagina. The deduction from this was that masturbation was immature, and a woman who could only reach an orgasm by masturbation was sexually and psychologically immature, whilst the woman who had a vaginal orgasm was sexually and psychologically mature. This error, although suspected for some time, was finally laid by Masters and Johnson who showed that an orgasm is an orgasm, and there is no difference in how it is produced, whether as a result of clitoral area manipulation, by movement of the penis in the vagina, by simply fondling the breasts, or even by listening to music.

In nearly all orgasms, the 'trigger' which starts the orgasm reflex is the stimulated clitoris, although additional messages may come from stimulation of the vagina. In all people an orgasm is expressed by contractions of the deep pelvic muscles including those of the vagina in women and is felt as pleasure by a special area of the brain. Many women believed, until recently, that men 'gave' them orgasms and if a woman failed to have an orgasm during coitus she was deficient in femininity and would make the man feel sexually inadequate. Because of this many women 'faked' orgasms so that the man would not feel inadequate or she unfeminine. With a more open approach to woman's sexuality, it is now known that women who fail to reach an orgasm during coitus are not deficient in sexual drive, and that to 'fake' an orgasm is folly.

Almost every women can have an orgasm either by masturbating, or by being sufficiently relaxed and confident in her relationship to let her partner know her needs, so that he helps her reach an orgasm by stimulating her. In a fulfilling relationship the man must be willing and happy to stimulate the woman sexually in the way she wishes.

Ideally, no woman should be embarrassed about asking her partner to do this, nor should a sensitive lover be resentful if asked. But many women are ashamed to ask, and because of this reduce their sexual pleasure.

Resolution Phase: In both sexes, the convulsive muscle contractions and the deep pleasure of orgasm are followed by relaxation. But in contrast to a man's penis, the clitoris is usually not tender and some women can have one orgasm after another without intermission. Other women find one orgasm is all that they want. In the first five to ten minutes of the resolution phase the tissues of the vagina and the vulva lose the fluid which had seeped into them; but if restimulated sexually a woman can be aroused and have other orgasms at shorter intervals than a man.

On the other hand, if a woman is stimulated to the plateau phase but is not helped to have an orgasm, or does not masturbate to give herself an orgasm, the resolution phase is often prolonged and the congestion of the tissues is slow to resolve. Repeated stimulation and failure to achieve an orgasm can lead to physical and mental frustration, and may be the underlying cause of several psychosomatic gynaecological complaints. For this reason, as well as for reasons of love and affection, the man should help the women to reach a climax if she desires this.

About 35 per cent of women reach an orgasm with every, or nearly every episode of sexual intercourse and one woman of every three in this group are able to have multiple orgasms. About 55 per cent of women occasionally reach a climax during sexual intercourse and consistently do so if the clitoris is stimulated with the man's finger or his tongue before or after he has had an orgasm, or if the woman masturbates. Only about 10 per cent of women reach an orgasm very occasionally or never.

MASTURBATION

Stimulation of the genitals by the fingers is almost universal in childhood, and in adolescence masturbation is general. Studies in several countries have shown that almost all young males masturbate, and three-quarters of females have masturbated by the age of 21. As the person gets older and heterosexual contacts are more readily available, the frequency of masturbation diminishes, although it continues throughout life. Masturbation is a normal part of sexual development, and does no physical harm whatsoever, however frequently or infrequently it takes place. The only harms which may result from masturbation are feelings of guilt, occasioned by the Judeo-Christian religious disapproval of masturbation.

Strange, nonsensical myths are still perpetuated: masturbation is said to make a person weak, to damage the eyesight and, in excess (whatever that is), to cause brain decay or insanity. Masturbation does none of these things, but these particularly pernicious ideas are still spread by ignorant people. In the female, masturbation has been said to lead to enlargement of the inner lips of the vulva, to 'congestion of the pelvis', and to venereal disease. Again, all these ideas have no foundation. Masturbation has been declared as evidence of immaturity, which is clearly not true, as people who are sexually well-adjusted and mature obtain sexual pleasure from masturbation, when married or when single. Masturbation is said to lead to sexual frustration and frigidity, but as other equally distinguished investigators declare that it leads to sexual excess, it is obvious that these objections are emotional not factual. It has been said that one cannot possibly get full emotional gratification through masturbation. Recent research has shown this to be false, and many people obtain as much, or more pleasure from masturbation as they do in sexual intercourse.

Masturbation has several positive values. Through it, in childhood and adolescence, a girl may learn to explore her body and not to feel shame or guilt about touching her genital area. It may help a girl become aware of her response to stimulation, and to recognize the stages of her sexual arousal. It may also enable a girl to develop the physical aspects of her sexuality, which should contribute to her later sexual fulfillment. Despite the positive value of masturbation, many parents still condemn their children if they find them masturbating. The effect of this is to increase the child's guilt, as 100 per cent of boys and over 70 per cent of girls masturbate, whatever their parents say.

As adults, both men and women continue to masturbate, although less often than when adolescents. Within a sexual relationship the couple may enjoy masturbation as another way of making love. During periods of separation or if one's sexual partner dies, women and men may prefer to masturbate rather than seeking a lover, when they become sexually tense or excited.

Most people – both men and women – fantasize during masturbation; that is, the person imagines a sexual situation with a lover, or some other sexual situation. Some people can fantasize unaided, but others need the added stimulus of erotic literature or pictures to enhance the fantasy.

As sexual desires continue into old age, as women tend to live longer than men, and as, in our society, it is easier for an older man to find a new partner than it is for an older woman, masturbation may be an older woman's only way of re-enacting an orgasm. No guilt should be experienced, as masturbation is a normal sexual outlet at any age. (See also p. 358.)

PETTING

Petting is an American term for love-making which reaches to, but stops short of, sexual intercourse. In other countries and at other times, other terms have been used; 'bundling', 'lolligagging', and 'smooching'. The activity is as old as tribal society, and is practised by tribes as primitive as those of New Guinea, or by people with a culture as sophisticated as that of the U.S.A. In Western countries, petting seems to be confined largely to adolescence. In 'light petting' or 'necking', the couple kiss passionately, their bodies (usually fully clothed) are in contact, but certain zones are 'forbidden' by the girl, who may refuse to allow her breasts to be caressed, and will not allow wandering hands to reach for her vulva. In 'heavy petting', passionate kissing, love bites, breast stimulation, caressing of the clitoris to orgasm, and of the penis to ejaculation, are accepted in varying degrees; but the girl remains a technical virgin, as she does not allow a man's penis to enter her vagina.

'Petting' plays an important role in the development of sexual behaviour as it offers the opportunity for body exploration, for genital exploration and for emotional interaction. The body exploration which petting permits is important, particularly for those people who obtain a great deal of pleasure from touch. Since this is conditioned by childhood learning, it is likely that men would be more willing to touch, and would obtain more pleasure from touching were they not taught to believe that touching is 'weak' and 'feminine'. Many women enjoy body contact for long periods of love-making before they want sexual intercourse, and many men would find that they too would get sexual pleasure from touch if they could overcome their inhibitions.

Petting was until recently a socially acceptable way of releasing sexual tensions in a society in which sexual intercourse outside marriage was condemned – at least for women. This has changed to some extent in recent years, as the prohibitions of the 'double standard' of sexuality have diminished. Today, when there is a more open attitude towards non-marital sexuality the question, 'what intensity of petting should be permitted' has been replaced by new questions. These are: whether to have (or to allow) sexual intercourse; with which partner or partners, and in what circumstances.

Information from surveys of sexual behaviour in Western nations suggest that by the age of 17, 55–65 per cent of single men and 25–35 per cent of single women have had sexual intercourse. By the age of 24, 85–90 per cent of single men, and 70–80 per cent of single women have had sexual intercourse. Even though sexual intercourse is increasingly usual amongst single people, so that petting as a substitute has become less common, the change should not diminish the importance of touch and of the arousal of sexuality by body exploration and contact, which was a feature of petting. To do so would reduce the pleasure women and men can obtain from sex.

SEXUAL INTERCOURSE

It is strange that there is no verb for sexual intercourse which can be used normally. Even the Latin term used in medical textbooks, *coitus*, is a euphemism. It is made up from the two words *co*, together and *ire*, to go, so that it means to go together.

The delicacy in language about a universal pleasurable activity may be due to the Judeo-Christian belief that coitus should be practised principally for the procreation of children, and only secondarily permitted as an expression of the love that exists between the two sexual partners. Today, with efficient contraception, these two functions can be separated, and it is increasingly accepted that sexuality and its active genital component, coitus, form a physical and emotional bond holding two people together in warmth, security and mutual pleasure. Sexual intercourse should not be a competitive indoor sport, nor a virtuoso performance to be boasted about later, but a physical and emotional expression of a warm relationship between two 'turned on' people, which may last permanently or may be temporary.

A sexual relationship implies more than sexual intercourse. It also includes enjoyment of being with a person, touching and mutually pleasuring. In the early years of a sexual relationship, coitus commonly takes place frequently, often one or more times a day. The frequency falls off after one or two years, to two or three times a week up to the age of about 35. As middle age approaches, coital frequency often falls to once a week or less. But there are very considerable variations, and some couples only have sexual intercourse at infrequent intervals in the early years, whilst other couples enjoy sex frequently and satisfactorily well into old age.

It is sometimes asked, can coitus take place too frequently? The answer is a firm No! There is no such thing as 'excessive coitus'. Provided the male can obtain and maintain an erection of his penis, and provided that he can do this as often as he and his partner desire to have sexual intercourse, coitus can take place as often as they wish. Frequent coitus does not lead to any weakness of either partner. Occasionally, frequent coitus does cause irritation to one or other partner's genitals from over-stimulation or friction. In such cases, a period of a couple of days' rest will restore the function to normal.

How often a couple have sexual intercourse is a matter for their joint decision. 'Excessive' coitus does not exist, and 'infrequent' coitus is equally harmless provided that this pattern is acceptable and not frustrating to either partner. Nor is there any truth in the belief that to be healthy a woman or a man needs to have sex at regular intervals. Neither a woman nor a man can have too many nor too few orgasms. Each individual has different needs and desires for an orgasm at different times in his or her life. When a person has no sexual partner, orgasms can be produced as often as the person desires by masturbation. With a partner an orgasm may be the culmination of sexual intercourse, which is the way a man usually prefers; or can be produced by one partner stimulating the other's clitoris or penis with tongue or finger; or by masturbating either during sexual intercourse, or afterwards.

As I have mentioned, because of culturally induced inhibitions, many women take longer to be aroused erotically than do men. For this reason, mutual pleasuring should take place before coitus is attempted. I prefer the term mutual pleasuring to the older word foreplay because foreplay has acquired a special meaning which is insulting to women. Many men believe that foreplay means that the man briefly fondles the woman's breasts and fumbles at her vulva whilst she caresses his penis. It is brief because it delays what he really wants: and that is to put his penis in her vagina, thrust and have an orgasm. Mutual pleasuring involves much more than that. It involves cuddling and exploring each other's body surface. It involves stroking, and it involves kissing and exploration of other parts of the body with lips and tongue. It involves stimulation of those parts of the body each person feels is erotic by fingers, tongue, lips, thighs and body.

The extent and sequence of mutual pleasuring is one which each couple evolves uniquely for themselves. They make their own formula, for what erotically stimulates a person is unique for that person, and has to be communicated to the partner either by using words or by body language. And in this communication each partner has to accept that the other knows what most excites him or her.

During the period of mutual pleasuring, both partners become increasingly stimulated by kissing, by bodily contact when they hug or cuddle each other, by stroking each other's bodies, especially the areas which arouse sexual desire – for example, the woman's breasts and thighs and the man's genitals. But each partner has to discover the erotic areas of the other. Mutual pleasuring goes on for as long as the couple wish, until each is aroused and ready for coitus. The man shows this by his erect penis, the woman by her lubricated vagina. Both acknowledge it by an increased sexual urge. Women, particularly, say that they can enjoy the closeness, the body contact and the intimacy of sexual intercourse, and obtain pleasure in 'pleasing' a man sexually. But the real overwhelming pleasure occurs when sexual pleasuring comes to a climax in an orgasm.

The first coitus, if neither partner is sexually experienced, or if the man is unaware of a woman's sexual needs, can be clumsy and frustrating to both partners, or painful to the woman. The psychological dangers of forceful, clumsy attempts at penetration on a woman who is not ready for coitus have been exaggerated. Even so, a traumatic first coital encounter with an insensitive man may create anxieties in the woman which even her love for him cannot resolve, and their sexual relationship may be marred. The full establishment of sexual compatibility may take some time.

The period of sexual arousal during the first time the couple have sexual intercourse is important, as it may be painful to the woman if her vagina has not become lubricated before her partner's penis enters it. Once she is sexually excited and her vagina is moist, she may wish to feel her partner's penis in her body. She should guide it so that it lies against her hymen, making sure that no strands of vulval hair are in between. If she lies on her back, the man on top of her, her legs apart, her knees bent, she will find it easier to guide his erect penis. In this position, as he lies over her, he slowly and gently presses his penis into the vaginal entrance, and then withdraws slightly. This movement is repeated, and each time he presses his penis a little further into the vagina, always moving slowly so that the muscles which surround the vagina have time to relax, and the hymen to stretch. Slowly he moves, and soon he finds that his penis has been introduced fully into the vagina. If he tries to introduce it too quickly, he may cause the woman pain, which could cause her vaginal muscles to contract against him causing her more pain. With careful penetration, coitus can proceed normally, the penis deeply inside the vagina and its thrusting movements bringing the man to orgasm. Immediately after ejaculation of semen, the tip (or glans) of the penis is exquisitely sensitive, and the erection subsides. The sensitivity lasts only for a few moments, but whilst this is occurring he lies relaxed and still.

The woman may reach her orgasm during the man's thrusting but if she has not, she may wish him to help her reach orgasm by stimulating her with his fingers or tongue. If they are aware of each other's needs and desires, there should be no problem about this. Embarrassment or resentment should have no place in a warm loving relationship.

Sexual adjustment between the two partners may occur quickly, may take time, or may never be fully achieved, depending on the sexual knowledge of the couple, their inhibitions towards sex and their ability to express their sexual needs to each other. The understanding between them required for the first coitus to be pleasurable to both partners, needs to continue into subsequent love-making. Unless a woman is sexually aroused and stimulated each time, so that her vagina is lubricated, intercourse may be painful because of soreness at her vaginal entrance. The cure for this is to improve the quality of the pleasuring, for the man to be sensitive when he inserts his penis and for the couple to use some other form of sexual expression, such as masturbation, until the woman's discomfort has subsided.

COITAL TECHNIQUE

Sexual intercourse can take place in a variety of positions. These have been described in the literature of all cultures, and ancient Indian literature is particularly informative, as shown by Vatsyayana's *Kama Sutra*, written in 200 BC, and in the sculptures on the temples of Khajuraho. Basically, the positions can be reduced to about half a dozen, all of which are normal.

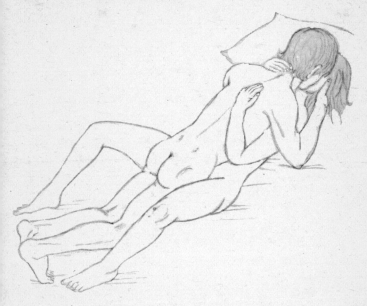

FIG. 5/1 Coital position. Face to face, man on top

Face to face, the man on top: The man lies on top of the woman, either putting his weight upon her, or supporting most of his weight on his elbows or hands. She spreads her legs apart, and may for variety flex her knees, sometimes placing them around her partner's waist. She may place a pillow beneath her buttocks to lift her pelvis. There are many variations of this basic position. The woman may keep her legs stretched out, her partner's legs inside hers, or she may bring her legs together, so that her partner's knees are outside. She may flex her thighs more so that her legs are clasped around his shoulders.

This position is the most usual, and has the advantage that it makes penile entry into the vagina easy. The bodies of the two partners are in close proximity, so that they can kiss and caress each other during coitus; it permits the male to set the pace and slow or hasten coitus, to reach an orgasm at a desired speed; and it is probably the best position for pregnancy to occur, as after ejaculation the seminal fluid bathes the cervix. The disadvantages of the position are that it restricts the woman's movements and thrusts; male orgasm is often reached too quickly; penetration may be painfully deep, and the male is unable to caress the woman's clitoris during coitus, which she may desire (Fig. 5/1).

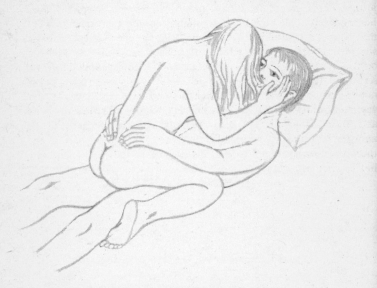

FIG. 5/2 Coital position. Face to face, woman on top

Face to face, woman on top: The man lies on his back, the woman squats over him and guides his penis into her vagina. Once this has occurred, she may lie upon him, her weight resting on his body; she may support her weight on her arms; or she may sit upright across his thighs. The man may lie flat, raise himself on his arms, or clasp his legs around the woman's waist.

This position has an advantage if the man is heavy and his partner light in weight. In it the woman has the greatest freedom of movement, and the male can caress her clitoris and vulval area during coitus.

The disadvantages are that some women cannot control the depth of penile penetration too easily, and it may be too deep and so painful. During coitus the man's penis may slip out of the vagina, which is uncomfortable for both and spoils smooth coital sequence. (Fig. 5/2)

Man's face to woman's back; rear entry: There are several variations of this position. The man may lie behind the woman, his hands around her to caress her breasts or clitoris. She lies in front of him, her legs bent at the hips, her body slightly curved away from his. The man's penis is inserted into the vagina from the rear, and once inside she presses her thighs together and pushes backwards so that her buttocks make a firm contact against his lower abdomen and scrotum. Alternatively, she may lie on her stomach with her pelvis raised and her legs apart. The man lies on top of her, entering her vagina from the rear. Or she may kneel on hands and knees, her head and breasts touching the bed, the man kneeling behind her. In another variation, the man sits on the edge of a chair, or the bed, and the women with her back to him, sits upon his penis and as it slips into her vagina, eases herself onto his lap.

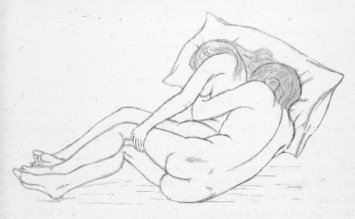

FIG. 5/3 Coital position. Rear entry

The advantages of these positions are that the contact of the woman's buttocks on the man's abdomen, legs and scrotum may stimulate them both; he can readily caress her breasts or her clitoris during coitus; and the couple can rest on their sides during coitus. In late pregnancy this position is the most suitable one. (Fig. **5/3**)

Face to face, side by side: This position is, in fact, not exactly side by side, for penile entry would be almost impossible if it were. Usually the couple's legs are interlocked, and the man may lie largely on his back, the woman resting on his chest, or alternatively, the woman may lie largely on her back, one thigh beneath him. (Fig. **5/4**)

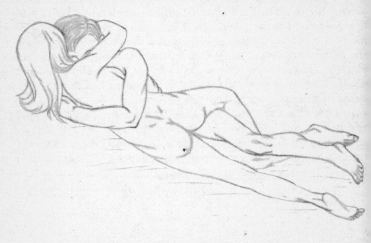

FIG. 5/4 Coital position. Face to face, side by side

Sitting positions: The man sits on a chair, or the edge of a bed, and the woman sits astride his lap, his penis within her vagina, his arms around her body, and hers around his. Alternatively, the woman can lie on her back, the man squatting between her thighs, her legs clasped around his hips, his penis in her vagina. He can then make thrusting motions, or she can pull her pelvis back and forth. Another alternative is for the woman to squat between the man's thighs, supporting her weight on her outstretched arms, whilst he lies on his back with his legs apart. Once his penis is inside her vagina, she moves her pelvis in a circular fashion. (Fig. **5/5**).

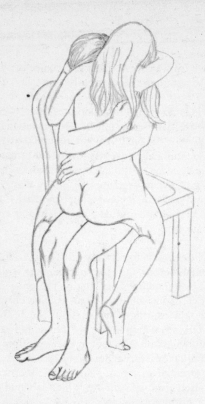

FIG. 5/5 Coital position. Sitting position

Standing position: By bending his legs, the man can introduce his penis either facing the woman, or from the rear. She may put her hands around his neck and clasp his hips between her thighs. The couple may move around during coitus, or coitus may take place in surroundings different from normal, such as during a shower.

The advantages of the sitting and standing positions are that they may be more exciting because they are unusual and not used routinely.

Extravaginal sexual stimulation

The man may obtain stimulation by rubbing his penis between the woman's thighs, or between her breasts. The advantage of these positions, apart from variety, is that the chance of conception occurring is remote, although ejaculation outside the vulva may lead to conception.

One 'notorious' extravaginal position is often followed by a deep emotional release. This is the simultaneous caressing of the woman's clitoris and vulva by the man's tongue (cunnilingus), whilst she puts his penis in her mouth and caresses it with her tongue (fellatio) until they both have orgasms. Although this position has been condemned by the clergy, and is whispered about by adolescents as the sixty-nine or soixante-neuf position, it is completely normal, and a couple need feel no guilt if they obtain mutual pleasure, happiness, sexual relaxation and release from it.

For sexual intercourse to be truly satisfying, after one partner has had an orgasm, or before, the other partner may wish to be helped to reach orgasm by cunnilingus or fellatio. The entry of the penis into the vagina, or caressing with the tongue, should only come at the end of a sequence of pleasuring activities (body touch, stroking, hugging, exploration, talking) which draws the bonds between the partners closer, surrounding them with feelings of warmth to each other, and joy in their mutual embraces. Sexual intercourse is not just a silent monotonous thrust of an urgent penis into an indifferent vagina. It is a complex, varied group of activities which can lead to the maximum sexual joy for both participants.

APHRODISIACS

Since the dawn of time, erotic stimulants have been sought by men who felt that their sexual performance was waning, and given to women who failed to respond to sexual advances. The oldest existing medical textbook, an undated Egyptian scroll from about 2000 BC, contains recipes for making 'erotic potions'. Shakespeare wrote extensively of aphrodisiacs. The great number of substances recommended as sexual stimulants indicates that none is of much value. Oysters are said to lead to amorous behaviour; rhinoceros horn powdered and drunk in wine is said to restore waning sexual function; whilst yohimbine, derived from the bark of an African tree, has long been used by the natives to increase their sexual powers. Cantharides, or Spanish Fly, which is an irritant of the urinary tract, also has an aphrodisiac reputation. All these beliefs are baseless, and none of the many foods, drugs or irritants recommended through the ages has any aphrodisiac property. Set apart, because of its frequent consumption in Western society is alcohol, particularly champagne, which is credited as being a considerable erotic stimulant. Alcohol, it is true, causes dilation of the skin blood vessels and a feeling of warmth which extends to the genitals, and in small quantities it acts as a narcotic of the higher centres, producing a light-hearted approach and reducing the 'moral' block to sexual behaviour. In larger quantities, its narcotic effect reduces rather than stimulates sexual desires and performance.

In summary, there is no such thing as a true aphrodisiac, and no drug exists that the eager male could give to the resistant female which would render her unresisting and so full of sexual ardour that she would welcome seduction.

THE NEW SEXUALITY

Sexual research, in recent years, has established that many of the beliefs which surround sexuality are untrue, and today a better attitude towards sexuality is evident, especially amongst younger people. The research has shown, amongst other things, the following important findings:

- The 'double standard' of sexual behaviour has diminished, and today women can behave sexually much more freely. Some people regret this sexual 'permissiveness', but they are usually wrong. The change does not mean that most sexual relationships are a sequence of 'one-night stands' (which are unusual, except in certain groups) but that women, as well as men, now feel free to express their sexuality in any way they choose.
- Many more unmarried men and women are living together, and most of these relationships, which may last for a longer or shorter period, are sharing, one to one relationships. This is something which those people who are anxious about today's sexual permissiveness and decadence fail to notice.

● Although some men and woman may still feel uncomfortable about explaining their sexual and emotional needs to their partner, this inhibition is beginning to diminish.

● There is more open discussion about sex between men and women so that each becomes aware of the other's sexual desires and needs. This is good. Only when there is open discussion between lovers, will they become aware of each others sexual desires and needs.

There are several other facets of sexuality which I believe should be emphasized. Many women have known about them, but male dominated society has largely rejected them until recently. They include the following:

● Women have no less enthusiasm for sex, no less enjoyment of sex and no less sexual drive than men.

● A woman's sexual response is not intrinsically different from that of a man, but many women are slower to reach full sexual arousal than men, probably because of the sexual attitudes they learned during childhood.

● Women should be able to say 'yes' without shame, and 'no' without guilt, to a request for sexual intercourse. A woman need no longer be anxious that she may lose the man's love if she refuses his request and should be able to talk with the man about her decision.

● Women should be encouraged to expect that their relationship with a man is one in which mutual respect for the woman as a person replaces the older expectation that a woman should be dependent financially, emotionally and socially upon him. It is a relationship in which the mutual respect extends to each person's sexuality.

These changes should create an atmosphere in which sexuality is more open, more honest and more fulfilling, and the relationship between the two people should be more rewarding. The changes will neither increase, nor diminish, the number of people who obtain sexual enjoyment in a series of 'one-night stands' or who have relationships with several partners simultaneously, not serially. Provided all the partners accept and enjoy this convention, no psychological damage results, but two physical problems may arise.

The first is that each of the multiple partners has a greater chance of contracting a sexually transmitted disease, usually gonorrhoea, from another partner than would occur in a one to one sexual relationship (see p. 345). The second consequence, which also applies to a one to one relationship, is that a woman runs the risk of becoming pregnant unless she or her partner take contraceptive precautions. Unfortunately, some women and men do not use birth control measures, and unwanted and unwelcome pregnancies continue to occur. With the change in society's attitude to single mothers, the problems of out of wedlock pregnancy have decreased, but sufficient disapproval and discrimination persists towards single parents to make the care of the child a burden to many unmarried mothers. Only if society provides sufficient financial and emotional support will the burden be reduced, and single parents be able to raise their children as satisfactorily as married parents.

Even so, an unexpected pregnancy can cause great stresses in a relationship, which may be so severe that the relationship is jeopardized. Today, with effective birth control measures (see Chapter 7) unwanted pregnancy should only occur rarely, provided adolescents and adults of both sexes have been informed about contraception and, if sexually active, have access to contraceptives. This means that all nations must implement the declaration their leaders collectively agreed to in 1974, at a United Nations Conference in Bucharest. They agreed that 'all couples and individuals have the basic right to decide freely and responsibly the number and spacing of their children and have the education and information to do so'.

The responsibility for avoiding un unwanted pregnancy is that of both partners. Unfortunately, at present, many women believe the man when he says he 'will be careful'. This is not enough. Contraception must be a mutual responsibility. If a woman is uncertain that her partner will use a condom, she must protect herself from becoming pregnant. A more permissive attitude to sex does not mean abandoning all sense of sexual responsibility.

Sexual responsibility should be part of a new sexuality. If religious prohibitions and traditional sexual attitudes to premarital sex are increasingly abandoned, they must be replaced by the much more difficult concept of personal sexual responsibility. The code by which people live together is something only they can decide for themselves, but it should surely be based on emotional harmony, which includes sexual harmony. There is no place for emotional and sexual exploitation.

People who desire a return to traditional values of sexuality, that is sexual exploitation of women by men and the double standard, appear to believe that the new sexuality will lead to greater sexual self-indulgence, to less sexual responsibility, to the disappearance of marriage and family life and to the rejection of the 'deeper, basic values of society'. They ignore the fact that many young people who are trying to find new sexual values, also reject other values which our society accepts as normal: deceit in government and business, greed for wealth and possessions, unequal opportunities for women, self-seeking by individuals and dishonesty by many individuals and companies.

Hopefully, these new sexual values will mean a sharing relationship with another person, in which the needs and desires of each are accepted. People accepting these values may not reject marriage, as over 90 per cent of people marry; nor will they reject the family as a social unit. But they may question whether the present family of 'legally' married father and mother and two children, living in relative isolation, is the best social unit, and ask whether other types of family may not produce better adjusted, happier, more 'sharing' people.

THE MARRIAGE PARTNERSHIP

It is often asked, 'if women become sexually liberated and if society accepts the new sexual values, will marriage survive?' The evidence is that it will; but no one really knows why, in our society, two people fall in love with each other and marry.

In many societies, love is not a factor in marriage; in India for example, marriages are arranged by the family, who select a suitable girl from one of several villages which traditionally supply brides to the village of the groom. The groom does not see his bride before the marriage. The evidence is that these marriages work fairly well; each partner knowing his or her duties and responsibilities, and the sexual aspect being limited. But in our society, the decision is made by the man and the woman that they will live together, will procreate and bring up children, will support each other, and will merge their personalities to some extent. This is not an inconsiderable undertaking, when one considers the different and unique background, training, experience, loves, hates, attitudes and personality structure of each partner. Studies have been made which show that, in fact, the choice of a mate is limited. The 'pool' of eligible males from which women select partners is usually determined by the race, the social class, the age, the level of education, the place of residence and also by religion. It is true that a few couples step over the expected boundaries and successfully marry outside their 'class' or 'race', but even in multi-racial societies, such as Malaysia and Fiji, inter-racial marriages are unusual.

As well as the 'social factor', there is a second, less understood factor which has been called the 'complementary need factor'. This factor is much more specific for each individual, and operates usually without their knowing it in their choice of a person with whom 'to fall in love'. A woman who needs to 'mother' another person may choose a man who has an obvious problem, and she gratifies her 'need' for mothering by looking after him and helping him to overcome his problem. An aggressive, demanding man may select a timid, passive woman, on whom he can vent his need for aggression, without receiving a rebuff. These are extreme examples, as many marriages are contracted for emotional rather than rational reasons. In these marriages, it has been suggested that the 'complementary need-factor' may operate. The strongly-sexed male may be attracted to a girl who refuses his sexual advances because her upbringing has led her to believe that premarital sex is prohibited, and his main reason for seeking the marriage may be that she refuses to permit sexual intercourse. Meanwhile he has had sexual intercourse with other girls, but because his upbringing has made him value virginity, he would not think of marrying one of them, although she might make him a more suitable partner.

In our society, sexual compatibility is an important factor in keeping a marriage stable but, of course, it is only one of many factors. If one of the partners to a marriage has been taught to believe that sexual intercourse is something shameful and dirty, and that for a woman sexual intercourse is something to be passively endured, rather than an activity for the mutual pleasure of the couple, problems will arise.

Clearly, incompatibility will not vanish even if both partners have received some education in sexual matters, but the problems will be reduced. Obviously, too, a knowledge of sex will not make a woman happier if her partner is an alcoholic or a philanderer. Nor will it keep the marriage stable if the male is brutal, emotionally disturbed or completely selfish. But then any attempt by one individual to bend or damage the personality of another is a sin, if not a legal one, certainly one against humanity, particularly in a relationship where the two personalities are in intimate contact over a long time. Since the sexual side of personality is an important one, perhaps this is the reason why sexual compatibility plays such an important part in a stable marriage. It gives even greater emphasis to the belief that 'marriage should be made harder to obtain, and divorce easier'.

Legalized marriage remains the most favoured institution for couples in most nations, despite the concern from some religious groups that so-called 'sexual permissiveness' will lead to the demise of the family.

SEXUAL PROBLEMS

It is impossible to calculate the frequency of sexual problems which may mar, or destroy a relationship as, until recently, people were ashamed to seek help.

The evidence suggests that in men two sexual problems predominate. These are premature ejaculation and impotence. The man with premature ejaculation is able to get a penile erection but, before or very soon after his penis is enclosed in his partner's vagina, he ejaculates. The speed with which this happens prevents his partner from obtaining sexual pleasure. The condition of the impotent man is more serious – he is unable to obtain or sustain an erection of his penis, so that sexual intercourse cannot occur. Whilst disease and drugs may cause impotence in a few men, most men with premature ejaculation and with impotence have psycho-sexual problems, which usually can be resolved with the help of their partner and, perhaps, a counsellor.

In women, three main problems occur. The first is that sexual intercourse is painful so that it is either abandoned or else causes such a severe upset that it is never pleasurable. This problem is called *dyspareunia*, which means painful coitus. When the woman finds it too painful to let the man put his penis in her vagina and resists by tightening the muscles surrounding her vaginal entrance, the condition is called *vaginismus*.

The second problem is failure of the vagina to become lubricated and the soft swellings around its entrance to develop, despite mutual pleasuring. The woman fails to become 'turned-on'. She derives little or no erotic pleasure or, worse, finds coitus repellent. This is called lowered libido or general sexual dysfunction.

The third sexual problem of women is failure to achieve an orgasm, or 'orgastic dysfunction'. This term needs to be interpreted carefully. Some sex therapists believe that all women who fail to have orgasms during sexual intercourse have orgastic dysfunction. This is too restrictive. A woman has not got orgastic dysfunction if she usually has an orgasm during love-making, whether she reaches an orgasm by masturbating, whilst her lover is thrusting in her vagina, or by being stimulated by her lover before or after the lover has had an orgasm. Nor does a woman who has orgasms by masturbating when she is alone have orgastic dysfunction, even if she does not have orgasms when she is with her lover. None of these women is sick, nor are they 'frigid'.

Only women who never reach an orgasm, whatever the stimulation, have orgastic dysfunction. It is important for everyone to remember this. It is also important to remember that many women obtain a great deal of pleasure and emotional warmth from the closeness and intimacy of sexual intercourse even though they do not have an orgasm. Magazine articles which stress the need for a woman to become a real woman by having orgasms do a disservice. What should be stressed, instead, is that those women who obtain emotional closeness and pleasure during sexual intercourse will obtain even more pleasure if they are helped to reach an orgasm by their lover.

If you can have an orgasm, by whatever method you reach it, you are normal. If you do not have an orgasm during sexual intercourse, but do reach an orgasm when your partner stimulates you, or by masturbation, you are normal. And the orgasm reached during sexual intercourse is no 'better' or more 'normal' than that reached in any other way.

But if you are unable to achieve an orgasm with your lover or are too ashamed to reach an orgasm by masturbating, and you are worried about this, you can be helped. Women with one or more of these sexual problems have been called 'frigid'. This term should be abandoned. It implies that the woman, because of some congenital condition, will never be able to respond fully sexually. This is untrue. With counselling and with the help of a lover, most women can become aroused sexually and nearly all can reach an orgasm. There is a difference in the speed of the change: women who are unable to become aroused sexually are harder to help than women who are aroused but who fail to reach an orgasm.

Failure to become sexually aroused and the inability to have an orgasm, like impotence in men, may be the result of ill-health and depression. The drugs used to treat many illnesses, or to counteract depression, may also reduce a person's sexual drive.

Fatigue is a cause of a reduced sexual drive and sexual capacity in many people and, in our society, women may become more fatigued than men. Because women are subjected to so much physical and emotional pressure, by the demands of rearing children, maintaining a house, often simultaneously working at a job, and by demands for companionship and socializing, they may be too exhausted to respond sexually.

It is likely, however, that in many cases, the underlying cause of most sexual problems is psychological, resulting from firstly, ignorance or misinformation about sexuality; secondly, shame about sexual activity and thirdly, a lack of communication and an inadequate relationship with the partner. These factors have been mentioned before but bear repeating.

IGNORANCE: Faulty childhood upbringing by 'strict', sexually inhibited, parents who condition the girl to believe in the double standard of sexuality, to submit to her partner's 'demands' passively, and to expect to receive no sexual pleasure, can lead to a reduced sexual drive, and foster the belief that sex is a duty to be paid to a demanding, sexually aggressive man, rather than a mutually enjoyed pleasure.

GUILT AND SHAME: Some parents may condition their daughters to believe that sex is a shameful activity in which a person 'indulges'. In these families, sex may never be discussed openly and such information (or more accurately, misinformation) as is obtained, is from the whispered confidences of girls of the daughter's own age. If the parents consider the human body, apart from the exposed face, arms and legs, to be indecent and punish the girl when she asks about it, or if they do not respond sensibly to the child's natural curiosity about sex and human reproduction, the child is likely to believe that sexual activity is indecent, shameful and something to be ignored as far as possible. These attitudes may influence her enjoyment of sex.

The opposite attitude towards sex can also occasion shame. A 'sophisticated' woman who reads books about sex and who openly discusses sexual matters may also have a deficient sexual drive. In Western society success is lauded, and if in sexual relations success

means reaching a consistent orgasm in each episode of sexual intercourse, success may elude many women. This is not because they are
inadequate for, as I have stressed, sexual desire and the ability to
achieve an orgasm vary very considerably over the years. But
because a woman fails to achieve sexual success by having orgasms,
she may become ashamed at what she believes is her sexual inadequacy. This shame can lead to a reduction in her sexual desire, as a
safeguard against 'failure'.

During sexual intercourse, a woman can increase her sexual
awareness by fantasizing about sexually arousing stimuli. But if she
keeps thinking how terrible it will be, and how inadequate she is if she
does not have an orgasm, she may reduce her sexual desire by her
over determination to be a 'normal' woman. This feeling of inadequacy is increased by the cinema and by literature. So many films
stress by implication, and so many books indicate explicitly, that
when a woman has an orgasm, bells ring, lights flash, music falls from
the air and the planets stop in their courses, that she believes she
should experience all these explosive sensations. If she has an orgasm
without fireworks or comets, she may believe that she is sexually
deficient, although with it, a warm delightful sensation sweeps over
her. The conflict created by this false belief may cause her subconsciously to reduce her sexual desires, so that she may avoid the pain
and shame of failure.

Her sense of sexual 'failure' may be compounded by the knowledge that she can reach an orgasm if her lover stimulates her erotically, or if she masturbates. Many women have been brought up to
believe that masturbation or stimulation is shameful. This myth is
also believed by many men. The truth is that an orgasm is an orgasm
however it is produced.

INADEQUATE RELATIONSHIP WITH HER PARTNER: This is probably as, or more, important than the other two factors, but is interlinked with and dependent upon them.

The lack of communication and ignorance of a woman's needs may
lead to a change of feeling between the couple and to the further
reduction of their mutual sexuality. This in turn may further reduce
the woman's sexual desire, or lead to her unwilling, often hidden,
acceptance of the man's sexual needs for fear of losing his affection.

WHAT CAN BE DONE? If the woman has dyspareunia there may be a local cause, and a doctor would be able to make sure that she has no infection such as monilia (see p. 341), which could make sexual intercourse painful.

In most cases of dyspareunia, and in all cases of vaginismus, the problem is a psychological one which may be aggravated by an unaware lover. Many women still believe that intercourse is painful or impossible because they are 'small made' – meaning that their vagina is too small or the man's penis too large. Their lover can reinforce the belief if he fails to stimulate the woman before he tries to insert his penis into her vagina, so that it is insufficiently lubricated. Many women are ignorant about the genital anatomy. They have no idea where their clitoris is, nor how the labia surround their vagina. Many women have never looked at their vulva in a mirror so that they could see what it looks like. These beliefs and failures produce the fear that intercourse will be painful and may damage the woman, and consequently it is painful.

But with counselling, understanding and the lover's help, every woman who has vaginismus can be cured, but only if she takes the first step to obtain help from a concerned, helpful counsellor. Unfortunately, doctors have as many sexual hang-ups as their patients, and the couple have to find a doctor who has been trained to manage sexual problems. Some doctors still use surgery to 'widen' a narrow vaginal entrance. In very rare circumstances this operation may be needed, but they are so rare that if a doctor suggests surgery the woman should at once obtain a second opinion.

The solution to the problems of lack of sexual arousal (general sexual dysfunction) and the failure to have orgasms (orgastic dysfunction) is rather more complicated. First, lack of sexual arousal.

If the couple do not relate adequately emotionally they may also not be able to relate sexually. If the woman is uncertain about her relationship and uncomfortable about her sexual desires, and has, as a partner, a lover who is sexually inhibited, uninformed and emotionally 'up-tight', neither will be able to communicate to the other about their sexual needs. Lacking insight, the lover is unable to perceive that the woman has a problem and she is unable to talk about it.

The lover knows when he is sexually excited and how to reach an orgasm, which he often does quickly; he forgets that he should be involved in helping his partner to become sexually excited, and ignores the fact that it may take her longer than him to reach the pre-orgastic stage of sexual arousal, so that it is all over for him before she is ready. Because of their inhibitions in communicating their sexual needs, the woman is unable to ask her man to help her reach an orgasm by stimulating her, and he is too inhibited or too ignorant to take the initiative. Masters and Johnson have pointed out that in the resolution of a sexual problem, there is no uninvolved partner. A woman's sexual problem will only be resolved if her partner is prepared to help willingly and lovingly.

With his co-operation and with informed guidance from a counsellor who may be a family doctor, a psychologist, a gynaecologist or a psychiatrist, cure is likely. The counsellor first makes sure that the woman has no disease which may reduce her sexual desire. The next step is to find out what excites the woman sexually and conversely what 'turns her off' sexually, so that she can become sexually self aware, and so that her partner can become aware of her sexual needs. The counsellor next tries to help the couple obtain a relaxing, erotically stimulating environment in which they can learn to pleasure each other sexually, giving pleasure to get pleasure. In this relaxed environment, where there is no pressure to perform sexually, the woman's sexual desires are usually aroused. At first the arousal may be small but with continued pleasuring it increases. Only when she is really aroused do the couple try having sexual intercourse.

If the woman's sexual problem is the failure to have orgasms, the couple use the same pleasuring techniques, but go through the learning stages more quickly. Often the man has to learn techniques of stimulating the woman erotically so that she reaches an orgasm. It is important that she tells him what gives her sexual satisfaction, rather than permitting him to do what he thinks will give her satisfaction. She is the director and the authority about what most stimulates her. When the problem is orgastic dysfunction, some women may find it easier to begin by masturbating when alone, using fantasy as an erotic stimulus, rather than to be stimulated erotically by a partner. If these methods fail to help the woman to reach a climax, the doctor may suggest that she uses a vibrator, which a woman can use to stimulate herself erotically so that she reaches an orgasm.

Once a woman has achieved one orgasm, by whatever method, she is well on the way to being regularly orgastic. With the help of a co-operative, gentle, sympathetic partner, most women who have failed to have an orgasm and a large number who could not be aroused sexually find their sexual response heightened and reach an orgasm regularly.

NYMPHOMANIA

Whilst increased sexual desire is the normal sexual make-up of some women, an incessant and overwhelming urgency for sexual intercourse, even in the most inappropriate circumstances, is abnormal. This condition is called nymphomania, and it has a psychological basis. Treatment is needed, and should only be given by a qualified psychiatrist who has an especial interest in sexual disturbances.

HOMOSEXUALITY

Over 90 per cent of women find companionship, a stable relationship and sexual fulfilment with a member of the complementary sex. Note that I have called men the complementary sex – not the opposite sex. This is what men are to women, and women to men – the sex of each complements that of the other partner. About 5 per cent of women, perhaps more, are bisexual; that is at some time, or for several periods of their lives, they choose to cease to have a sexual relationship with a man and form a relationship with a woman. In both kinds of relationship they give and receive sexual pleasure, so that they obtain emotional contentment from both. Bisexual women say that they relate differently to a male lover and to a female lover. Sexual relationships with a man may be conditioned by the man's cultural belief that he must be the initiator, that he is the sexual expert and that his sexual needs are paramount. The woman may be conditioned to be passive, to aim to 'please' the man sexually, to adjust her response to his and to hope, but not expect, that he will help her reach her sexual fulfilment including an orgasm. By contrast, bisexual women say that when their lover is a woman, the mutual pleasuring is slower, more innovative and lasts longer. They have a total body response rather than a genital one, and feel a warmer, deeper, reaction to their lover, because each is more sensitive to the other's needs. The information is fragmentary at present, but in the next few years, more may be discovered and the social constraints towards bisexuality may diminish.

About 5 per cent of women have no sexual interest in men, although they may have friends who are men, and their sexual interests, their need for companionship, are met by alliance with another woman. These women are homosexuals: their sexual desires are directed to members of their own sex. They are also called lesbians, because a group of homosexual women, prominent amongst whom was the poetess Sappho, lived on the island of Lesbos in the time of the ancient Greek civilization. This civilization, lauded as one of the peak periods of human creativeness, incidentally was relatively permissive in regard to sex.

Until recently it was thought that a homosexual tendency was in-born, in other words, it was there from before birth. Although it is true that there are shades of femininity and masculinity in every person, it is now known that homosexual attitudes are *acquired* during the child's upbringing. It was also thought at one time that feminine men and masculine woman were so because the man manufactured too much female sex hormone, and the woman too much male hormone. It is true that women do manufacture some male hormone in a gland called the adrenal, but the quantity is small, and there is no difference in the amount of hormone secreted by homosexual or heterosexual women. A similar consideration applies to men, and the much-derided 'pansy', 'fairy' or 'queer', although different in character, has the same amount of male sex hormone (or androgen) circulating in his blood as the bovine football hero. Very rarely a woman may develop a tumour which manufactures androgen, and as the concentration of androgen increases in her blood, she becomes physically less feminine: hair appears on her body and face, her breasts become smaller, her clitoris enlarges, but her feminine attitudes do not change.

Small children have no particular thoughts about sex—except perhaps to note that little girls do not have a penis – and until parental attitudes direct them into one sexual role or another, they are content, each seeing the other merely as a playmate. However, the cultural attitudes of our society towards sexual differences are soon imposed on the child. A girl should be quiet, play with dolls, help mother, wear 'pretty dresses', be demure; a boy is expected to be untidy, play 'rough' games, like toys which are destructive, to be 'manly' and to imitate father. Most societies recognize that a distinction between the sexes is needed for survival and each sex is trained to believe that certain activities are predominantly theirs – housework and cooking are for girls; car-cleaning, wood-cutting, painting are boys' work. Ultimately, then, the sexual inclinations of the child are determined by the attitudes of its parents, and some parents unwittingly encourage homosexuality in their children. These parents would be shocked to learn that this is what they have done, for they are often more rigid in their attitudes, more puritanical towards sex, and more derogatory about homosexuality than average. A brutal father may make his son fearful of men and drawn to his oppressed, humiliated mother, so that he identifies himself with her, and in adult life becomes a passive, 'female type' homosexual. Oddly enough, opposite parental attitudes can encourage homosexuality. The mother who perpetually pampers her son, who never lets him out of her sight, who forbids his playing with 'common, dirty' companions, who surrounds him with 'smother love', may turn him towards homosexuality. This is even more marked when the sex of the child is in some doubt at birth. Since most of these children look like girls, they are brought up as girls, and find that they are quite happy in the female role. Later it may be found that the 'girl' was in fact genetically a male – she had the Y chromosome in all her body cells – but by this time it is almost impossible for her to exchange roles, and unwise for her to be forced to do so unless she wishes it herself.

As far as girls are concerned, it appears that the mother is the dominant parent in the child's sexual development, although a poor relationship with the father is an important factor. The mother who 'wanted a boy but got a girl' may consciously or unconsciously impose her disappointed desire on her daughter, so that in life she has many masculine attitudes. This does not mean that she will become homosexual, but she may. Similarly a mother who has an unhappy relationship with her husband, may influence her daughter to hate men, and later seek affection and companionship only with women.

The importance of a stable, warm family life as a means of preventing the possible development of homosexuality is shown by a study in Britain of over 120 lesbians. Children reared in families which have only one parent, which are disturbed by distortions in the relationships of the parents to each other or to the child, or whose sexual attitudes are repressive or ignorant, are particularly vulnerable.

In these ways homosexuals are created. Of course, only some children whose backgrounds resemble the ones described become homosexual. Most are heterosexual, although their sexuality may be impaired or damaged, so that they find it difficult to achieve a happy relationship with their chosen partner.

Ultimately it is the sensible attitude of the mother to the upbringing of her child which counts. But, as always, the behaviour of both parents towards each other and towards the child influence the way she will develop.

In the normal sexual development of a child, psychiatrists consider that there is a period when homosexual alliances are normal. This period is usually of limited duration during early adolescence, and is marked by a special closeness for a friend of her own sex. For a period, life away from the chosen one is intolerable, the clothes they wear must be the same, they must do the same things, they are miserable when separated. The intense homosexual friendship wanes as the child grows older and forms heterosexual companionships. Often it is replaced by a more emotionally stable friendship, which persists throughout life. In some 10 per cent of cases of adolescent homosexual friendship, the sexuality of the girls is stronger than usual, and they mutually masturbate by stimulating each other's clitoris. There need be no parental anxiety about this, as mutual masturbation is without any consequences, and certainly does not predispose to homosexuality in adult life. Another form of the adolescent homosexual phase is the development of a 'crush' or 'pash' for an older person. Again this is a normal phase, and may be less traumatic to the child, and to its parents, than the heterosexual 'crush' on the latest 'pop' or T.V. star which replaces or follows it. Hero-worship is a normal development in which the child, beginning to be independent, sees in the hero a substitute, stronger and more romantic than either a dominating or a cold indifferent parent. By the age of 15, the homosexual phase has waned in most girls. They are now more interested in boys, their friendships for other girls lingering on, but with much less intensity. A few remain homosexual.

In our society, female homosexuals are condemned and persecuted far less than male homosexuals. There are several reasons for this. Homosexuality in the male is thought more of a danger to a male dominated society, where 'men are strong and dominant' and women 'weak and submissive', than is lesbianism. In our culture, women are permitted to show greater physical intimacy between each other than men: girls habitually hug and kiss; if men do this, it is considered improper. For these reasons, female homosexuals may live together in complete intimacy, rarely incurring the disapproval of the community. Male homosexuals living together are sometimes sneered at and attacked. It is true that male homosexuals appear to be less able to form stable associations with each other, and tend to change partners or seek new sexual contacts more frequently than female homosexuals, who are generally monogamous with one partner. This may give some point to society's condemnation of male homosexuals, even if most of it is due to ignorance, prejudice and perhaps to unsolved sexual problems amongst those who condemn. Those who protest too much, may themselves be latent homosexuals, or so some psychiatrists believe.

Many female homosexuals can form a stable, happy relationship with another woman, and can lead full, contented lives. These women need no help, and are not a cause for anxiety. Not all are as lucky as this, and some lesbians have considerable emotional problems. These arise partly because of their own impaired personality development, but more because society's condemnation increases their insecurity, and they need compassion and tolerance rather than derision and disapproval. Many heterosexuals have personality problems which cause distress in their sexual relationships, but they are not singled out for disapproval on legal, social, moral or religious grounds. It seems unjust that homosexuals should be, when understanding for the woman as a person, not as a homosexual, is needed.

Chapter 6

The Infertile Marriage

It is a strange thing that in a world where one of the main problems facing mankind is the 'population explosion', or the birth each year of too many children, a fairly large group of women are seeking desperately to become pregnant. In times past barrenness was always blamed on the wife, but today it is known that in many cases the reason for the childlessness lies with the husband.

If a couple are normally fertile, and have sexual intercourse reasonably regularly, a pregnancy will result within one year of marriage in 90 per cent of cases. For this reason, a couple is considered to be infertile after this time, and will require investigations, tests and treatment if they wish to have a child. With treatment about 35 per cent of the infertile couples will achieve their desire – a pregnancy, resulting in a healthy child. The majority of women becoming pregnant do so within one year of the investigations and treatment, but pregnancies occur up to 10 years after the investigations have been completed. In recent years the numbers of tests, investigations and suggested treatments have increased very considerably, but the success rate after the investigations has remained stubbornly at the same 35 per cent.

This is not to say that an infertile couple should not be investigated. It is well worth while, but neither the enthusiasm of the doctors, nor the couple's desire to clutch at every straw should lead them on the round of visits to many doctors in many places to receive a variety of treatment to achieve nothing.

Careful investigation of the causes of infertility has shown that in about 25 per cent of cases the wife is at fault, in about 25 per cent of cases the husband. In the remaining 50 per cent of cases factors which affect them both are present.

It is usual for the wife to consult the doctor first when pregnancy fails to occur. This is correct and proper, for it is she who will carry the growing baby in her uterus for the 40 weeks of pregnancy. At this first visit the doctor enquires about the past operations and illnesses she may have had, about her present health, and about her menstrual history. He will want to know when menstruation first started, of its duration, the interval between periods, and if the periods were painful. Also he will enquire about the couple's sexual habits. The patient should not be embarrassed at this, for it is essential for the doctor to know the frequency of sexual intercourse, and whether the wife felt it to be satisfactory. It is then usual for him to examine the woman thoroughly, firstly to make sure she has no disorder which would make pregnancy hazardous to her, and secondly so that he may perform a pelvic examination to make sure that her genital organs are normal, as far as he can tell from this examination. In several surveys of infertile couples, it was found that in 3 per cent sexual intercourse had not taken place properly, and the wife was still a virgin. It was hardly surprising that pregnancy had not resulted!

The doctor will now outline what he intends to do. He will explain that investigation of infertility usually takes several visits, and that as the problem concerns the husband as much as the wife, he would like to see him as well as her at the next visit.

INFERTILITY FACTORS

The factors which may lead to infertility are rather complex, but can be understood if a little thought is applied. The male seeds, or spermatozoa, have to be ejaculated into the upper vagina. They then wriggle their way through the cervix, swimming up between the seaweed like strands of mucus which stretch downwards from the cells which line the cervical canal. They have to negotiate the cavity of the uterus, and by the time they have done this, of the millions ejaculated, only hundreds remain active. They then have to get through the narrow opening joining the cavity of the uterus and the hollow tube of the oviduct. Only a few dozen spermatozoa succeed in doing this. They then swim along the oviduct, against the current as it were, to reach the outer portion. If this occurs just at the time when the ovum has been expelled from the ovary, and if the ovum has been taken up by the fine finger-like projections at the end of the oviduct, conception may occur. If it does, the fertilized egg has to pass down the oviduct again, spending three days in the process, during which time it has divided and the one original cell is now a collection of cells, still within the shell of the *zona pellucida*. The fertilized egg reaches the cavity of the uterus three days or so after conception, and then by shedding the zona pellucida, implants itself into the soft, juicy lining of the uterine cavity. If all goes well, it now grows and becomes a baby; if all does not go well, an abortion occurs, which may or may not be noticed by the woman. It has been calculated that where no bar to conception is present and where every chance of becoming pregnant has been taken, in any one month of 100 fertile women, 60 will become pregnant and 40 will not. Of the 60 who do become pregnant, 45 deliver a live baby and 15 abort, but in 6 the abortion is undetected as it happens so early.

Considering the long journey made by the sperm to fertilize the egg, and the long journey made by the fertilized egg to reach the uterine cavity and implant itself there, it is surprising how readily pregnancy occurs. This description of how fertilization takes place enables a list of factors which prevent fertility to be made.

The male factor

The husband may fail to manufacture any spermatozoa, or because of illness which has damaged the tube (the *vas deferens*) linking his testicles to the collecting areas (or *seminal vesicles*) in his prostate gland, the spermatozoa may fail to reach the collecting areas (Fig. 6/1). The spermatozoa may be few in number or weak in activity, so that they have not the strength to swim up the genital tract of the wife. Finally, the husband may not be able to ejaculate, or even to practise sexual intercourse properly. Because of these possibilities, the doctor enquires from him about any illness he may have had, particularly mumps which may have damaged the testicles, and gonorrhoea which may have damaged the vas deferens. He will also ask about his smoking and drinking habits, for excessive smoking and too much alcohol both reduce sperm production and reduce the frequency of coitus. He will require to know his occupation, for some jobs reduce sperm production; and about his sexual habits. He will perhaps require to examine the husband, although this can be avoided if the husband is embarrassed provided that the doctor is supplied with a specimen of the husband's semen. This can be obtained if the man goes to the laboratory and masturbates, but many men find this inhibiting. The other ways are for the couple to masturbate or to have

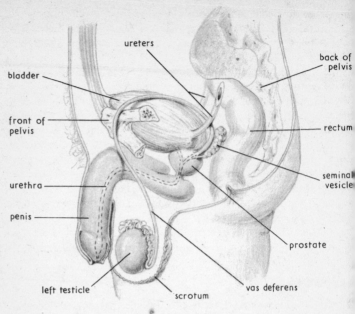

FIG. 6/1 The male genital tract

sexual intercourse. If they choose the latter, just before ejaculation, the husband withdraws his penis from his wife's vagina, and ejaculates into a dry, wide-mouthed jar placed beside the bed. His specimen is then brought to the laboratory by the wife, if this is more convenient. The wife should note the time the specimen was produced and bring it to the laboratory within two hours. Another method is not quite so satisfactory, but is preferred by some patients and some doctors. In this method, the husband and wife have sexual intercourse normally. Six hours later the wife goes to the doctor, who introduces a speculum into her vagina and takes a sample of the semen which is in her vagina (Fig. 6/2). This method, called the 'post-coital' test, has one particular advantage, it *proves* that normal coitus takes place and that the man ejaculates into the woman's vagina; but it is impossible to determine the quality of his semen from this method.

The main purpose of all the methods I have mentioned is to determine the quality as well as the quantity of the sperms in the

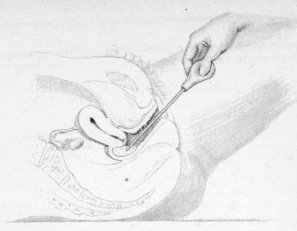

FIG. 6/2 The post-coital test

seminal fluid. If the test shows that the man's sperm has a poor quality, the test is repeated at least twice, sometimes after giving antibiotics, before any final decision about its quality can be made. Unfortunately, if no spermatozoa are found in any of the tests, the husband is sterile and nothing can be done. If, however, there are spermatozoa but they are of poor quality, certain treatments are available. The man may have varicose veins around his vas deferens, for example. It has been found that the surgical treatment of these varicose veins is often effective in producing a better quality semen. If the husband has no varicose veins, changes in living habits, in tobacco and alcoholic consumption may help. Unfortunately, none of the many hormones, drugs and vitamins which have been prescribed in the past to improve a man's fertility have any effect, whether given by injection or by mouth.

Because it is so easy to check the male factor by examining the semen, this is usually one of the first tests made when infertility is investigated. Indeed, logically, a semen analysis should be made before any complicated tests are made on the wife. For example, if the husband were found to be sterile, it would be pointless and heartless to perform tests on the wife.

The ovulation factor

Quite obviously if the wife fails to produce an egg, pregnancy cannot occur. Although in the years before the age of 18 and after 38 ovulation occurs less regularly, between these years most women ovulate each month. This can be checked by the wife herself, after consultation with her doctor. Usually she is asked to take her temperature each morning on waking, before she gets out of bed or drinks anything. In a menstrual cycle during which ovulation occurs, the temperature rises in the second half of the cycle. If the daily temperature is charted, this rise can be seen, and the fact of ovulation can be established (Fig. 6/3). The doctor may use other methods to determine ovulation, and if lack of ovulation is confirmed over several months, one of the special new 'ovulating drugs' may be prescribed, provided no other reason for the couple's infertility has been found. The use of the 'ovulating drugs' is fairly complicated, and most doctors insist that they are only given by specialist gynaecologists who have access to special laboratories, so that the exact dose required for the particular patient may be determined.

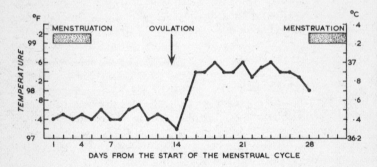

FIG. 6/3 A temperature chart showing that ovulation has occurred on day 14

The oviductal factor

The sperm has to pass upwards along the oviduct to reach the egg, and the fertilized egg has to pass downwards along the oviduct to reach the uterine cavity. If the oviduct is blocked, these essential events cannot happen. The next step in the investigation, after the husband has been found to be normal, and the wife to be ovulating, is to determine if the oviducts are clear. The most informative way of finding out is to ask the woman to come to an X-ray department which has an image-intensification unit. This apparatus enables the doctor to obtain the most information with the least discomfort to the woman. No anaesthetic is needed for this investigation.

In the X-ray department, the doctor inserts a speculum into the woman's vagina and puts a narrow tube into her cervix; this tube is connected to a syringe which is filled with an oily substance opaque to X-rays. The doctor injects the oil slowly so that it fills the uterus and then passes along the oviducts. He watches what he is doing on the television screen of the image-intensification apparatus. The woman can also watch what is happening and a sensitive doctor can explain to the woman what he sees.

The test will show if the oviducts are normal and unobstructed so that sperms can wriggle along them to reach the ovum. If the test suggests that the oviducts are blocked somewhere along their course obviously the chance of pregnancy is reduced. All tests have errors so that it is usual to repeat the test, which is called a hystero-salpingogram, after a one to two month interval. Should this second test still suggest that the oviducts are blocked, many doctors try to find out if surgery would be of help by using a laparoscope. This instrument, which is like a very narrow telescope, is gently inserted into the abdomen through a tiny cut at the lower edge of the umbilicus. Once inside the abdomen, the uterus and oviducts can be seen and any abnormality observed. At the same time a dye is injected into the uterus through the cervix and the doctor looks through the laparoscope to see if it emerges from the finger-like outer ends of the oviducts.

Laparoscopy is currently fashionable and, in properly selected situations, the doctor can obtain much helpful information using the instrument. However, the woman undergoing laparoscopy has to have a general anaesthetic; she has her abdominal cavity blown up with gas, and will have some discomfort for 24 to 48 hours after the operation. For these reasons, I believe that laparoscopy should only be used if the simpler, easier hystero-salpingogram gives doubtful results.

Surgery in infertility

If tests show that the woman's oviducts are blocked, surgery is possible. Because the oviducts are so narrow and delicate, the surgery should be undertaken by a gynaecologist who has made a special study of infertility surgery. Even in these circumstances only one woman in every five operated upon becomes pregnant later and delivers a live healthy baby.

Other tests

Certain other tests are frequently made although their practical value is doubtful. As I have mentioned, some doctors believe that the mucus secreted by the cervical glands is sometimes 'hostile' to spermatozoa. If this really does occur, then obviously pregnancy is less likely. To test this, the doctor takes a specimen of the mucus at ovulation time, as this is the only time when the spermatozoa can wriggle easily through the strands of mucus. He places the mucus on a glass slide and adds some of the husband's spermatozoa so that the two touch. He then measures how many spermatozoa penetrate into the mucus and how far. For convenience, he can do this test at the same time as he does the 'post-coital' test using the spermatozoa which are still in the vagina. If few spermatozoa penetrate the mucus he says that the mucus is 'hostile' and suggests treatment. The reservation I have about the test is that many couples who have been found to have poor sperm penetration of the mucus get pregnant with no treatment at all. This suggests that the treatment has little real value.

Recently, tests have been made to see if a woman has made antibodies to the man's spermatozoa which either make them immobile or cause them to clump. In either case they would not be able to make the journey through the uterus and oviducts. Whilst studies have shown that more infertile couples have sperm antibodies than are found in fertile couples, it is not clear if they are of any real significance in preventing pregnancy and there is no effective treatment if they are found.

ARTIFICIAL INSEMINATION OF DONOR'S SEMEN

It may be that the only reason for the barrenness of the couple is that the husband is sterile. In these circumstances, some couples decide that they would prefer to let the wife bear the child of an unknown donor's semen, rather than adopting a child or doing nothing at all. The procedure is called A.I.D. (artificial insemination of a donor's semen). In recent years fewer babies have become available for adoption and the waiting time has increased, often lasting for 3 years. For this reason A.I.D. is becoming increasingly popular. The physical characteristics of the husband are matched as closely as possible to the unknown donor. He is never seen, or known, by the couple, nor does he know to whom his donated semen has been given. At about ovulation time, the wife goes to the doctor's surgery and each day for three or four days the donor's semen is injected into her upper vagina to bathe the cervix. On average, three inseminations a month for three months are needed to obtain a pregnancy, and about two-thirds of the women inseminated become pregnant and deliver a live child. This child is brought up as the natural child of the father. The legal position of the child is not quite clear, and a couple who decide after careful thought to try A.I.D. should take legal advice.

Infertility investigations take time and pose problems. Because of this, the couple must co-operate fully and should seek a doctor who has an interest in infertility, who is sympathetic to the patients, and who is careful never to do too much to little purpose. Although 35 per cent of couples will achieve a pregnancy, it is kinder to tell some of the others that pregnancy is impossible, and to suggest adoption whilst they are still relatively young. An adopted child can give as much joy to a family as a natural child.

Chapter 7

Birth Control and Family Planning

Of the many interlinked problems facing humanity in the last quarter of this turbulent century, that of the rapid rate of population growth is a major one. Because of the reduction in the deaths of infants and children due to better sanitation and the control of diseases, increasing numbers survive to reach their reproductive years and, being human, they reproduce. The scale of population growth is immense. In 1776, the population of the world was about 1,000 million. In 1885, one hundred years later, it had risen to 1,500 million. In 1975, it reached 4,000 million and by 2005, it is likely to reach 6,500 million, unless global disaster occurs before that time (Fig. 7/1). All these people need to be able to eat adequately, to receive some education, to find some form of employment and to have some enjoyment of life.

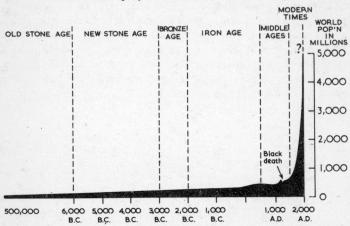

FIG. 7/1 The growth of the world's population, redrawn from Population Bulletin, 18, 1, 1962

In the rich, developed nations of the world, the population growth rate has diminished as women (and men) have chosen to have fewer children and, by using birth control methods, have been able to have smaller families. By contrast, in most of the poor, hungry developing nations, the birth rate remains high, and only a few couples limit the size of the family. This is because children are seen as valuable in societies in which social welfare measures are few and provision for old age almost impossible because of poverty. Children are also esteemed as they demonstrate the masculinity of the man, and are useful extra hands in rural communities. But even in these nations, surveys show that women want fewer children than they actually have, so that the desire to limit the size of the family is present. There is also the realization that if children are 'spaced' so that an interval of between two and three years separates each birth, the health and welfare of each child, as well as that of the mother, benefits.

In all nations, for one reason or another, women are beginning to realize that they are no longer condemned to a life of constant childbearing and childrearing, but are increasingly able to choose how many children, or how few children, they really want to have.

The choice of method may be to prolong breast-feeding, which considerably reduces the chance of another pregnancy, or to use contraceptives which effectively prevent a new pregnancy occurring, or to have an abortion which ends a new pregnancy. Obviously, it is better to prevent a pregnancy than to terminate it – better on medical and social grounds. Yet, induced abortion is still the most usual way by which women limit the size of their family, although the use of modern efficient contraceptives is rapidly replacing it. However, even in the most sophisticated society, induced abortion remains as an important method of birth control. For this reason I will discuss it later in the chapter.

FAMILY PLANNING OR CONCEPTION CONTROL

Family planning is available to help individuals and couples to choose if and when they will have a child (family planning), or to choose the number of children that they will have (family limitation). The choices depend on a complicated mixture of social, cultural and psychological influences; and today for the first time in history, men and women have reliable methods to enable them to make that choice freely and relatively easily.

This principle of choice is important, as it includes not only the choice of using family planning, but the choice of the birth control method most suited to the particular circumstances of the couple. But neither the man nor the woman can make an informed choice until each has the basic knowledge of the different methods, their efficiency in protection against pregnancy and their advantages and disadvantages.

The choice may be that the man uses contraceptive measures; or that the woman chooses the contraceptive. Both should know of the available methods so that the decision is made carefully. The choice is helped if each partner has an idea of how efficient the method chosen is in preventing an unwanted pregnancy. A measure of contraceptive efficiency which is used by many people is the Pregnancy Index or the Pearl Index (from the name of the man who first used it). The Pregnancy Index, is calculated in the following way:

$$\frac{\text{The number of pregnancies} \times 1,200}{\text{Total months of exposure to pregnancy}}$$

The result is expressed as the number of pregnancies per 1,200 months of exposure, or preferably as the number of pregnancies per hundred 'woman years'. This shows how many of every 100 women making use of the particular method chosen are likely to become pregnant if the method is used for one year.

Contraceptives for men

The choices available to a man are for him to use a temporary method, so that he remains fertile; or a permanent method so that he becomes sterile. Compared with the contraceptives available to women, those available to men are limited. This is not due to lack of research but to the fact that sperm production in man is infinitely greater than the production of ova in women, and methods of hormonal or chemical suppression of sperm development are consequently much more difficult to discover. It will be some time before a male contraceptive pill or injection is available which is both effective and acceptable.

At present, two temporary contraceptive measures are available to

en. These are coitus interruptus (withdrawal) and the use of the
ndom. One excellent permanent method is currently available.
his is vasectomy.

OITUS INTERRUPTUS: For many years withdrawal of the penis
om the vagina just before ejaculation has been used to avoid
egnancy. In several investigations, made in the days before the Pill
came available, it was found to be the most usual method adopted.
relies, of course, on the ability of the man to recognize the sensa-
ons which occur in his genitals just before ejaculation, and for him
pidly to withdraw his penis from the vagina and ejaculate outside.
is requires great self-control, as the man will often want to keep his
nis in the woman's vagina for as long as possible to obtain the
eatest amount of pleasure. As the first spurt of semen, which
ntains the most spermatozoa, may either be ejaculated during
thdrawal or may spurt into the vaginal entrance, the risk of preg-
ncy is high, and the pregnancy index is 35 per 100 woman years.
Coitus interruptus is said to lead to pelvic discomfort in a woman,
o is stimulated but not relieved (unless she reaches a climax first),
d in the man who has to withdraw at a moment when he would
netrate more deeply. Over long periods it was said to cause mental
sorders. There is no evidence that coitus interruptus leads to either
these conditions, or indeed to any disease at all, but it is not a very
tisfying method for either sexual partner. Better methods are
ailable. If a couple have used coitus interruptus successfully for
ars and it suits their particular sexual needs, no pressure should be
t on them to change, but they should be told of the other more
liable methods now available.

IE CONDOM: If the male covers his penis with a sheath, which is so
in that it is not noticed by either sexual partner, but so strong that
ither the movement of the penis in the vagina, nor the ejaculation
semen tears it, pregnancy will be prevented as no spermatozoa will
deposited near the cervix. The sheath (or condom), which today is
ade of fine latex rubber, has been used since Roman times
ig. 7/2). In the past century its use has been widespread, and
hough primarily used to prevent conception, the condom was
ued to soldiers who were going to fornicate with prostitutes as a
ethod of reducing the chances of catching venereal disease. If the
nis was 'protected' by the condom, the germs which lived in the

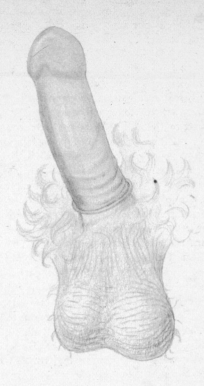

FIG. 7/2 The condom drawn onto the erect penis

genital tract of many prostitutes were unable to get into the delica
tissues of the opening of the 'eye' in the glans of the penis, or
invade the glans itself. In this way the spread of gonorrhoea an
syphilis was to some extent prevented.

The disadvantages of the condom, or French letter, as a method
contraception are that the male must put it on, usually waiting un
he has an erection of his penis. The need to do this may interfere wi
his love-making, and he may therefore decide 'to take a chance'. Th
disadvantage can be avoided if the woman puts the condom onto th
man's erect penis during love-play.

The advantages of the condom are several. First, modern condom
are prelubricated by adding silicone and are individually packed

hermetically sealed aluminium foil sachets which enables them to be kept for a long period. The quality of the condom and its prelubrication makes it easy to put it on to the man's penis by unrolling it. Provided the man makes sure that no bubble of air is left in the closed end, it is very efficient. Air, together with the ejaculated semen, can lead to the condom bursting. Because of this slight risk, many doctors recommend that the woman puts some spermicidal cream in her vagina if the man uses a condom. Secondly, the condom is probably the most suitable contraceptive if sexual intercourse takes place infrequently and unpredictably. In such circumstances a man may choose always to carry a condom in his wallet, and a woman may either have a condom or a vaginal diaphragm available should erotic stimulation lead to sexual intercourse and the man has not a condom available. Thirdly, there are no side-effects, because no hormones or chemicals are used, and the condom protects by acting as a mechanical barrier, preventing the spermatozoa reaching the cervix.

The assumed disadvantage that the condom reduces sexual pleasure is untrue. Modern condoms are usually unnoticeable to either partner, and a reduction in sexual pleasure is not so much due to the physical presence of the condom, as to psychological 'hang-ups' about its use.

Because of its cheapness, its reliability, its ease of purchase and of use, the condom continues to be a popular method of birth control in all nations. Its reliability in protecting the woman against an unwanted pregnancy is more difficult to estimate and depends on the motivation of the couple always to use a condom during sexual intercourse. Amongst highly motivated couples a pregnancy rate of less than 5 per 100 woman years is reported, but most reports show a pregnancy rate of about 15 per 100 woman years.

VASECTOMY: Increasing numbers of men are becoming interested in vasectomy as the operation provides an easy, relatively painless method of making a man sterile without interfering with the couple's sexual enjoyment. Vasectomy must be clearly differentiated from castration, in which the man's testicles are removed surgically. Vasectomy merely prevents the sperm from being ejaculated. The testicles remain and function normally so that a man who has had a vasectomy is no less masculine, nor does he have any fewer sexual desires. He is able to perform and enjoy sex as much as, or more than a man who has not had the operation.

The operation is relatively simple. The principle is to cut a small segment out of the vas deferens, the narrow tube which carries the spermatozoa from the testicles, where they are made, to the area of the prostate gland where they mature (Fig. **7/3**). If you gently palpate a man's scrotum, at the level where it joins his body, by putting your thumb in front and your index finger behind, you will feel a cord-like tube as you roll the folds of skin between your thumb and index finger. This is the vas. There is a vas from each testicle, so you will feel one on each side.

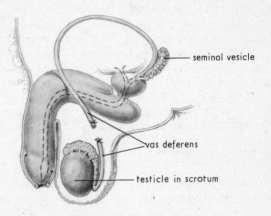

FIG. 7/3 Ligation of the vas deferens

The operation is made through a tiny cut into the skin, and can be done under local anaesthesia or using a general anaesthetic if the man prefers it. Each vas is identified and a small segment is cut out, after which the cut in the skin is closed. The operation takes about 15 minutes, and throughout the world about 10 million operations are done each year.

Sexual intercourse can be resumed as soon as the man wishes, but the couple must continue using some form of contraception until the man has had about twelve ejaculations. This is because he has to ejaculate all the spermatozoa which have been stored in his prostate gland. Once all these sperms have been ejaculated, the man is sterile although he continues to ejaculate fluid which is made in the prostate gland so that neither he nor his partner notice any difference in their sexual pleasure.

What happens to the spermatozoa which are produced in the testicles but cannot escape because of the cut vas? They cease to be produced after a short time, so there need be no anxiety about the testicles becoming bloated with sperms!

The effect of the operation on the sexual pleasure of a couple has been investigated sufficiently to establish that over 70 per cent of men find that after vasectomy their sex life is improved, and only 2 per cent find it to be worse. The remainder said there was no change.

Methods requiring co-operation

'THE SAFE PERIOD': In a woman with a normal cycle, ovulation will occur approximately 14 days before the anticipated menstrual period and the ovum can only survive for 2 days unless it is fertilized. After intercourse, the ejaculated spermatozoa survive, and are able to fertilize the ovum, for 4 days at the most. From these facts you can deduce that if coitus is avoided from 4 days before to 4 days after ovulation pregnancy should not occur. Coitus should therefore be restricted to the days of menstruation, to the 4–6 post-menstrual days and the 10 pre-menstrual days. The physiological concepts of ovulation were independently observed in 1929 by Dr Knaus in Austria, and Dr Ogino in Japan. The so-called Ogino-Knaus method was enthusiastically adopted by Roman Catholics who could argue that they were not preventing conception, but were regulating births in a 'natural way'. The original observations have been developed in recent years but the principle is the same: that is, the couple have to restrict coitus to the time of physiological infertility. Unfortunately, the method, despite the improvements, requires considerable motivation and is not particularly safe, as the average woman does not have an exactly regular cycle, and ovulation may occur at other times of the cycle, especially if the emotions are stirred.

Since the method is the only one permissible to Roman Catholics who accept the Church's dictates, it requires further, and rather detailed, consideration in its three rhythm techniques: the 'calendar method', the 'temperature method' and the 'mucus method'.

The calendar method: If a woman is prepared to use a calendar, and over a period of 6 menstrual cycles to record the duration of each cycle, she can determine her own safe period by calculating the date

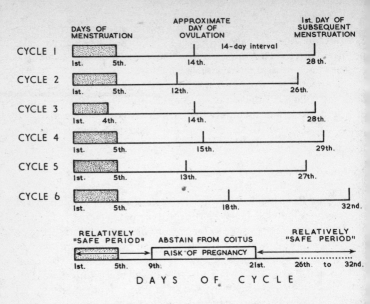

FIG. 7/4 The Rhythm Method: calculation of the 'Safe Period'. In this example the shortest cycle was 26 days, the longest was 32 days. Ovulation in the shortest cycle was calculated to take place on day 12, in the longest on day 18. Three days each side of ovulation are potentially fertile (as the spermatozoa and ovum live for 3 days). For this particular woman, the days on which coitus should be avoided are from day 9 (i.e. the day of ovulation in the shortest cycle, less 3 days) to day 21 (i.e. the day of ovulation in the longest cycle, plus 3 days)

of ovulation in each cycle, and then subtracting 3 days from that day in the shortest cycle and adding 3 days in the longest cycle (Fig. 7/4). Coitus should be avoided during the danger period. If a woman has a cycle of less than 20 days, or if the duration of her cycle varies by more than 10 days, she will only be able to have 'safe' sexual intercourse at infrequent intervals and sexual frustration is likely to occur. A careful study in Washington D.C. of 30,000 cycles in 2,316 women showed that only 30 per cent of them would qualify for the calendar rhythm method on the basis of a cycle range of 8 days or less. The cycle range varied with age, the smallest variation being in the age group 30 to 34, when 40 per cent had a cycle with a range of 8 days or less. However, if the couple are prepared to accept that coitus takes place in accordance with the calendar, not with desire, then the method is reasonably successful.

The temperature method: This is a more accurate method of pinpointing ovulation. It is based on the physiological observation that when ovulation has occurred the body temperature rises slightly. To detect this temperature rise a woman has to be sufficiently motivated to take her rectal, or vaginal, temperature each morning on waking and before she gets out of bed (which may be difficult for a woman with a young family), or has any food or drink. From the daily reading she makes a chart, and can have coitus safely 3 days after the temperature rise has occurred. The problems are that not all cycles show 'ideal' temperature rises and if the woman has a cold, flu or some other infection, the method cannot be used. It also requires considerable motivation to remember to take the temperature each day (Fig. 6/3).

The mucus method: In this method, which was developed by an Australian physician, the woman learns to examine her vaginal orifice for the presence of mucus. Immediately after a menstrual period the vaginal orifice feels dry, but as ovulation time approaches mucus can be detected. Initially, it is cloudy and sticky, but as the level of oestrogen rises, the cells of the neck of the womb (the cervix) are stimulated to secrete more mucus and its character changes. It becomes clearer, strands stretch without breaking and it 'feels slippery'. The peak of the clear mucus is reached on the day of ovulation, after which the mucus becomes cloudy again. The physiological concept of this sequence is correct, but the detection of mucus at the vulva requires considerable motivation, and perhaps the eye (and finger) of faith. As well as this, vaginal secretions, either physiological or pathological, can confuse the issue. The motivated woman is given a chart and enters her findings each day using differently coloured stickers for different types of mucus. Coitus is 'safe' when there is no mucus, and more than 3 days after the last day of the clear mucus. Between these times coitus should be avoided. Patients trained by Dr Billings claim considerable success with his method, but in the two investigations reported, the failure rate was between 15 and 25 per 100 woman years, which is about the same rate as that of the other 'safe-period' methods. The problem is one of motivation. If the couple avoid coitus whenever there is any mucus, the woman will avoid pregnancy; she may also have to avoid coitus for most days of the month, which can be frustrating to both sexual partners. However, when a couple choose one of the 'natural' methods of birth-control, they only have to avoid *sexual intercourse* on the 'dangerous days'. They can still enjoy cuddling, kissing and body contact and if aroused sexually, can be helped to orgasm by oral or digital stimulation of the woman's clitoral area and the man's penis.

Contraceptives for women

DOUCHING: Many women believe that if they douche immediately after coitus, they will prevent pregnancy occurring. There is no truth in this belief, as the spermatozoa enter the cervix almost immediately after ejaculation. The douche only washes the vagina, and clears the semen left there. As the woman has to go and douche immediately after the man has ejaculated, she may not have an orgasm herself and the need to leave can interfere with their mutual pleasure considerably. Douching is not a method of contraception, and has other disadvantages (see p. 345).

VAGINAL JELLIES OR CREAMS: These are preparations containing chemicals which will kill spermatozoa if the sperms are in contact with the chemical for sufficient time. Used alone, the jelly or cream (which may foam) is introduced high into the vagina with a tube and plunger, just prior to coitus. It is a poor method of contraception about 35 women in every hundred using it for a year become pregnant. Spermicidal jellies and creams are also used in conjunction with vaginal diaphragms, or when the man uses a condom. Used in these ways they add to the protective value of both methods against an unwanted pregnancy.

THE VAGINAL DIAPHRAGM: As its name implies, the vaginal diaphragm, or Dutch cap, consists of a thin rubber dome which has a coiled metal spring in the rim. The diaphragms are made in various sizes, and the woman must be examined vaginally and given the size most suitable for her vagina. She is taught to smear spermicidal jelly in the dome and around the rim of the cap, and to insert it into her vagina by squeezing the sides of the diaphragm together. Usually she squats, or stands with one foot on a chair, to introduce the cap, and

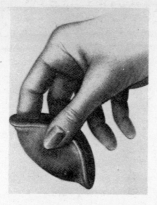

(a) Holding the diaphragm

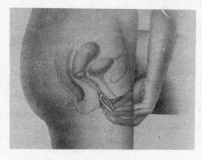

(b) Insertion

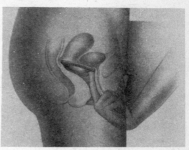

(c) Placing it correctly

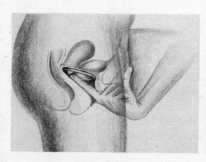

(d) Ensuring that the cervix
is covered

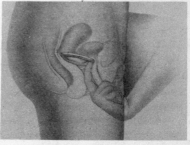

(e) Removing the diaphragm by
hooking the index finger under
the spring rim

FIG. 7/5 The technique used in inserting the diaphragm

inserts it into her vagina in an upward and backward direction. Inside the vagina, it regains its shape and fits snugly across the vagina covering the cervix (Fig. 7/5). After childbirth, the capacity of the vagina may increase to some extent and the woman should be refitted if she intends to continue to use the diaphragm as a contraceptive method.

. The advantage of the diaphragm is that it is completely without side-effects (although a few spermicidal creams may cause a mild vaginal irritation, which disappears when the cream is changed).

Its disadvantage is that it should be inserted each day whether coitus is anticipated or not. The psychological problem to a sexually aroused couple of the woman having to go away to put in her diaphragm is obvious. The alternative is for the woman to put the diaphragm into her vagina during love play, helped by her partner. Once inserted, the diaphragm should be left in the vagina for six hours after the last time the man ejaculated, and then removed, washed and stored.

If a woman chooses this method of birth control she needs to be seen by a doctor so that the size of the diaphragm most suited to her can be chosen and so that she can learn how to introduce it into her vagina and how to remove it. Since it is essential that a spermicidal cream is used in conjunction with the diaphragm, she learns to place a large blob in the centre of its upper surface and additional cream around the rim. This also makes its introduction easier. She learns how to be sure that the diaphragm is in place, and to know this she must feel her cervix through the rubber. A woman generally needs to have some knowledge of her anatomy, many quite incorrectly believing that the vagina runs vertically upwards rather than upwards and backwards, and she should practise introducing and removing the diaphragm at home (Fig. 7/5). If she can, she should revisit her doctor a few days later, wearing the diaphragm, so that she can be reassured that her technique is good, and so that her additional questions can be answered.

It will be realized that the complexity of fitting the diaphragm, the necessity for the patient to use intelligence in its insertion, and the need for her to be so motivated that she makes sure it is in place every time she expects coitus, has limited its popularity. The pregnancy rate is 3 per 100 woman years when a motivated couple use the method but unfortunately the average pregnancy rate is 15 to 25 per 100 woman years.

The place of the diaphragm as a method of birth control should not be minimized, as it has no side-effects, is perhaps protective against cervical cancer, and if maintained properly can be used for one to two years before being changed. In the past few years, the popularity of the vaginal diaphragm as a contraceptive method has increased, and more women are using this method.

HORMONAL CONTRACEPTIVES: To most women, hormonal contraceptives mean the Pill. Since it was first used in 1955, the number of women taking the Pill at any one time has increased to over 65 million. Nor is the Pill used today the same as that used more than 20 years ago. Today's Pill contains less oestrogen and less gestagen than the original Pill and so is a much safer product. And although the Pill is a method of contraception most favoured by women, the two hormones may be used singly, or together, given by mouth or by injection to suit the needs of different women.

The two hormones which are used in the Pill are laboratory made substitutes of the two female sex hormones, oestrogen and progesterone, which we discussed in Chapter 4. The hormones give a woman her feminine contours, they prepare her uterus each month to receive a fertilized egg and they encourage it to develop into a child.

You may remember (if you don't you can find out again by rereading Chapter 4) that ovulation is controlled by a special area of the brain – the hypothalamus. From cells in this area, hormones travel to the pituitary gland, at the base of the brain, and stimulate it to release a hormone, called follicle-stimulating hormone, into the blood. This, in turn, stimulates between 12 and 20 egg cells (or follicles) in the ovary to grow. As they grow they produce oestrogen. The oestrogen levels rise and 'feed-back' to the hypothalamus. This has the effect of reducing the amount of follicle-stimulating hormone released, and of causing the release of a second hormone, the luteinising hormone. The sudden surge of this hormone in the blood causes an egg, and usually only one egg, to escape from one of the growing follicles. The egg is expelled and the follicle, which looks like a tiny thick-walled balloon, collapses. It quickly undergoes conversion into a yellow-coloured structure which produces not only oestrogen, but also progesterone. If pregnancy occurs the yellow-coloured structure continues to live, but if pregnancy does not occur it ceases to produce hormones after a life of about 12 days. When this happens, menstruation starts.

The hormonal contraceptives upset this sequence. There are two main types. In the first, both oestrogen-substitute and progesterone-substitute are given from soon after menstruation. At the dose chosen, the hormones 'feed-back' to the hypothalamus and prevent the release of the follicle-stimulating and of the luteinising hormones, so that ovulation is prevented. In addition, they alter the lining of the uterus so that it is not receptive to a fertilized egg; and they alter the secretions of the cervix so that they become thick and sticky. This prevents most spermatozoa from travelling upwards from the vagina and entering the cavity of the uterus. The 'combined' hormonal contraceptives protect a woman against an unwanted pregnancy in these three ways. But if a woman takes the Pill by mouth, she must remember to take a pill every day as the hormones are rapidly inactivated in her body, and the level may fall too low for the protection to occur, should she miss more than two days. The Pill is taken each day for 21 days and then stopped for 7 days, but in some formulations sugar pills are given for the 7 days so that the woman takes a pill every day.

The second type of hormonal contraceptive avoids the use of oestrogen, and contains only the progesterone-substitute, which is called gestagen. The gestagen hormonal contraceptives do not prevent ovulation consistently, but do alter the secretions of the cervix so that sperms have difficulty in wriggling through. The hormone also alters the lining of the uterus so that the egg, if fertilized, is unable to implant itself. The gestagen hormones can be taken by mouth each day, or can be given by injection at one-monthly, three-monthly or six-monthly intervals.

The 'injectables' are increasing in popularity. A single injection, every three months, is felt to be more convenient than having to remember to take the Pill each day, and since the injectables do not contain oestrogen many of the side-effects of the Pill (which are due to oestrogen) do not occur. Against these two advantages are the disadvantages. In the first six months, about one woman in four has quite irregular and unpredictable episodes of bleeding, and one woman in six ceases to menstruate. After six months an increasing number of women (up to 50 per cent) cease menstruation. Medically, there is no need for a woman to menstruate at all, unless she wants to have children when menstruation usually indicates that ovulation has occurred. Absence of menstruation does not damage a woman's health, and many women may prefer not to menstruate, although some will worry that a pregnancy has occurred. The other disadvantage (which is only temporary) is that if a woman stops having injectables because she wants to become pregnant, fertility is usually delayed (in other words ovulation and menstruation fail to occur) for 9 to 12 months.

As I mentioned, the gestagen can also be taken by mouth, each day. The advantage of this type of hormonal contraceptive, which has been called the 'mini-pill' is that it increases the flow of milk in some lactating women. Unfortunately, the gestagen mini-pill disturbs the menstrual cycle in a large number of women, so that it is not so convenient or acceptable as the combined pill, and its main use is for women who are breast-feeding but want the added security that a new pregnancy will be avoided.

When a woman weighs up the advantages and disadvantages of the hormonal contraceptives, she has to know how efficient the various hormonal contraceptives are in protecting her against an unwanted pregnancy. The combined oral contraceptive, the Pill, is the safest and provided it is taken daily as recommended, gives nearly 100 per cent protection. In a study in Sweden, only 17 pregnancies occurred in 4 million months of use – a pregnancy rate of 0.005 per 100 woman years. The 'injectables' are associated with a pregnancy rate of about 0.25 per 100 woman years; and the 'mini-pill' with a pregnancy rate of about 2 per 100 woman years.

When given the choice, most women prefer, at least initially, to use one of the combined oral contraceptives, rather than one of the other types. Because of concern about side-effects, (which we will discuss later) the majority of formulations of the Pill now contain only a tiny amount of oestrogen (which is two or three times less than the amount contained in the original Pill). As well as this, the amount of gestagen has been reduced over the years and today's Pill contains considerably less than some years ago.

Recently, a new lower dose formulation has been developed which should probably be the first choice for most women. This formulation is effective in preventing pregnancy and has a low incidence of side-effects. For those people who want precision, this formulation contains 30 mcg ethinyl oestradiol (the oestrogen) and 150 mcg norgestrel or 1,000 mcg norethisterone (the gestagens).

The side-effects of the Pill prevent it from being the 'perfect' contraceptive and reduces it to being a very good contraceptive. Since contraception is such an emotional matter, the incidence and severity of the side-effects are influenced by gossip and by sensational articles in women's magazines, which are often rich in speculation if poor in scientific observations.

The side-effects most often reported are listed in Table 7/1. This table does not prove that a side-effect is due to the Pill as many of the complaints are found in women not taking the Pill. But if you believe that the Pill is causing a particular side-effect which distresses you, you should consult a doctor and if necessary change to another method of contraception.

Table 7/1.

The side-effects attributed to oral contraceptives (The Pill)

Acne	Some increase in some women who take the combined Pill.
Blood pressure	About one woman in every 20 taking the Pill, experiences a small rise in blood pressure. A few susceptible women, generally over the age of 35, get a rather greater rise in blood pressure. The newer low-dose Pill does not seem to affect the blood pressure as much as the older higher-dose Pills.
Depression, mood changes	No increase, except amongst women who were depressed before taking the Pill, or who feel guilty about taking the Pill. A few women who have depression when taking the Pill find that it is relieved by taking tablets of pyridoxine (Vitamin B6).
Headaches and migraine	In carefully controlled investigations, no increase has been found. However, if a woman taking the Pill develops severe migraine which is localized, she should consult a doctor.

Menstruation	Tends to be reduced in amount, and often the colour changes from red to dirty brown. This is unimportant and does not mean that toxic substances are collecting in the body. Menstruation occurs on a predictable date, but a few women have spotting of blood, or a small bleed, on an unexpected day. If this is repeated in another cycle, a doctor should be consulted.
Nausea and vomiting	Fairly common in the first and second cycles on the Pill, thereafter unusual.
Pain with periods	Women taking the Pill usually have painless periods; this is a beneficial side-effect of the Pill.
Sexuality	Despite a good deal of anecdotal information, sexuality, sexual desire and enjoyment are usually unchanged.
Thrombosis in veins	There is evidence from investigations in Britain, the U.S.A. and other countries that women taking hormonal contraceptives (especially if they contain oestrogens) are more likely to develop clots in deep leg veins (deep venous thrombosis) than women using other methods. The risk is not great, but is increased if you are overweight, oversmoke and are over 40 years of age.
Vaginal discharge	The vagina is normally kept moist by secretions from the cervix. Women taking the Pill may expect increased vaginal moisture, and some discharge. If this is not irritating it is of no consequence. If it is irritating, a doctor should be consulted at once, as you may have developed monilia, which is slightly more common amongst women on the Pill.

Weight gain   Most women, whether taking the Pill or not,
                   gain weight from retaining fluid in the few days
                   before menstruation. This disappears when
                   menstruation starts. Some women taking the Pill
                   gain weight after a few months of use. This may
                   be due to the hormone, gestagen, or to an
                   increased appetite when the fear of pregnancy is
                   lifted. Weight gain is usually controlled by
                   a proper diet.

This information should help you decide if you would prefer to use oral contraceptives to the other methods available. Perhaps it will help even more if some questions often asked are answered.

Are there any women who should not use the Pill? Because of the reported side-effects, which in turn are due to complicated biochemical changes in the body, some women should not use the Pill. These include some women who have infrequent menstruation; women who previously had a clot in a deep vein or a pulmonary embolism; women who have liver disease; women who have severe migraine, especially if it localizes to a small area of the head; and women who have certain blood disorders. As well, women with a very high blood pressure or women with severe diabetes would be wise to use another method of birth control as both conditions may worsen when taking the Pill.

Does a doctor have to prescribe the Pill? The answer is yes, at least in most countries. Before prescribing the Pill, the doctor should find out if a woman has any of the diseases just mentioned. He should take her blood pressure and check her urine for sugar. Since she is well, and seeking protection against pregnancy, he should offer her protection against breast or uterine cancer by palpating her breasts and taking a 'cervical smear' (see p. 351).

The problem is that many young women are deterred from obtaining the Pill because they have to go to a doctor, and so fail to obtain protection against pregnancy. If they become pregnant, they seek an abortion. Because of this and because many doctors fail to do the examinations I have mentioned, and because in young women the diseases mentioned are unusual, I believe that a young woman should be able to obtain the first supply of the Pill without having to go to a doctor, provided she has regular periods, but should be encouraged to go to a doctor to obtain a repeat prescription.

Does the Pill lead to promiscuity? Some people believe that a woman avoids intercourse because of fear of pregnancy, and fear of venereal disease. The Pill has removed the first fear but has done nothing to reduce the risk of getting venereal disease. It happens that a relaxation of the double standard of sexuality and so a more liberal attitude to woman's sexuality has coincided with the availability of the Pill. There is no evidence that the Pill increases promiscuity, whatever may be written or said.

Should the Pill be stopped for a month or two each year? This idea originated from the belief that as the Pill suppresses ovulation, it was wise to give the ovaries a chance to function normally each year. It is nonsense and is dangerous because an unwanted pregnancy can occur unless some other efficient contraceptive method is chosen. A woman can take the Pill, without a break, for as long as she wants. But if she is told to stop taking the Pill she must make sure that she uses some other reliable contraceptive method.

If a woman takes the Pill before she is married, will it prevent her from having a baby when she marries? This is a particularly insidious, nasty myth. In Chapter 6, I pointed out that about one couple in seven is unable to have a baby. It is true that after ceasing the Pill (and sometimes when taking the Pill) the periods do not always come on time. In the first month after ceasing to take the Pill, ovulation is often delayed for 2 or 3 weeks, but after this most women ovulate regularly. In a few women, ovulation and menstruation takes longer to return, but by six months 99 out of every 100 ex-Pill takers ovulate regularly. In only 2 in every 1,000 does lack of ovulation and lack of menstruation persist for more than one year. The women who develop post-pill amenorrhoea are of all ages, have been taking the Pill for a short or for a long time, and have had infrequent or normal periods before using the Pill. There is no way of detecting which women will menstruate immediately and in which women ovulation and menstruation will be delayed. But should this happen, treatment is available which generally enables a woman to ovulate, should she want to become pregnant.

When can a woman start using the Pill? She can start using the Pill from the time she becomes sexually active and at risk of becoming pregnant provided her periods are regular. If her periods are irregular, some other method of contraception may be preferred.

When should a woman start contraceptives after childbirth? If she is not breast-feeding she should start within 4 weeks. If she is breast-feeding it is unlikely that ovulation will occur for about 20 weeks, although it sometimes does. For this reason, many women do not want to take the chance and decide to take hormonal contraceptives. The gestagen-only pill is to be preferred as it stimulates, rather than reduces milk flow, and can be started when leaving hospital after the birth of her child or at the postnatal check-up.

When should a woman cease using the Pill? It is not certain for how many years a woman past the age of 40 should use contraceptives in order to avoid any possibility of pregnancy. Ovulation occurs less frequently after the age of 40, and rarely after the age of 47. At the moment, then, it would seem wise for her to continue with contraception until the age of 50. If she is taking the Pill she will, of course, continue to bleed each month, and will not know when she has reached the natural menopause, or 'change of life'.

Because of the increased risk of deep vein thrombosis, pulmonary embolism and stroke in women over 40 who are overweight and are also heavy smokers, it has been suggested that such women should use other methods of contraception. This belief has been extended by some doctors to apply to all women over 40. I do not agree, particularly as the new low-dose Pill is available. The amount of oestrogen (30 mcg) in this Pill is little more than the amount many women are recommended to take by doctors to avoid menopausal symptoms.

What is the morning-after pill? This is a method of preventing pregnancy in a woman who has had sexual intercourse at ovulation-time when neither she nor the man have used contraceptives. In this case oestrogens in large doses are given for 5 days starting no later than 72 hours after the coital experience. The morning-after pill has also been suggested for women who only have intercourse once a week or less frequently and in this instance a large dose of a gestagen is taken *within 3 hours of each coital episode*.

Large doses of oestrogen make one woman in four nauseated and vomit, but the gestagen seems to have few side-effects. The protection against pregnancy is very high when oestrogens are used after a single coital episode, but when gestagens are taken after each episode, the pregnancy rate is about 3–5 per 100 woman years.

Fear has been expressed that hormones used in this way may cause abnormalities in the fetus should pregnancy occur despite the drugs. There is no evidence for this, but if a woman requests an abortion it should be given to her.

The alternative method in the situations I have mentioned, is for a woman so exposed to pregnancy, to wait for her period and if it fails to arrive 4 to 7 days after the expected date to seek help from a doctor who uses 'menstrual regulation' (see p. 135) or to seek an abortion.

What are the long term effects of taking the Pill? The Pill has now been available and used, for over 20 years. No long term side-effects have been found. It does not increase the risk of cancer of the breast or uterus. It does not lead to the birth of abnormal children to women who have taken it for some years. It does not increase the incidence of diabetes or liver damage.

Isn't the Pill dangerous? No. The dangers of oral contraceptives have been exaggerated. Newspapers, women's magazines and the media find that a scare headline sells more copies than an item about the value of the Pill. The truth is that the Pill is not perfect, but no other 'drug' has been subjected to so much careful investigation in the whole of history, and the safety:efficiency ratio of hormonal contraceptives is equal to or better than that of any other known drug.

The benefits of the Pill The use of hormonal contraceptives does have real advantages. The obvious one is that they enable women to control their fertility with ease and, in general, with little upset. But the Pill confers other benefits. A woman taking oral contraceptives is unlikely to have dysmenorrhoea, her menstrual flow will be reduced, (which in turn helps to prevent anaemia) and she is likely to have a reduced amount of premenstrual tension. In addition women taking the Pill have a lesser chance of developing ovarian cysts. Recent work suggests that a woman has a lesser chance of developing the lumpy condition of the breasts which is called by various names, usually benign mammary dysplasia (see p. 300). These benefits are usually not publicized, but they are real.

In the end, *you* have to choose whether or not you want to take oral contraceptives to prevent an unwanted pregnancy. You may prefer to use another method – a popular choice is to use an intrauterine device – an I.U.D.

The intrauterine contraceptive (The I.U.D.)

The I.U.D. is being chosen increasingly by women who wish to avoid pregnancy. It has an advantage over the Pill, in that once it has been placed inside the uterus and has been accepted, the woman has not got to do anything else to protect herself. She does not have to remember to take the Pill each day. She can have sexual intercourse with reasonable safety and without worry.

There is nothing new about the I.U.D. Arab camel drivers in Biblical times used the method. They used to introduce a round stone, the size of a pea, into the uterus of their female camels, which then repulsed the advances of the male camels, and worked harder! In the 1920s, a German gynaecologist used a silver or gold device which he introduced into the womb. Unfortunately it caused many complications and was abandoned by most doctors as unsafe! A revival of interest in this form of contraception occurred after the discovery of polythene. Polythene is a plastic, which easily regains its shape after stretching, is not irritating to the tissues, and can be made free from germs quite easily. Because of the urgent need for some cheap form of contraceptive device, various shapes of polythene were devised to see if they would prevent pregnancy when inserted into the uterus of a woman. Of the bewildering and fanciful shapes which have been produced over the past two decades, three remain the most popular. One, the Lippes Loop, is the most successful of the 'first generation' of I.U.Ds. The others, one of which is an I.U.D. to which fine copper wire has been added, and the other an I.U.D. containing progesterone, are examples of the 'second generation' of I.U.Ds. (Fig. 7/6).

No one yet knows how the I.U.Ds work. The most recent evidence suggests that they cause a change in the environment inside the womb which makes its lining 'hostile' to the egg. It is known that the larger the device, the lower the pregnancy rate. Unfortunately, the larger the device, the more likely is the woman to have cramping pains and to have heavy periods, which are a considerable disadvantage. This was the reason for adding copper wire to the device. Inside the uterus

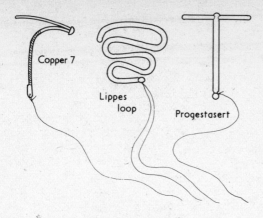

Fig. 7/6 I.U.Ds. in common use

the copper slowly ionizes, and this affects the lining of the uterus so that it rejects the egg. Copper has permitted scientists to make the device smaller, and consequently to reduce the side-effects whilst giving the same protection against pregnancy as with the larger devices (Fig. 7/7). The smaller device is also easier to introduce into the uterus of a woman who has never had children. There is one problem with the copper-containing I.U.Ds. It is that as the copper slowly ionizes, the device becomes less efficient. At the moment, scientists think it should be changed every 24 months, whilst the Loop can stay in the uterus and give protection against pregnancy for as long as a woman wishes. The newer progesterone-containing I.U.D. has to be changed each year.

It is quite surprising how many women are misinformed about their anatomy. Before the I.U.D. is inserted it is important that the woman should talk with the health worker – doctor or nurse – so that she can learn about her genital anatomy and have the opportunity to ask questions. The health worker will examine her vaginally so that the size and position of the uterus can be determined. Once this has been done, the I.U.D. is put into the womb painlessly and easily. Modern devices are prepacked in sterile packs and it is simplicity itself to introduce it into the patient's uterus. Usually she lies on her back with her legs apart. The health worker puts a small instrument into her vagina so that the cervix can be seen. It is cleaned with a

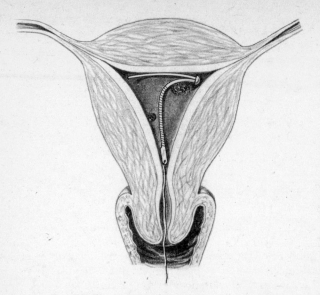

FIG. 7/7 The intra-uterine contraceptive device

gentle antiseptic, and then the introducer, preloaded with the I.U.D.
is slowly pushed along the canal of the cervix so that its tip lies in the
cavity of the uterus. The plunger is pushed, and the device is expelled
to lie in the womb. There is no need for an anaesthetic, and the
woman can go home immediately after.

The best time to put an I.U.D. into the uterus is in the last days of
menstruation; at a postnatal visit, which usually takes place six to
eight weeks after childbirth; or just after an abortion. At these times
the canal of the cervix is wider and it is easier to introduce the I.U.D.
A few women feel a little faint during the procedure, and some have
cramping pains for a few hours, as the uterus adjusts to its new
occupant, but most have no trouble at all. A few women bleed for a
day or so after the insertion, but the amount is slight.

In the first months after an I.U.D. is inserted, most women report
an increase in the amount and duration of menstruation. It tends to
start one or two days earlier than usual. At first, the blood loss is slight
but it becomes heavier and some clots may be expelled. The heavier
bleeding goes on for about four days, after which the period ceases

or spotting may continue for 2 or 3 days. Usually menstruation returns to the pattern normal for the particular woman within 3 or 4 months. The smaller copper-containing I.U.Ds cause fewer menstrual disturbances than do the loop. Women who continue to have heavy periods with an I.U.D., find that the new progesterone-containing I.U.D. reduces the blood loss.

Apart from cramp-like pains experienced by some women when the I.U.D. is inserted and some discomfort during menstruation when clots are expelled, pain is unusual. Should a woman have pain in her lower abdomen and this is associated with an increased discharge from her vagina and perhaps pain during intercourse, it may be a warning that she is developing a low-grade infection in her oviducts. She should go to her doctor and have the I.U.D. taken out. Luckily, this is a rare problem.

Two other problems should be mentioned. About two women in every hundred find that the presence of the I.U.D. increases the contractions of the uterus so that the device is expelled. This usually takes place during menstruation but it can occur at other times. Of course, if the I.U.D. is not in the uterus the woman is not protected against an unwanted pregnancy. This is one of the purposes of the nylon thread attached to the tail of the I.U.D. A woman should examine herself vaginally after each menstrual period to make sure the thread is there. If it is, all is well. She need not worry that the nylon will injure her sexual partner. The nylon is soft and there is no danger that it will spike his penis! In a very few women, the contractions of the uterus propel the I.U.D. in a different direction – the I.U.D. being pushed through the wall of the uterus to lie in the peritoneal cavity. This occurs in one insertion of every 1,000 made. Once again, the nylon thread can no longer be felt when the woman examines herself. The woman should see her doctor so that he can decide if the device has been expelled or has been pushed through the uterine wall.

As a method of contraception, the I.U.D. is not as efficient as the pill or the injectables. About two women in every hundred become pregnant whilst wearing an I.U.D. and the rate seems to be the same whichever device is chosen. If pregnancy occurs the woman has two choices. She can ask to have an abortion, and her request should be granted without any difficulty, as in a few cases of pregnancy occurring with an I.U.D. in the uterus, a spontaneous abortion (or miscarriage) occurs in the second quarter of pregnancy. Rather a high proportion of these abortions are accompanied by infection which may reduce the woman's chance of becoming pregnant later, when she wants to have a baby. Alternatively, she can continue with the pregnancy. She should visit her doctor as early as possible, after she knows that she is pregnant. The doctor will try to pull out the I.U.D. without disturbing the pregnancy but if he fails the pregnancy may continue. But should signs of a 'threatened' spontaneous abortion arise (see p. 274), she should see the doctor again, and be checked for signs of infection.

Provided she does not abort she can be reassured that the I.U.D. will not harm her baby in any way – there is no truth in the story that a copper-containing I.U.D. causes abnormalities in the fetus.

TUBAL LIGATION

Increasingly, couples who have completed their families are seeking permanent methods of birth control. In many cases the man chooses to have a vasectomy, as the operation is simple to do, relatively painless and highly efficient. In other cases the woman chooses to take the permanent measure. In her case the operation consists of cutting out a portion of the oviducts. These are the tubes which stretch from the upper corners of the uterus towards the ovaries. The egg, whether fertilized or not, passes along the oviduct. The sperms swim through the cavity of the uterus and along the oviduct where, when conditions are favourable, one of them fertilizes the egg. If a segment of the tube is excised, and the cut ends tied, the sperms cannot reach the ovum and pregnancy will be prevented (Fig. 7/8).

This is the principle of the operation of tubal ligation. It is also called sterilization, as the woman is permanently prevented from having children. Unfortunately, many women believe sterilization means castration, and confusion occurs. The ovaries are never removed in tubal ligation operations and after the operation continue to function normally, producing the hormones which help to make a woman a woman. Neither her femininity, nor her sexuality are diminished. Some women who contemplate having tubal ligation are anxious lest the eggs, released from the ovary each month, collect in the abdomen 'like frog spawn', as one of my patients said graphically. This fear is unfounded. At the most, only one egg is released each

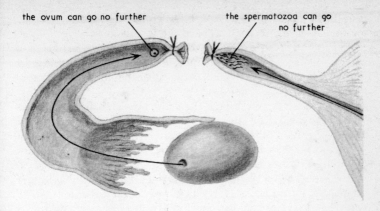

the ovum can go no further

the spermatozoa can go
no further

FIG. 7/8 Ligation·of the oviducts (Fallopian tubes)

month, and it at once migrates into the oviduct where it is destroyed
by other body cells.

Before deciding on the operation a woman should talk it over with
her doctor, who will be able to answer all her questions. He will also
need to examine her vaginally as certain conditions make tubal
ligation inadvisable. These conditions include uterine 'fibroids', a
marked prolapse, or a history of irregular menstruation which has not
responded to hormones. If a woman has any of these conditions, and
also wants permanent birth control, a hysterectomy is the preferable
operation.

Nowadays, tubectomy (as the Indians prefer to call the operation)
is a relatively simple procedure requiring only a short stay in hospital.
The operation can often be done very conveniently in the first days
after childbirth, or it can be done apart from childbirth. Many doctors
refuse to do the operation if the woman has less than four children.
This is, of course, arrogant of the doctors. If a couple decide they
want no more children, and are aware that the operation produces
permanent sterility – so that if they change their minds later it cannot
be readily reversed – then they should have the right to choose.

The usual method is to make a small cut just below the umbilicus
when the operation is done just after childbirth, or just below the
pubic hair-line when the operation is done apart from childbirth. The
cut need only be 2 to 4 cm in length. Each tube is brought up into the
cut and a wedge removed. The alternative method is to use an

instrument called a laparoscope which is introduced into the peritoneal cavity through a 1 cm cut at the lower edge of the umbilicus. An electric current then burns each tube. Each method has its advocates and probably there is little to choose, although I prefer to see the oviduct and to cut it rather than to use the laparoscope and burn it.

Tubal ligation is a most successful and appreciated method of birth control provided the woman is aware that it is permanent. It is true that an operation to reverse the procedure can be attempted, but at present only a few pregnancies occur after it. In the future, with new methods of microsurgery, this may change, but at present a woman must have made up her mind that she does not ever want a further pregnancy. In certain cases the doctor may suggest that it would be preferable to remove her uterus, which is called hysterectomy, rather than performing a tubal ligation. In these cases the woman may have 'fibroids' or have consistently heavy periods. Before the woman makes a decision whether to choose a hysterectomy she should expect her doctor to discuss the matter with her fully. Provided the woman has had the opportunity to discuss the operation with her doctor and has been counselled properly, few problems occur whether tubal ligation or hysterectomy has been chosen. After tubal ligation more than 99 per cent of women are very pleased they had the operation. There are no side-effects and the couple need take no other contraceptive precautions, confident that pregnancy will not occur.

A few myths persist about tubal ligation. These are that after tubal ligation (or 'sterilization' as it is sometimes wrongly called), the woman loses her sexual urge, her periods stop, she gets fat, and after a few years the oviducts open up and pregnancy becomes possible once more. These 'folk-tales' are all untrue. After tubal ligation a woman has the same sexual desires and urges as before the operation.

Usually a woman's periods are unchanged in amount or in frequency, but if she was taking the Pill before tubal ligation she may find that her periods are heavier. This is because the hormones used in the Pill usually cause a reduction in menstruation so that when the Pill is no longer taken the periods seem heavier. There is also some evidence that a woman's periods are a bit heavier if she has chosen to have tubal ligation done through a laparoscope. A woman does not get fat after tubal ligation – unless she overeats; and the operation does provide permanent protection against pregnancy.

THE EFFICIENCY OF CONTRACEPTIVES

Most sexually active people use contraceptive measures to enable them to enjoy the mutual pleasuring of sexual intercourse without the fear of a pregnancy occurring at an inappropriate time.

Table 7/2

Failure rates over a period of 12 months

	per cent
No contraception	70
Vaginal douche	45
Vaginal foam, jellies, etc.	30
Rhythm method	30
Withdrawal	25
Condom	15
Vaginal diaphragm + spermicidal jelly	10
Intrauterine contraceptive device	3
Oral contraceptives:	
Continuous gestagen	4
Sequential	2
Combined	0.25

In her reproductive years a woman may spend periods of time using one form of contraceptive, periods when she uses no contraceptives, periods when she is pregnant and periods when she returns to contraceptive use. She will want to know which of the contraceptive measures available is the most efficient in preventing a pregnancy so that she can make a choice, (Table 7/2). It may be that she will choose one of the most reliable methods (such as the hormonal contraceptives or the I.U.D.) despite the side-effects. It may be that she will choose a less efficient method (such as the vaginal diaphragm or condom) which has few or no side-effects. This choice may be made as a woman grows older, when her fertility is reduced, secure in the knowledge that should an unwanted pregnancy occur she can obtain an abortion with safety. But it would be irresponsible for a woman to choose not to use any form of contraception and rely on abortion to end her unwanted pregnancies. A single abortion poses little danger to a woman, but repeated abortions increase the danger of damage to her body. This is why I have written that when a woman desires to limit the frequency of pregnancy she should use contraceptives, relying on abortion as a 'back-stop' if the contraceptive fails to prevent pregnancy or when an unwanted pregnancy unexpectedly occurs.

INDUCED ABORTION

Induced abortion has been practised by women since people collected in groups for their mutual protection. When food was plentiful children were welcome; when food became short, either because of famine or population pressures, an additional child could mean disaster. As no contraceptive methods were available (apart from sexual abstinence), abortion was used to end an unwanted pregnancy. Few of these abortions were performed under ideal conditions, but most women survived, although many were injured or made sterile by infection following the abortion.

The toll which induced clandestine abortion took of the health of women has led enlightened legislators, in the past few decades, to change the laws which made abortion illegal, replacing them by laws which permit abortion to be performed with dignity and safety. The change is due to several factors. First, it was apparent that even in nations where abortion was illegal, large numbers of women continued to seek and to obtain abortions. Second, a wealthy woman could always obtain an abortion without humiliation and with considerable safety but her poorer sister was often humiliated and her health placed in jeopardy when she sought the services of a backstreet abortionist. The dangers of back-street abortions are demonstrated by the finding that the majority of deaths following abortion occurred if the woman had tried to abort herself or had used the services of an unskilled person; and by the statistic that in certain Latin American countries, between 25 and 50 per cent of beds in maternity hospitals are occupied by women suffering from the effects of illegally induced abortion. Third, the existing laws did not prevent induced abortions from occurring; the more liberal laws, it was hoped, would reduce the dangers of abortion. This has proved to be so.

The change to legal abortion has spread rapidly since 1970 and today 60 per cent of the world's women live in nations where a legal abortion can be obtained, usually with relatively little difficulty or loss of dignity. Experience of legal abortion in the U.S.A. and Britain has been carefully documented and analysed. These investigations show that since legal abortion has been introduced, the number of deaths due to abortion has dropped dramatically, so that a woman who has an abortion of a pregnancy which is no more than 10 weeks advanced, performed in an appropriate place by a skilled medical attendant, has only one chance in 100,000 of dying as a result. This is twenty times less than the deaths associated with childbirth. The studies also confirm that the longer the duration of the pregnancy the higher are the possibilities of complications.

In nations where abortion laws have been made less restrictive, opponents of reform have declared that if abortion was permitted more freely than previously, women would abandon other methods of birth control and would rely on abortion. They foresaw a continually rising frequency of abortion. They were wrong. In Britain the number of abortions did rise for the first 5 years after the more liberal laws came into operation, but the rate has since fallen. Moreover, fewer than 5 per cent of women who have had an abortion, have returned for a second abortion. The remainder have either become pregnant and have delivered a live baby, or have used contraception to prevent another unwanted pregnancy.

The women, and men, who campaigned for abortion law reform correctly believed that the majority of sexually active women would be protected by contraceptives; that abortion would be used as a 'back-stop' for those women who became pregnant through ignorance, ill-luck or great misfortune; and that most of those women who had had an abortion would subsequently avoid an unwanted pregnancy by using contraceptives. This belief has proved true, and it epitomizes a rational attitude to abortion. This is that women and men should be informed about contraception, that contraceptives should be easily obtained, and couples would use one of the contraceptive measures currently available to prevent an unwanted pregnancy occurring. But should an unwanted pregnancy happen, the woman should be able to have an abortion performed without delay, without the need to beg or risk being humiliated, and in a place where the abortion can be performed by a skilled medical attendant. It also implies that all the people with whom she comes into contact should be sympathetic and understanding helpers, and should give the woman counsel so that any guilt she might feel would be minimized, and inform her about contraception so that she might prevent another unwanted pregnancy.

Organizations, such as Preterm in the U.S.A. and in Australia, and similar organizations in Britain, as well as many hospital clinics, meet these criteria. More will do so if women continue to make their voice heard.

It is true that organizations opposing abortion have also become increasingly vocal. They point out that the fetus has a right to life, and if aborted its mortality is 100 per cent. Unfortunately, they also tend to publish selective, inaccurate statistics which make induced abortions appear far more dangerous that they really are, and some of their propaganda induces strong feelings of guilt amongst women who have had an abortion. This is an affront to the integrity of a woman who has sought an abortion only after careful thought, as most women do. If you want to know more details about the medical and sociological aspects of abortion, you might care to read one or both of my books *Human Reproduction and Society* or *People Populating*.

Before abortion law reform in Britain, fearful women who wanted an abortion resorted to the most useless and sometimes the most desperate methods. Many were misled by friends and friendly pharmacists, when they tried to obtain drugs to induce the abortion of an unwanted pregnancy. An investigation by Dr Martin Cole in Britain in 1964 showed that 'female remedies' could be purchased in 12 out of 15 pharmacies chosen at random, and in 17 out of 22 shops selling condoms or diaphragms. Most of the drugs claimed to bring on menstruation suppressed 'due to colds, shock, fright, strain, etc.'; but they were sold as abortifacients, and were not cheap. The drugs studied contained iron, quinine, purgatives or herbals such as aloes and pennyroyal which tradition held brought on menstruation. They are, of course, all quite useless if a woman is pregnant. None will procure an abortion.

The lack of efficacy of these drugs led women, who could not afford proper care, to try to induce an abortion using the easily available enema (or vaginal douche) apparatus. With considerable contortions, women have introduced the nozzle of the douche into their cervix and have tried to fill their womb with mixtures of soapy water or caustics. In all too many cases this led to a medical disaster, and often to the death of the mother. In other instances desperate women have introduced a domestic instrument – crochet hooks, button hooks, knitting needles, or pieces of wood – into their womb in the hope that it would bring about an abortion. Often it did – but often the woman also became infected.

When a woman went to a back-yard abortionist, her chance of obtaining an abortion, whilst avoiding death from haemorrhage, or sterility from infection, varied with the training and skill of the abortionist. The best trained were fairly efficient and used gynaecological instruments skilfully. Others used an enema syringe, or introduced an object into the womb to start bleeding so that the woman could then go to the hospital claiming that she was aborting spontaneously. This situation has now changed, and although some women still hopefully and ineffectually try 'home remedies', and some still go to back-street abortionists, most have access to the services of skilled medical helpers. In their hands abortion is very safe, provided it is undertaken in the first quarter of pregnancy.

The safest abortion is that which is performed on a healthy woman, whose pregnancy is less than 10 weeks advanced, by a skilled medical attendant, in a well-equipped clinic or hospital. The earlier the abortion, the safer it is. This has led some doctors to suggest the method of 'menstrual regulation'. In this a woman who is at risk of being pregnant, waits to see if her menstrual period comes on time and, if it does not, seeks help within 7 days. At this time it is impossible to diagnose pregnancy clinically, and laboratory tests (except for a special test) are not helpful. The doctor empties the uterus with a small tube attached to a syringe. The woman may or may not be pregnant so that no moral question is raised and the doctor is only regulating her menstruation.

Menstrual regulation is very safe, but the pregnancy continues in one woman in every hundred on whom the procedure is used. Menstrual regulation can be performed painlessly without any anaesthetic. A possible 'disadvantage' of the simplicity of the procedure is that it may prevent some women from using contraceptive methods, although I believe it doubtful. Large numbers of women have been treated by 'menstrual regulation', and the reported results show that only one woman in every 250,000 treated has died – a rate three times less than the deaths which follow an injection of penicillin! The safety of menstrual regulation emphasizes the importance of seeking help as early as possible if you think you may be pregnant and do not want to continue with the pregnancy. Even so, it is better, safer and less distressing to prevent pregnancy by using a contraceptive than by resorting to abortion, whether menstrual regulation or some other method is used.

The method of suction is also used by doctors who end an unwanted pregnancy in its first 10 weeks. An injection of local anaesthetic is made into the cervix, which blocks all pain; or else the woman may choose to have a general anaesthetic. A narrow glass, metal or plastic tube, the size depending on the number of weeks the woman is pregnant, is pushed gently through the cervix, so that it lies in the cavity of the uterus. The tube is connected, through a second tube to a vacuum bottle. The vacuum created in the uterus sucks the tiny embryo in its sac (see p. 146) from its attachment to the lining of the womb with no damage to the uterus itself. Usually there is no more bleeding after the operation than there is with a normal menstrual period and often there is far less. The woman can go home within a hour or so of the procedure and usually has no further problems, although she is counselled what to do should problems occur.

After the 10th or 12th week of pregnancy suction curetting, as it is called, is not recommended, and if the pregnancy is over 14 weeks complications may be frequent and serious.

Because of these dangers, most gynaecologists recommend that if the pregnancy has lasted for more than 12 weeks after the last menstrual period, surgery should be avoided. Instead, substances called prostaglandins, should be used. These substances are injected into the uterus and after a period of time (which lasts on average 16 hours) bring on strong contractions of the uterus, rather like a 'miniature labour' which, after some hours, lead to an abortion. During the interval between the injection and the abortion, the woman may feel nauseated, or develop a fever, as prostaglandins have these side-effects. The process of the abortion is not very pleasant and can be painful though pain relieving drugs are given. It is associated with more complications than occur when the abortion takes place in the first ten weeks of pregnancy. Both the discomfort and the greater danger of late abortion confirm what I have written earlier in this chapter. This is that abortion is most safely performed in the first 10 weeks of pregnancy.

As the duration of pregnancy increases abortion becomes increasingly dangerous to the woman. The mortality rises (Fig. **7/9**) and the complications increase. If the abortion is performed before the 10th or 12th week, only 2 per cent of women have complications, usually heavy bleeding requiring a curettage, or fever. When the abortion is performed between the 12th and 15th week, heavy bleeding complicates 5 per cent, and fever 4 per cent of the abortions. As well, there is some concern that abortions performed in the second quarter of pregnancy, between the 10th and 19th week, may damage the cervix of the uterus causing 'cervical incompetence'. This complication is rare.

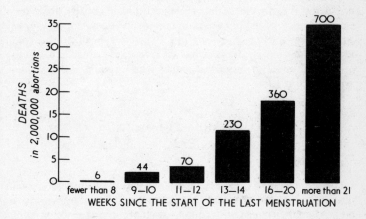

FIG. 7/9 Deaths from abortion. Two million abortions reported in the U.S.A. 1972–1975

For these reasons when a woman has made the decision, and discussed it with a counsellor, that she wishes to have an abortion, the operation should be done with the least delay, with consideration for her feelings, and in an appropriate place.

Chapter 8

A Slight Touch of Pregnancy

Most women have a pretty good idea that they may be pregnant before they consult a doctor to confirm their suspicions. For most, the confirmation is an occasion for joy; for some an occasion for anxiety and sorrow. A few women, desperately wishing to become pregnant, can mimic many of the signs of pregnancy, and believe themselves to be pregnant when in fact they are not. Even after the doctor has told the patient that she is not pregnant, she refuses to believe him. These patients have a 'phantom pregnancy', and require sympathetic psychiatric attention.

THE SYMPTOMS OF EARLY PREGNANCY

Amenorrhoea

The first symptom of pregnancy is usually that the menstrual period fails to occur on the expected date. If a woman has regular periods and has had the chance of becoming pregnant, the absence of menstruation (or amenorrhoea) suggests that she is pregnant. But a woman who has regular periods should wait at least 10 days before consulting a doctor, as before this time he will not be able to tell if she is pregnant. If her periods are not regular, amenorrhoea is less helpful in making a diagnosis of pregnancy.

Pregnancy is the most usual cause of amenorrhoea in women aged 16 to 40, but it is not the only cause. Menstruation may be delayed or suppressed by the emotions, in certain illnesses and when certain drugs are taken. Emotional stress is the most usual cause of amenorrhoea, apart from pregnancy, in a woman who has previously menstruated normally. The emotions act on the part of the brain which controls the release of hormones. Fear of an unwanted pregnancy; a fight with a loved one; a new and difficult job; or a journey, all can cause amenorrhoea.

Breast changes

Many women experience breast fullness and discomfort just prior to their menstrual period. If pregnancy occurs, these symptoms persist and are increased. The breasts become fuller, firmer and more tender. Occasionally they throb and the nipples tingle. The degree of these symptoms is quite variable, but as pregnancy advances the fullness of the breasts increases, and the nipples become larger and darker. The area around the nipple, which is called the areola, also becomes larger, darker and rather swollen. In this area there are tiny openings to milk ducts and minute glands. In pregnancy the minute milk glands and ducts enlarge to form small protuberances or follicles – which are named Montgomery's follicles after an Irish obstetrician who first described them. These are rarely noticeable until the pregnancy is 8 weeks advanced.

The changes in the breasts are caused by the female sex hormones oestrogen and progesterone produced by the placenta. These hormones cause growth of the ducts and milk sacs of the breast, and lead to fat being deposited around the milk apparatus to cushion it. The tingling and throbbing occasionally felt is due to the increased flow of blood through the blood vessels which supply the breasts.

Nausea and vomiting

In about half of pregnant women some degree of nausea or vomiting occurs. Usually this is quite mild, and occurs in the morning. Occasionally, however, it is more severe, and vomiting may occur at any time of the day. When this occurs, it usually starts about 2 weeks after the first missed period, and lasts for about 6 to 8 weeks. The cause of the nausea is not known, but it seems probable that it is due to the increases in the amount of sex hormones produced in pregnancy. It usually goes by the 12th week of pregnancy as the body adjusts to the higher hormone levels.

Bladder 'irritability'

In early pregnancy the kidneys function over-efficiently, and the bladder fills with urine more quickly. This leads to frequency of urination, which is an early symptom of pregnancy.

WHAT THE DOCTOR LOOKS FOR

The patient visiting her doctor in early pregnancy will be asked about the symptoms just mentioned, and will then be examined. As will be described in the chapter on antenatal care, the examination includes a careful assessment of the patient's general health, in which the heart is listened to, the breasts are examined, the abdomen is palpated, and an 'internal', or pelvic, examination is performed. This examination need not be feared, as it is quite painless. The patient lies on her back with her legs bent and her knees apart. She breathes slowly and relaxes all her muscles. The doctor first examines her vulva and then gently introduces a small instrument, called a speculum, into the vagina so that he may look at the cervix. Many doctors take this opportunity to take a sample of the cells which cover the cervix, so that these may be examined in the laboratory. This is called the 'Pap smear' (cervical smear) test, after Dr. Papanicolaou who first described it. Abnormal cells are found in about 1 sample in every 200 examined. These patients have to be investigated further in case the abnormal cells indicate a very early cancer of the cervix.

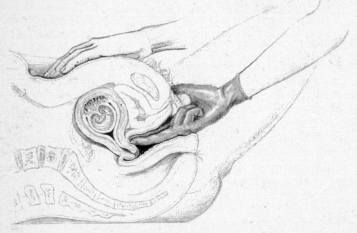

FIG. 8/1 The diagnosis of early pregnancy

The doctor then removes the speculum and putting on a plastic glove, inserts two fingers into the vagina. With his other hand he presses gently on the abdomen just below the umbilicus (Fig. **8/1**). In this way he can feel the shape of the uterus and tell if it is enlarged, as would be expected in pregnancy, or if there are any other swellings which may require treatment. The pelvic examination is most informative when made between the 6th and 10th week of pregnancy.

TESTS FOR PREGNANCY

Immunological tests

After the general and pelvic examinations, the doctor may still be unsure if the patient is pregnant, so he may make a test on the patient's urine. This test depends on the fact that within 40 days of the last menstrual period, a large amount of a special hormone called

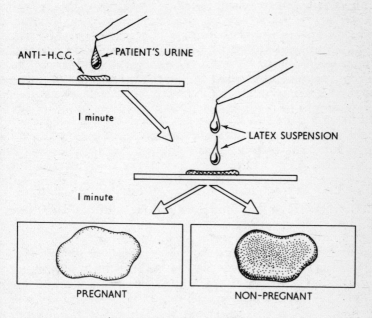

FIG. 8/2 How pregnancy is diagnosed by a 'slide test'

HCG, made by the placenta, circulates in the blood. This hormone is then excreted in the urine and can be measured by a simple test. A drop of a substance which neutralizes HCG (anti-HCG) is put on a glass slide, and a drop of the patient's urine is added. The two drops are mixed, and after a minute two drops of a milky substance made of latex rubber particles covered with HCG are added. If the patient is not pregnant, the anti-HCG substance will fix onto the HCG covering the latex, and they will clump together to form 'curds' in the milky substance. However, if the patient is pregnant, all the anti-HCG will have joined with the HCG present in her urine. Because of this, the particles will not clump and the milky solution has no curds when examined. The test takes two minutes to perform, and is 95 per cent accurate after the 40th day of pregnancy. It is called the 'agglutination-inhibition test for pregnancy' (Fig. 8/2).

Ultrasound

An even more exciting development is a machine which uses 'radar' to detect if a pregnancy is present. The machine uses ultrasound (that is, sound waves of a very high frequency). The sound waves 'echo' off different tissues and can be translated into a picture. The machine has many uses in obstetrics, as well as diagnosing early pregnancy. In early pregnancy it can detect an ectopic pregnancy, in which the embryo is in the oviduct, not the uterus. In late pregnancy it can detect the position of the baby, the presence of twins, the position of the placenta, and by taking readings at intervals, it is possible to determine the speed of growth of the baby. The machine is expensive, but as time passes more and more hospitals will be able to offer this diagnostic service to patients.

THE SYMPTOMS AND SIGNS OF LATER PREGNANCY

As the uterus grows, its size becomes obvious, however much a woman may desire her dressmaker to hide it! After the 16th week of pregnancy, other symptoms and signs also indicate pregnancy, although by this time it should be pretty obvious to any intelligent woman that she is pregnant.

'Quickening'

At about 18 to 20 weeks in first pregnancies and two weeks earlier in subsequent pregnancies, the first faint fluttering movements of the baby are felt. This is called 'quickening' because once it was believed that the baby only became alive at this time. It is reflected by the Biblical reference to the 'quick and the dead'.

Movements of the fetus become strong and more frequent as pregnancy advances, and the mother may notice that her baby has periods of activity and periods of rest. In the rest periods, it probably sleeps. Provided the periods of activity and rest coincide with the same periods in the mother, all is well; but some babies seem to take a perverse delight in having their active periods at night, to the annoyance of the mother! If the movements are very active, lumps appear and disappear on the uterus and are noticed by the mother. They are caused by the baby's limbs stretching the muscles of the uterus. Many babies are less active, and sometimes a day or more passes without movements being felt. This does not mean that the baby is dead, but if the patient feels no movements for a longer period, she should consult her doctor, who will listen for fetal heart sounds. Recently a machine, called a Fetal Heart Detector, has been developed which relies on the 'doppler principle' of sound waves. This machine can detect the baby's heart beats as early as the 12th week of pregnancy, and is nearly 100 per cent accurate after the 16th week.

Frequency of urination

Frequency of urination, which was a symptom of early pregnancy, ceases after the 12th week, to reappear in the last weeks of pregnancy. In late pregnancy the symptom is due to the pressure of the baby's head on the bladder, and can be quite disturbing, especially at night.

WHAT THE DOCTOR FINDS IN LATE PREGNANCY

The growth of the uterus

To some extent the doctor can tell how much the pregnancy has advanced by noting the height of the top of the uterus in the patient's

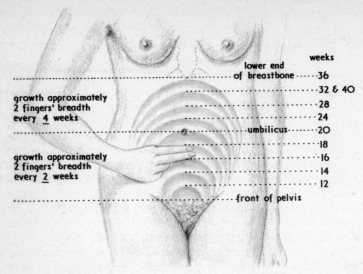

weeks

lower end
of breastbone ⋯⋯ 36

⋯⋯⋯⋯⋯⋯⋯⋯⋯⋯⋯ 32 & 40

growth approximately
2 fingers' breadth
every <u>4</u> weeks

⋯⋯⋯⋯⋯⋯⋯ 28

⋯⋯⋯⋯⋯⋯⋯ 24

umbilicus ⋯⋯ 20

⋯⋯⋯⋯⋯⋯ 18

growth approximately
2 fingers' breadth
every <u>2</u> weeks

⋯⋯⋯⋯⋯⋯ 16

⋯⋯⋯⋯⋯⋯ 14

⋯⋯⋯⋯⋯ 12

⋯⋯⋯ front of pelvis

FIG. 8/3 The growth of the uterus in pregnancy

abdomen (Fig. **8/3**). The method is not very accurate, and various factors such as tenseness of the abdomen or obesity can lead to false readings. At the same time, the doctor gently runs his fingers over the uterus to determine the position of the baby. He should always tell the patient where her baby is lying, outlining the position for her. He usually listens for the baby's heart sounds, but if the patient is feeling the 'movements' of the baby, this is not really necessary.

The growing uterus stretches the patient's abdominal skin, and by the 20th week it will be obvious that she is pregnant. From this time on small pinkish streaks, about 4 cms (1½ in) long, appear over the lower abdomen, especially in the flanks. These 'streaks of pregnancy' are due to small breaks in the lower layer of the skin which is less well able to stretch. They also sometimes appear on the thighs. After the birth of the baby, the colour fades to silvery-white, but remains permanently. There is no known way to prevent them, although some women believe that massage of the skin with olive oil helps.

In dark-haired women, another change may be found. This is a brownish pigmented line stretching in the midline from the umbilicus to the pubic bone. It is of no consequence, and fades after delivery, almost disappearing in time.

X-rays

Occasionally the doctor has to make use of X-ray examinations to clear up an obscure point. X-rays have a slight potential danger if overused and, in general, doctors avoid taking X-rays in pregnancy unless they are absolutely necessary. The reason is that if X-rays are used excessively the baby has a slightly greater chance of developing leukaemia. However, I should stress that the risk is very low and that today X-rays are used very much less than formerly. The modern tendency is to use them only when really necessary. For example, the doctor may be unable to decide whether the baby is lying as a breech, or if there are twins present. In these cases an X-ray may be necessary. In other cases the patient may have felt no movements of the baby, and the doctor fails to hear the baby's heart. If he does not have a fetal heart detector, he may suggest an X-ray examination to try to determine if the baby is alive or not. Occasionally an X-ray examination of the shape of the pelvis is required if the baby's head does not settle properly into the mother's pelvis in late pregnancy.

Mothers sometimes ask if an X-ray can be taken to determine the sex of the unborn baby. Since X-rays only show up bones, it is impossible to tell the sex of the baby in this way.

Chapter 9

A Most Wondrous Growth

THE FETUS

Fertilization occurs in the outer part of the oviduct, when a single spermatozoon penetrates the 'shell' (or zona pellucida) of the egg and enters its substance. The sperm's tail is stuck in the 'shell' and drops off, leaving the sperm head free in the egg. The part of the sperm head, called the nucleus, which contains in twisted strands the information needed to make a new individual, joins with the nucleus of the egg, and they fuse. The first step towards a new individual, who will take half of its characteristics from its father and half from its mother, has been taken. Inside the zona pellucida, the fertilized egg with its fused nucleus divides into 2 identical cells, then into 4 cells, then into 8 cells, then into 16 cells, and again until it looks like a mulberry made up of 64 cells. These divisions take place during the 3 days that it takes the fertilized egg to gently move along the oviduct to reach the cavity of the uterus. Inside its cavity, the fertilized egg develops further, fluid appearing amongst the mulberry cells, and eventually splitting them into two parts: an outer shell of cells, and a collection of cells at one side. The outer cells will form the placenta; the inner mass will form the embryo. Quite soon after this, on the same or the next day, the zona pellucida dissolves and the fertilized egg, now called a blastocyst, plants itself into the juicy, soft lining of the womb (Fig. 9/1). Nine days after fertilization the blastocyst has burrowed deeply into the lining of the womb and has grown to the size of a pin-head. Four days later, at the time the menstrual period is expected, it has enlarged to be just visible to the naked eye. From now on the growth of the embryo and the placenta proceeds apace. From the very earliest time, a fluid-filled space develops around the embryo. This space is lined with a thin, glistening membrane, and this in turn is surrounded by a thicker membrane. The membranes with

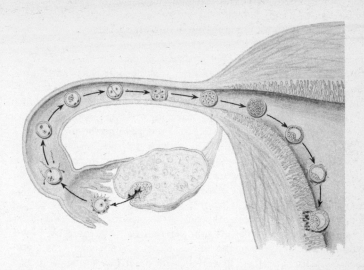

FIG. 9/1 The beginning of pregnancy
The diagram shows fertilization of the egg in the oviduct,
and its development as it journeys through the oviduct to
reach the uterus and implant

the contained water are called the amniotic sac, or the bag of waters.
By the 36th week of pregnancy, 1,000 ml (1¾ pints) of water surround the fetus. The fetus (until the 8th week of pregnancy, it is
called the embryo) is able to move about freely within the amniotic
sac, but it is prevented from being injured should the expectant
mother fall, as the water absorbs all the shock.

Within two days of implantation, the outer cells of the blastocyst
are sprouting in finger-like projections all round the sphere of the
egg. Quite quickly most of them die, and only the disc of cells lying
deep in the lining of the uterus continue to grow. This disc forms the
placenta, through which the fetus obtains all its nourishment. The
placenta is connected to the fetus by the umbilical cord. At first the
umbilical cord reaches from the placenta and joins the embryo near
its tail, as can be seen in Fig. **9/2**, but quite soon the tail curls round
and the umbilical cord joins the fetus in the centre of its abdomen, at
the place which after birth is the navel, or umbilicus. This is shown in

Fig. **9/3**. In many ways the placenta and the fetus work together, which is understandable as they form from the same fertilized egg. The placenta acts as the lung, the liver and the kidney of the fetus. Oxygen for its energy needs is transferred from the mother's bloodstream, where it is carried by the red blood cells, to the blood in the fetus. Carbon dioxide, and the other waste products of energy production, are transferred from the fetus to the mother's blood. This reduces the work which the fetal liver and kidney have to perform.

The fetus and the placenta work together to produce various hormones, which are so important in maintaining the pregnancy.

All these activities take place through the cells which form the placenta, and at all times the mother's blood and the blood of the fetus are completely separated. The two bloods never mix. The mother's blood bathes the placental cells, which permits them to take oxygen and nourishment from it, and to transfer them across the placenta into the network of tiny blood vessels on the fetal side of the placenta. These tiny vessels join together to form three big blood vessels, which pass along the umbilical cord to join up with the blood vessels inside the fetus. The umbilical cord is in fact a tube composed of a kind of thick jelly, though which the three vessels (two arteries and a vein) pass to link the fetus with the placenta.

It is easier to understand the further growth of the fetus and placenta by describing it at intervals: first at 6 weeks, then at 8 weeks, and then every 4 weeks to 40 weeks. In this description, the period is calculated from the first day of the last menstrual period, so the actual age of the embryo is about 2 weeks less. The new individual is called an embryo until week 8, and a fetus thereafter. During the embryonic period, all the structures which make it a normal human are formed; and subsequent development, during the fetal period, consists of growth and development of structures already formed.

To see the embryo and fetus, you have to imagine yourself inside the dark, warm, soft womb, where it grows throughout the pregnancy enclosed in the amniotic sac.

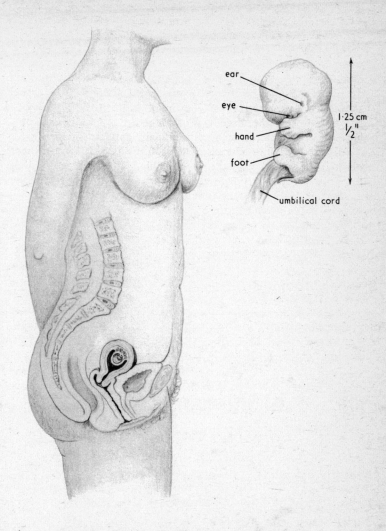

FIG. 9/2 Pregnancy at 6 weeks. The embryo is not recognizably human. It is only 28 days old, as conception occurs 14 days after the first day of the last menstrual period

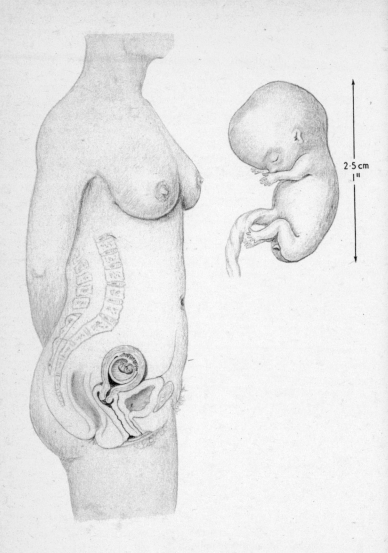

2·5 cm
1"

FIG. 9/3 Pregnancy at 8 weeks. The fetus is becoming
more human in appearance

6 weeks
(Fig. **9/2**)

The womb has enlarged, but it is still difficult for the doctor to tell if his patient is pregnant. It has enlarged rather more than is necessary for the size of the embryo; in fact it has *anticipated* its needs. The embryo is 1.25 cm (½ in) long. Its eye socket has formed, it has a reptile-like head and a tail. Its arm and leg buds are visible, but small and spade-like in shape. The placenta is larger and weighs more than the embryo.

8 weeks
(end of the
2nd lunar
month)
(Fig. **9/3**)

The womb has enlarged still more, and on a pelvic examination the doctor can tell that his patient is pregnant. Her breasts may be tender, and she may have some nausea.

The embryo is now much more like a human. It is 2.5 cm (or 1 in) long. The head is large compared with the body, and the external ears are forming. The limb buds have become arms and legs with tiny fingers and splayed toes. The eyes have become covered with eyelids which close across them, and remain shut until the 24th week. By now all the main organs of the body have formed, the heart beats sturdily, blood circulates through its vessels, its stomach is active and the kidneys are beginning to function. The only changes in the organs from now on will be an increase in their size and the sophistication of their function.

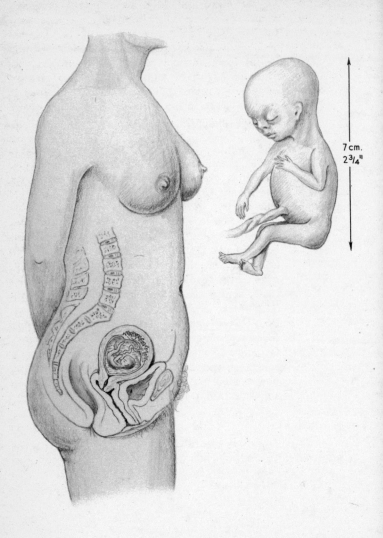

7 cm.
2³/₄"

FIG. 9/4 Pregnancy at 12 weeks

12 weeks (end of the 3rd lunar month) (Fig. 9/4) The uterus can just be felt peeping out of the pelvis, above the symphysis. The patient is sure that she is pregnant, and the nausea is almost gone.

The fetus, as it is now called, from the Latin, meaning a 'young one', is 9 cm (3½ in) long, and weighs 14 g (½ oz). The body has grown, but the head is still over-large. Nails are appearing on its fingers and toes. The external genitals are appearing, but it is still difficult to tell its sex. By the end of this week, the mechanical movements of legs and arms have changed into movements which are far more graceful and purposeful, as the nerve and muscle co-ordination improves, although the movements are tiny. The fetus can now swallow, and begins to swallow the amniotic fluid in which it lives. At the same time, it begins to pass drops of urine into the amniotic sac. The placenta has also grown, and now weighs about six times that of the fetus.

Babies 'breathe' long before they are born, probably from as early as 12 weeks after conception. Of course, no oxygen as such goes into their lungs, but blood does spurt through the lung blood vessels rhythmically, at about 80 'breaths' a minute. Babies can also get 'hiccups' in the last weeks of pregnancy, as many expectant mothers know. It is likely that this 'breathing' is the way in which babies prepare their lungs for life outside the uterus, and it has been found that babies who have a regular breathing pattern adjust to 'proper' breathing of air after birth more easily. This is being studied in research units and the 'breathing' pattern of babies in the uterus can be investigated by special machines. In the next few years this research may enable doctors to detect which babies are likely to have trouble adjusting to life after birth.

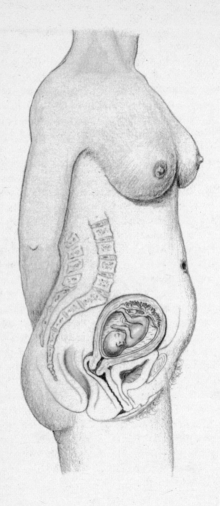

FIG. 9/5 Pregnancy at 16 weeks

16 weeks
(end of the
4th lunar
month)
(Fig. **9/5**)

The uterus is easily palpable, and reaches almost halfway to the umbilicus. It is beginning to make a bulge!

The fetus is now 18 cm (7 in) long, and weighs 100 g (4 oz). The head is still large for its thin body, which is bright red because the blood vessels glow through its transparent skin. Its heart is beating strongly, and its muscles are becoming active. Its sex can be distinguished. The growth of the placenta has slowed down, although its efficiency has increased, and now the weight of the placenta and the fetus are about equal.

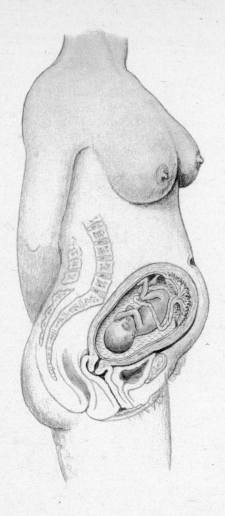

Fig. 9/6 Pregnancy at 20 weeks

20 weeks
(end of the
5th lunar
month)
(Fig. **9/6**)

The uterus reaches to the level of the umbilicus and the bulge is obvious, so pregnancy can hardly be concealed. But why conceal it, the expectant mother feels so well? What is more, she has probably felt the first small 'flutters' of her baby moving in the uterus.

The fetus is now clearly human in appearance, and has 'quickened'. It is about 25 cm (10 in) long, and weighs about 300 g (11 oz). Its skin is less transparent and is covered with a fine, downy hair (called lanugo), which covers its whole body. Some hair is appearing on its head; it has developed eyebrows, but its eyelids are still completely fused. It is very active in its weightless condition within the amniotic sac. Its internal organs are becoming more mature, but as yet its lungs are insufficiently developed to cope with life outside the uterus. It is a bit like an astronaut in space! It swims weightless in its heat-controlled capsule. Its food and oxygen are conveyed to it and its waste products excreted through its lifeline – the umbilical cord. The placenta and the mother act as its life-survival pack. From this stage of pregnancy onwards, the growth of the placenta slows down, whilst that of the fetus increases, so that by 40 weeks the placenta only weighs one-fifth the weight of the baby. However, its efficiency as an exchanger for oxygen, nutrients and waste products continues to increase up to the 40th week of pregnancy.

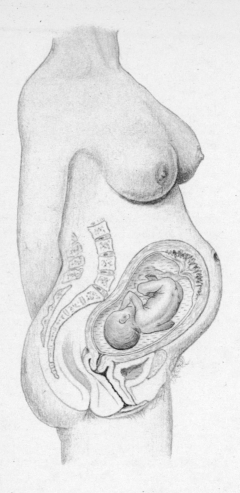

FIG. 9/7 Pregnancy at 24 weeks

24 weeks
(end of the
6th lunar
month)
(Fig. 9/7)

The expectant mother is now obviously pregnant! Her fetus measures 32 cm (13 in), and weighs 650 g (1 lb 7 oz). Its skin is now less red, and is covered with lanugo, and wrinkled because it lacks fat. From this month on, fat will be deposited in the skin. Its eyelids have separated, but a membrane covers the pupils, which are dull. The head is comparatively large. If the fetus is born at this stage, it will attempt to breathe, but its lungs are not properly developed so that it will have great difficulty in breathing. Its survival will depend on expert care.

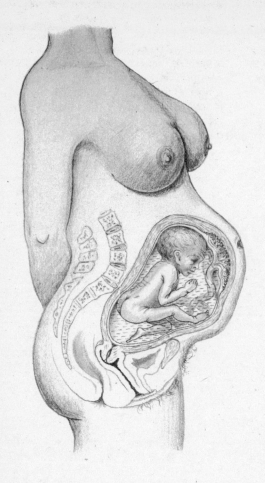

FIG. 9/8 Pregnancy at 28 weeks

28 weeks   The uterus now reaches 4 finger-breadths above
(end of the   the umbilicus.
7th lunar   The fetus moves around vigorously within the
month)   uterus, and its heart can be heard distinctly by
(Fig. **9/8**)   the doctor. Its length is 38 cm (15 in), and
its weight 1,000 g (2 lb 2 oz). Its body is thin; its skin
still reddish and covered with a protective coating of a
creamy, waxy substance, called vernix caseosa, which
is manufactured by small glands in the skin. It can
open its eyes, and the membrane covering the pupils
has gone. If born at this stage, it can now breathe (but
with difficulty), cry weakly, but move its legs
energetically. In the past most of these babies died,
but today more are being saved by treating them in
special neonatal intensive care units. In the best units,
one baby in every four now survives.

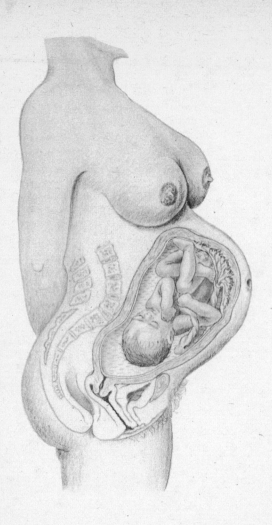

FIG. 9/9 **Pregnancy at 32 weeks**

32 weeks
(end of the
8th lunar
month)
(Fig. **9/9**)

The fetus is now 43 cm (17 in) long, and weighs about 1,800 g (4 lb). The skin is still reddened, rather wrinkled, but some fat is being deposited. The bones of its head are soft and flexible. Its lungs have developed and can now support life. If born at this stage, it has a good chance of surviving, provided it receives expert care.

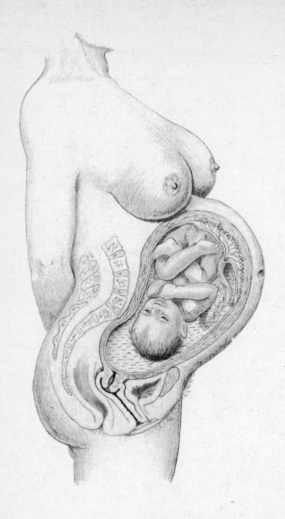

FIG. 9/10 Pregnancy at 36 weeks

36 weeks
(end of the
9th lunar
month)
(Fig. **9/10**)

The uterus now reaches up to the ribcage, and may cause some discomfort. The expectant mother throws her shoulders back to keep her balance.

The fetus measures 46 cm (18½ in), and weighs 2,500 g (5½ lb). It has put on a great deal of weight, 700 g (1½ lb) in the preceding four weeks. This is because fat has been deposited beneath its skin and around its shoulders. It has filled out; its body has become rotund, and its face has lost its wrinkled appearance. Its finger-nails reach to the end of its fingers.

If the baby is born at this time, it has over a 90 per cent chance of surviving.

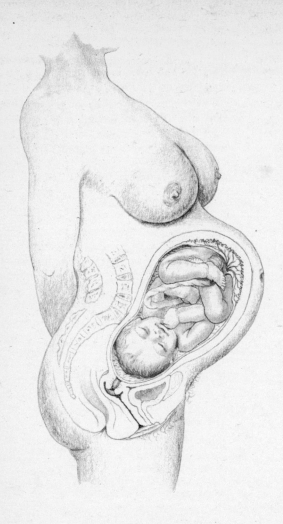

FIG. 9/11 Pregnancy at 40 weeks

40 weeks
(end of the
10th lunar
month)
(Fig. **9/11**)

The pregnancy is now at its full term. The expectant mother awaits the birth of her child with some degree of impatience.

The child is 50 cm (20 in) long, and weighs about 3,300 g (7 lb 4 oz), boys being about 100 g (3 oz) heavier than girls. There are very wide variations in the birth weight of the baby, and a normal, healthy, full-term child may weigh as little as 2,500 g (5½ lb) or as much as 4,500 g (10 lb). Occasionally the baby weighs even more. Its skin is smooth, and the lanugo which covered it has disappeared, except over the shoulders. The skin is still covered with the greasy vernix caseosa. Its head is covered with a variable amount of hair. The bones of the head are much firmer and are closer together, but the diamond-shaped soft area above the forehead and the Y-shaped area at the back of the head can still be felt. The head is now proportionate to the body, measuring about one-quarter of the body's length. The eyes are open, but usually a dull, slate colour – the permanent colour appears later. The ears stand out from the head, and the nose is well formed. The genitals are well formed, and if the infant is male, the testicles are in the scrotum.

CHANGES IN THE EXPECTANT MOTHER

Whilst the development of the embryo and fetus is progressing in the dark confines of the uterus, all the functions of the expectant mother's body are adjusting to the needs of pregnancy. The basis of all these changes is the effect of the sex hormones oestrogen and progesterone, which are manufactured by the cells of the placenta from its earliest days. The changes start very early in pregnancy, and most of them anticipate the demands that the fetus will make on its mother for oxygen, for food and to get rid of its wastes. In the early embryonic weeks, when the embryo's organs are forming at an incredible rate, the mother easily supplies the required oxygen and foods; in the later fetal weeks, when its growth is increasing even more, the fetus needs larger supplies of oxygen and nutrients for a longer period. The mother's body adjusts to these demands by quieting-down her own functions, so that nutrients (especially sugars) stay longer in her blood, and are more easily extracted by the placenta for the use of the fetus. Further energy is spared by the placidity which is common in a pregnant woman; her muscle tone is reduced, she does less, and because the energy is not burned-up, it is stored as fat deposited in her breasts, on her thighs and on her hips. But the slowing of her body functions has some disadvantages. Her gut is less active, so that her stomach empties more slowly and constipation is common; her kidneys receive a higher concentration of nutrients in her blood stream, and more are filtered out to be lost in the urine. This is part of the price she pays, but it is not difficult for her to compensate for this loss by eating a balanced diet.

The need for the placenta to receive a large quantity of blood, from which to extract the nutrients required by the baby, is met by a 40 per cent increase in the volume of the mother's blood, and by its more rapid circulation through her blood vessels. She manages to achieve this by increasing the amount of blood that the heart pumps out with each beat, and by increasing the rate at which the heart beats. This is why some women are conscious of the action of their heart in pregnancy, and complain of palpitations. More blood is pumped around the body more rapidly. The red blood takes up more oxygen in the lungs, and as nutrients are held longer in the blood stream, these and oxygen can be more readily given to the baby across the placenta.

As has been noted, this exchange takes place through the special cells which form the placenta, and the mother's blood and that of her

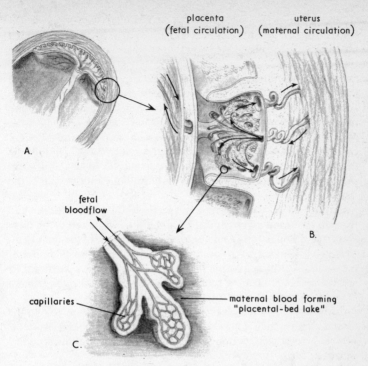

placenta
(fetal circulation)

uterus
(maternal circulation)

A.

fetal
bloodflow

B.

capillaries

maternal blood forming
"placental-bed lake"

C.

FIG. 9/12 A diagram showing (A) the placenta lying
attached to the wall of the uterus; (B) a section of the
placenta in detail; (C) how blood from the 'placental
lake' bathes the villus

baby are kept separate at all times. The blood of the fetus passes
through its body, then out along the vessels of the umbilical cord and
through the network of fine vessels (called capillaries) in the placenta, which you will remember is composed of cells of the outer part of
the fertilized egg (see page 146). The tiny vessels are covered by the
cells which make up the placenta. Although the placenta resembles a
soup-plate when seen after birth, under the microscope it is composed of hundreds of tiny finger-like projections (called villi), each
containing the network of tiny capillaries (Fig. 9/12) through which
the baby's blood flows. The surface area of these villi is enormous. It
has been calculated to be 11 square metres, or 12 square yards. The

villi hang into a lake of blood. The lake is filled with blood which comes from the mother's circulation, reaching it by passing through the blood vessels which supply her uterus. The lake lies deep within the uterus, and is in fact lined with tissues made by the placenta, rather as a swimming pool is separated from the garden by a concrete basin. Each time the mother's heart beats, her blood is pumped in spurts into the placental-bed lake, carrying with it the nutrients and oxygen. As it flows between and around the weed-like fronds of the placenta, the oxygen and nutrients are taken from it by the placental cells, and the waste products from the fetus are discharged into the mother's blood stream through the placental cells. In fact, as you can see, the placenta acts as a very efficient lung, kidney and bowel for the fetus.

Cleaned of its waste products and enriched with nutrients and oxygen, the blood in the capillaries of the villi is returned to the fetus along the umbilical vein, and enters its body again at the umbilicus. Meanwhile the mother's blood, with its extra load of waste products, is pumped out of the placental-bed lake and re-enters the mother's circulation to be cleaned by her kidneys, to take up more oxygen from her lungs and nutrients from her gut and liver.

In this way the fetus takes the first pick of what is available to the mother, and even in a famine when the mother is starving, the fetus will get a reasonable amount of food and will not be much under-weight at birth.

Other substances also pass across the placenta. For example, if the mother drinks alcohol, some of this crosses the placenta, but does not seem to do the baby any harm. Drugs cross the placenta, so that if the mother is given an antibiotic or an anaesthetic, some of this will appear in the fetus quite quickly. Perhaps more important are the antibodies which cross the placenta. If a person is infected by a germ, he forms substances in his body which attack and destroy the same germ if it infects him again. These substances are called 'antibodies'. Antibodies made by the mother cross the placenta all the time in the second half of pregnancy, so that when the baby is born it has a fair number of antibodies. These protect it against infections which lurk in the environment, until it starts to manufacture its own antibodies, which it does remarkably quickly.

The growth and development of the baby is an astonishing and prodigious event. From a single cell, containing in code all the information needed to make a new individual, growth occurs over a mere

266 days. At the end of this time, a new human being has formed, which is 8 million times heavier than the original fertilized cell. The cells have developed and differentiated to form special tissues and organs, all of which are co-ordinated and working, so that the child can breathe, digest food, move its muscles, hear sounds, taste flavours, react to stimuli, and develop further. A most wondrous growth!

Chapter 10

And Bears Healthy Children

It is only in this century that as much attention has been devoted by doctors to the care of the patient during the 40 weeks of pregnancy as was previously paid to the 14 hours of labour. This emphasis on antenatal care has resulted in a very considerable reduction in maternal deaths during childbirth, and a very considerable salvage of babies who might otherwise have died. Good antenatal care is so important that the World Health Organization has had two expert committees consider it. In one report the experts said that the object of antenatal care 'is to ensure that every expectant and nursing mother maintains good health, learns the art of child care, has a normal delivery, and bears healthy children'. In other words, good antenatal care is preventive medicine at its best. But the co-operation of every expectant mother and of her medical adviser is needed to achieve this high standard.

During the antenatal period, the fetus relies upon its mother for all functions, and the healthier the mother, the stronger and healthier will the infant be. Indeed, its health in the first years of life, and maybe even longer, is influenced considerably by the condition of the mother during the prenatal months.

For antenatal care to be effective, the patient must go to her doctor as early as possible in pregnancy, and be seen at regular and increasingly frequent intervals during pregnancy. A good doctor will not only examine the patient, but will provide time so that he may explain the changes occurring in her body, may answer her questions, and banish any anxieties she may have. The patient must always feel that she can ask her doctor about anything that is bothering her. She is not wasting his time, and it is part of the doctor's duty to try and help her, for her emotional condition is as important as her physical condition. Some of the problems about which she may worry are mentioned in this book; but conversation with her doctor is as important as reading, for points which are not properly understood can receive an explanation in conversation.

THE FIRST VISIT

The first visit to the doctor should be made at about the time of the second missed period. Whether the patient chooses a specialist, or a general practitioner (a personal physician, as he is more properly called) or a doctor in an antenatal clinic, is immaterial. What is important is that she has confidence in her doctor, and that he, for his part, is prepared to seek the opinion of a specialist should this be required. If the patient chooses her personal physician, he will already know a great deal about her general health, and many of the investigations mentioned in this chapter will not be required.

Many women dread the first visit, feeling embarrassed that they will be asked 'personal' questions and examined vaginally. Whilst the questions and examination are necessary, the patient need not be embarrassed, and the doctor will do everything to make the embarrassment as slight as possible. The patient can be reassured that the examination is quite painless.

The questions

The doctor first inquires about the date of the last menstrual period and the duration of the average menstrual cycle. This is measured, as has been mentioned, from the first day of the menstrual period (which is called day 1) to the first day of the next menstrual period. He will also need to know the duration of the menstrual period and whether the character of the bleeding has changed. From this information he can give the patient a prediction of the approximate date of her confinement. The patient can make the calculation herself in this way: to the date of the first day of the last menstrual period add 10 days (counting each month as having 30 days), subtract 3 months from the month in which the period occurred, and add one year. For example, a patient whose menstrual cycle is normal has started her last menstrual period on 12th September, 1977. When will the baby be expected?

Last menstrual period	12 / 9/77
Calculation	+10−3+1
Estimated date of delivery	22 / 6/78

The baby is due on 22nd June, 1978.

Another example: the patient's last menstrual period was 24th April, 1977. When is the baby due? Here the calculation is a bit more complicated, as the addition of 10 days brings the date into another month.

Last menstrual period	24 / 4/77
Add 10 days	+10
	= 4 / 5/77
Subtract 3 months,	
add 1 year	−3+1
Estimated date of delivery	4 / 2/78

The baby is due on 4th February, 1978.

The estimated date of delivery is accurate to within 14 days in over 80 per cent of women (four women in every five), and is a great help to the patient in planning for her confinement.

Having told the patient when her baby is expected to be born, the doctor asks how the pregnancy is progressing, and about any complaints the expectant mother may have. He then inquires about her past health, and lists the illnesses and operations which may have occurred. The purpose of these inquiries is to bring to light any conditions which may affect the course of the pregnancy, and for which treatment can be given. If there have been previous pregnancies (including abortions), the doctor should be told about these, and indeed he will inquire searchingly about them in detail. The purpose once again is to try to anticipate complications, and to find out how well (or badly) the patient was able to cope with her previous pregnancies.

The examination

The remainder of the visit is taken up with the examination. For this it is usual for the patient to strip completely and to put on a gown provided by the doctor. This is important, as the doctor tries to find out the general health of the patient. Usually he first notes her height and records her weight. Then he examines her breasts, and determines if the nipples are normal. If she proposes to breast-feed her baby, he may prescribe certain manipulations which are done by the patient herself during pregnancy. These manipulations encourage milk production and make the establishment of breast-feeding easier. He then listens to the patient's heart with a stethoscope, gently palpates her abdomen, and observes her legs to see if there are any varicose veins. In early pregnancy, the abdominal palpation is merely to check the tone of the abdominal muscles and to see whether there is any enlargement of the liver or spleen. After the 12th week of pregnancy, the doctor also palpates the enlarging uterus to determine if the baby is growing normally, and after the 28th week to check the position of the baby in the womb. After these examinations, and prior to the pelvic examination, the doctor takes the patient's blood pressure. It is left until this stage as emotions can often cause a rise in the blood pressure, and the doctor is trying to obtain a baseline blood pressure against which to measure changes. The estimation of the blood pressure is a most important investigation and is made at every visit, since a rise in blood pressure in pregnancy warns the doctor that 'toxaemia of pregnancy' may be starting. Its exact cause is not known, but it is known that the arteries which supply the uterus and the kidneys go into a spasm. If the spasm becomes severe, the blood supply to the placenta is reduced, and the baby may fail to grow properly, or may even die in the womb. The severity of the spasm can be reduced if 'toxaemia of pregnancy' is detected early. Appropriate treatment at this time will control the disease before it becomes a danger to the well-being of the baby.

Finally, the doctor performs a pelvic examination. It was noted in Chapter 8 that this examination is neither painful nor embarrassing if the patient co-operates. The doctor first introduces a speculum into the vagina to inspect the cervix and to take the cervical smear. He then gently performs a pelvic examination with two fingers introduced into the vagina.

Laboratory investigations

No first antenatal visit can be considered complete until the doctor has made certain laboratory tests. Just before the pelvic examination, the doctor will have asked his patient to empty her bladder of urine.

Many doctors ask for the urine to be passed in a special way. The patient is given a small moist cotton-wool swab with which she cleans the entrance to her vagina, wiping from the front backwards. She then starts to urinate, and when the flow of urine is running, she collects the 'midstream' specimen in a sterile container which has been given to her. This method is only necessary at the first visit. At all other visits, the patient either brings the urine specimen with her, or passes it into a container in the normal way. The purpose of the midstream specimen is to enable the doctor to find out if the patient has a hidden infection of the urinary tract. This hidden infection often becomes obvious in pregnancy, causing kidney infection, and many doctors believe in giving prophylactic treatment. The specimen of urine is also examined for the presence of protein and sugar. The presence of the former is another sign of impending 'toxaemia of pregnancy'. If sugar is found in the urine, investigations are made to find out if the patient has sugar diabetes.

Several important tests are made on a sample of blood taken from a vein in the arm. Patients tend to fear this procedure, but the discomfort is only momentary and the information obtained is very valuable. The blood is examined by a special test to determine if the patient has syphilis. This disease, which is spread by coitus, is increasing in incidence. It is important to detect the disease early in pregnancy when its cure is relatively easy. If left untreated, syphilis can damage the baby severely. In late pregnancy, the germs which cause syphilis pass through the placenta and multiply in the fetal tissues, either killing the fetus or damaging some of its organs. Those children who are the victims of congenital syphilis can be treated after birth, but treatment is not always successful. But if the disease is detected in early pregnancy and treated adequately, congenital syphilis will be prevented.

The specimen of blood is also examined to find out the mother's blood group, particularly whether she is Rhesus negative. Rhesus disease is considered in Chapter 16.

Finally, a sample of the blood taken, or else a further finger-prick specimen of blood, is examined to estimate the haemoglobin concentration. The haemoglobin concentration measures the amount of iron in the red blood cells, and so is an index of anaemia. It is important for the doctor to know if anaemia is present, as the expectant mother requires extra iron because the fetus also has to obtain a considerable amount of iron from the mother during pregnancy. If the haemoglobin concentration is low, the doctor will be able to treat it before it has any serious effects. Since the baby takes most of its iron requirements in late pregnancy, the haemoglobin estimation is repeated twice more during pregnancy, at the 32nd week, when the baby is beginning to increase its demand for iron, and again at the 36th week. Thus if the mother has become anaemic, she can be treated adequately before her confinement.

The summing-up

The examination and tests are over, the expectant mother has dressed again, has made-up her face, and now sits talking to her doctor so that he can discuss the diet she should eat, the exercise she should take, and can clear up any doubts she may have. She should not hestitate to ask her doctor about any matter which is bothering her. All too often, alas, women obtain misinformation about pregnancy from acquaintances, whose experiences invariably seem to have been gruesome. Just as after surgical operations, many women revel in exaggerating their experiences or, what is worse, misinterpreting the experiences they think that their friends have had. These women are all too ready to offer gratuitous information and advice to expectant mothers. Much of the information is erroneous, much of the advice harmful, so that the expectant mother is anxious, bewildered and confused. The person to clear up her confusion is the doctor. She should ignore the gossip of well-meaning busybodies, and should feel able to ask her doctor for accurate information at all times. He, for his part, should always be ready, and have time, to discuss the pregnancy with the expectant mother.

SUBSEQUENT VISITS

If she is otherwise normal, the expectant mother will make an antenatal visit to her doctor every 4 weeks until she is 28 weeks pregnant (7 lunar months), every 2 weeks from then until she is 36 weeks pregnant (9 lunar months), and every week from then until she has been confined. If any complication arises, or if the patient has previously had some illness, such as diabetes, 'blood pressure' or a heart condition, the doctor will want to see her more frequently.

At each of the visits during pregnancy, the doctor is concerned about two people – the expectant mother who is carrying the baby, and the fetus as it floats weightless in its heat-controlled, waste-disposal and food-intake controlled capsule (the amniotic sac) within the uterus. At each visit the doctor will seek to find out how the patient is progressing, and how she is enjoying her pregnancy. He will answer any queries, and if he detects that all is not progressing normally, will give advice. At each visit the expectant mother's weight is noted, and a weight gain of more than 4.5 kg (9 lb) in the first 20 weeks, or more than 0.5 kg (1 lb) a week in each of the last 20 weeks is usually frowned upon. Some doctors get most upset if the weight gain between visits exceeds these figures. The ankles and legs are examined for swelling and varicose veins, the blood pressure is recorded, and the urine tested.

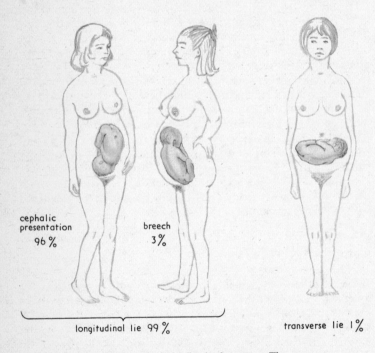

cephalic presentation 96 %

breech 3%

longitudinal lie 99 %

transverse lie 1%

FIG. 10/1 How the baby lies in the uterus. The percentages given for the different presentations are those found just before labour begins

The doctor then turns his attention to the baby. He estimates the height of the uterus, as was described previously, and he palpates it gently to find out the exact position of the baby. He will probably find that up to the 28th week (7th lunar month), the baby will be in a different position each time. It may be head down (called a cephalic presentation), or with its head in the upper part of the uterus and the buttocks in the lower part (a breech presentation), or it may be cross-ways (a transverse or shoulder presentation) (Fig. **10/1**). This is because at this early stage of pregnancy there is a relatively large volume of 'water' (really amniotic fluid, which does not have quite the same composition as water) in the amniotic sac, and the baby can therefore move about easily. After the 30th week of pregnancy, the great majority of babies settle with their head over the mother's pelvis, and their buttocks in the wider upper part of the uterus. By the 40th week, also called 'term', 96 per cent of babies lie in this position, as cephalic presentations, and between 3 and 4 per cent lie as breech presentations. In some cases the back of the baby is on the right side of the uterus, and in others on the left. It makes little difference to the progress of labour, and the baby can change positions between two examinations. The gentle palpation of the uterus distinguishes these points, and enables the doctor to determine whether the baby is lying as a cephalic or a breech presentation (Fig. **10/2**). This is of some

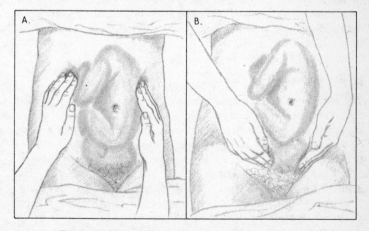

FIG. 10/2 How the doctor finds the position of the baby.
(A) Feeling the back; (B) Detecting the baby's head

importance at about the 34th week, as the doctor may wish to try to 'turn' the breech baby into a cephalic presentation with head down. At every visit the doctor should tell the expectant mother where the baby is, and should help her to feel it if she wishes. If he listens to the baby's heart, and she wishes to hear her baby's heart beat, he should try to arrange for her to do this using his stethoscope. The baby's heart beats much faster than the mother's, averaging 120 beats a minute, but varying a bit.

Lightening

By the end of the 36th week, most women carrying their first baby (primigravidae) feel 'lightening'. This is because the baby's head 'drops' into the pelvic cavity; consequently the upper part of the uterus drops, relieving the pressure under the ribs and making breathing easier. Lightening often occurs suddenly, the expectant mother waking up one morning relieved of the pressure and discomfort she has experienced previously. Unfortunately, the descent of the head into the pelvic cavity is often associated with pressure on the pelvis, and an increased vaginal discharge, so that she exchanges one set of mild complaints for another. At this time, too, the painless uterine contractions which have been felt for some weeks become more frequent.

In women who have had previous children, 'lightening' takes place later, either in the week or 10 days before labour starts or in the early stages of labour.

Pelvic examination

The descent of the fetal head into the pelvic cavity is a good indication that the pelvic size and shape are normal. The doctor uses this information to be sure that this is so. It is usual for him to make a pelvic examination at the 37th week. At this examination, he assesses the size of the pelvis, the relationship of the fetal head to the pelvic brim, and the softness and degree of opening of the cervix. The examination is delayed until this stage of pregnancy for two reasons: firstly, the fetal head has usually descended into the pelvis (doctors call this 'engagement' of the fetal head); and secondly, the pelvic tissues at this time are soft and stretch easily, so that the examination is painless. Just as she did during the pelvic examination at the first antenatal visit, the patient must relax her muscles completely in order for the doctor to obtain the maximum information.

The last weeks of pregnancy

The antenatal visits are made at weekly intervals; the patient has learned what signs show that labour has started; she is confident about her doctor; she is fit and well; she has a knowledge of what happens in labour; she has prepared the baby's clothes; she has visited the hospital; and the doctor has answered all her questions. In short, she is a healthy, knowledgeable mother, who has learned the art of child care, who knows the sequence of events she may expect in labour, and she is about to have a normal delivery and bear a healthy child.

Chapter 11

An ABC of Hygiene in Pregnancy

The conditions discussed in this chapter are all 'minor', that is they are minor in that they do not cause serious disease. To the expectant mother they may be major problems. Since so many body systems may be involved, it seems appropriate to list the conditions alphabetically for more ready reference.

Pregnancy and adjustment to parenthood are periods of emotional stress for all women, although the amount of stress varies very considerably. Some women find pregnancy a joyous period of their life, others become emotionally distressed. Still others are concerned about the mood changes they experience. Stresses which would be coped with easily when the woman is not pregnant may become distressing during pregnancy and an expectant mother may over-react emotionally to a real or imagined insult. Other women, who are usually mentally active, find that during pregnancy they become mentally lethargic and thinking is an effort.

In the early weeks of pregnancy most women identify with the tiny fetus; they talk about 'my' pregnancy rather than 'the' pregnancy or 'it'. This is because the fetus is perceived as part of the woman's body, and has no separate identity. Between the 15th and 20th week of pregnancy, a change occurs. The fetus begins to move, and to develop an identity of its own. The woman's enlarging abdomen tells her, and her friends, that she is really pregnant and she now begins to be interested in the fetus as 'her baby'. In late pregnancy, from about the 35th week, a further change occurs. Now most women become impatient with the pregnancy, bored with their swollen abdomen, anxious to give birth and to see, touch and care for the newborn baby.

As pregnancy advances, with its attendant minor discomforts, many women are concerned that their increased fatness, lethargy, distended abdomen and pendulous breasts may adversely affect their husband's love. The way a man can reassure his partner is to kiss and cuddle her and to be interested (as he should be) in the continuing pregnancy and the growth, in the mother's uterus, of their baby. After all, the start of pregnancy was a joint pleasure; its continuation should be shared too!

ALCOHOL

There is no reason why the expectant mother should not drink alcohol in moderate amounts if she so wishes. It has not been found to affect the course of pregnancy adversely, and indeed there is some evidence that alcohol prevents premature labour. However, this is not a reason for recommending alcohol for other than moderate social drinking.

BACKACHE

In late pregnancy particularly, the pelvic joints and ligaments relax. At the same time the growing weight of the uterus changes the centre of balance, so that the expectant mother has to stand with her shoulders further back than normal. This position has been called 'the pride of pregnancy'. However, it and the relaxed ligaments produce backache to some extent in most pregnant women, but more so in multigravidae (pregnant women who have previously had one or more pregnancies). The backache increases during the day and is felt most towards evening, and at night when it may prevent sleep. The pain is usually felt low in the back or over the sacro-iliac joint. Treatment is largely to prevent the condition from becoming severe. If the expectant mother's posture is bad, she should seek advice. High heels tend to aggravate the strain on the back, and should be avoided except when going out. 'Flatties' are fine in the house. If the backache is marked, analgesics may be needed, but the doctor should be consulted first.

BATHING

Showers are recommended in preference to long baths, or tub baths, as the Americans call them, in the last four weeks of pregnancy, when the bath water may conceivably enter the vagina. Before this time long baths are perfectly safe and pleasantly relaxing! Swimming in general is permissible, and may be continued as near term as the expectant mother wishes.

BREASTS

Care of the breasts in pregnancy helps the establishment of breast-feeding. The nipples should be stroked and drawn out gently for about two minutes a day from early pregnancy. If the expectant mother wishes, she may rub in some bland lanolin ointment, particularly if the nipples are dry. From about the 32nd week (8th lunar month), the breasts should be 'expressed' by placing both hands with the palms widely spread around them, and pressing towards the nipples. It will be found that a yellow secretion appears. This manipulation is thought to keep the ducts of the breasts open (Fig. 11/1).

CLOTHING

What should a pregnant woman wear? She should wear the clothes in which she is her most attractive, but which are comfortable at the same time. She will need a larger sized, well-fitting brassière because of the enlargement of her breasts due to pregnancy, and may wish to wear a maternity girdle, but expensive, complicated pregnancy 'foundation' garments are quite unnecessary. An ordinary elastic maternity girdle is all that is needed, and even this is not essential if the expectant mother feels comfortable without one. She should avoid constricting garters or elastic-topped stockings, as these may interfere with the return of blood from the legs in pregnancy, so increasing the risk of varicose veins, but a panty-girdle or pantyhose is quite suitable. When at home or working, she should wear low-heeled shoes, but if she goes out to some special event, she can wear normal high-heeled shoes. The pregnant woman should aim to look as attractive as possible, and not be a frump!

CONSTIPATION

You have two kinds of muscle in your body – the voluntary striped

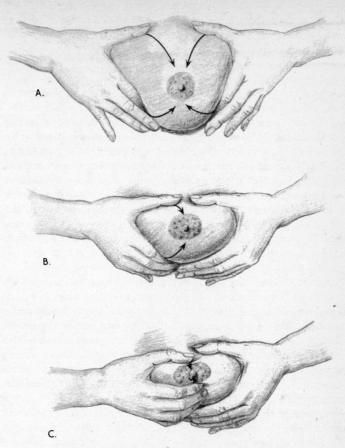

FIG. 11/1 The care of the breasts in pregnancy
A. How the hands are placed at the start of expression,
to enclose the breast at its margin
B. The hands move inwards towards the areola, firm
pressure is exerted on the whole breast. The movement
is repeated about 5 to 10 times
C. The breast is fixed by one hand and the milk ducts are
compressed with the other hand, the thumb above and
the fingers below. The pressure empties the milk ducts.
At the end of the expression, the nipple is drawn out with
the fingers

muscles, and the involuntary smooth muscles. The striped muscles make up the muscles of your arms and legs, and respond to your control. If you want to pick up a saucepan, a message goes from your brain and your arm muscles move your hand forward. If you find the saucepan is too hot, you voluntarily stop the movement! The smooth muscles make up the muscles of your heart, your gut, and your womb. These muscles work without voluntary control, and you cannot voluntarily alter their action. However, they do respond to some drugs and hormones. Progesterone, the special hormone of pregnancy, relaxes smooth muscle. In one way this is useful, as it enables the uterus, which is mainly composed of smooth muscle, to grow without attempting to expel the fetus prematurely. In other ways smooth muscle relaxation can be annoying. The muscle tone of the gut is lowered throughout pregnancy, which leads to constipation. In late pregnancy, the tendency is aggravated by pressure on the lower bowel by the enlarged uterus. If the expectant mother is worried about constipation, she should increase her fluid intake, and re-establish the 'habit' by attempting to open her bowels regularly just after a meal. Many doctors now recommend that women who are constipated eat about two tablespoonsful of coarse bran daily and choose wholemeal bread instead of white bread. These two measures have the effect of making the stool bulkier and reduce the time it takes for food to pass from the mouth to the time the residue is passed out as stools. Both these changes reduce constipation and eliminate the need for drugs. But if a woman does not want to eat bran and the other suggestions I have made fail, her doctor will give her 'Senokot' (standardised senna) or the contact stool-softening laxative, bisacodyl. She should avoid self-medication with strong laxatives, or oily laxatives.

DENTAL CARE

Care of the teeth does not differ in pregnancy from that at other times. The old notion that each child cost a tooth is a relic from the time when regular visits to the dentist were not made. Unfortunately, particularly in Australia, this still applies. In areas where fluoride is not added to the drinking-water, the use of one tablet per day containing 1 mg fluorine taken from the 20th week of pregnancy will protect the infant against dental caries. A few women develop swelling of the gums at the base of the teeth (marginal gingivitis, as it is called). This is not abnormal, and disappears after childbirth, but if in any doubt the expectant mother should consult a dentist.

DIET

More rubbish has been written about diet in pregnancy than on almost any other medical subject. In the years before World War II, the influence of diet on the growth and survival of the baby was thought to be considerable. Recent studies have cast doubt on this, and present opinion is that within the normal range of diets available, their influence on the birth weight and survival of the baby is minimal. As far as the obstetrical efficiency of the expectant mother is concerned, the diet she ate in her own infancy and childhood has much more importance. This is the reason the World Health Organization's Expert Committee on Maternity Care said that one of the objectives of antenatal care was to help the expectant mother 'learn the art of child care'. This includes giving her child a properly balanced diet, rich in protein.

By and large then, the effect of diet on the outcome of pregnancy has been exaggerated in the past. Fanciful, vague, complicated diets have been ordered which had little value and were often confusing. I do not suggest that a pregnant woman should not pay attention to what she eats. She should! In pregnancy she has to provide the nutrients necessary for the growth of her child, as well as for her own needs. This does not mean that she needs to 'eat for two', and as will be seen later, *excessive weight gained in pregnancy is very hard to take off*. It does mean that she should understand what she is eating and why.

Basically the diet provides *carbohydrates and fat*, which produce the energy needed for life; *protein*, needed for the formation of new tissues; *vitamins and minerals*, which help in the complex chemical processes in the body. All foodstuffs contain one or more of the above nutrients. Unfortunately, the cheaper foodstuffs are the energy-supplying carbohydrates, whilst the tissue-building protein, the vitamins and some of the minerals come from relatively expensive foods, like meat. Because of this, poorer people, and most of the people in the developing countries, eat too little protein, vitamins and minerals, and barely enough carbohydrate to provide the energy

needed for their daily tasks. This energy is measured in a unit called a
calorie, and the average pregnant woman needs about 2,500 calories
a day. In the affluent lands, most women eat too much, particularly
carbohydrates such as bread, cakes, sweets and sugar, but often eat
only just enough protein. Their calorie intake is excessive for their
needs, and the excess is stored in the body as fat.

Pregnancy puts an increased demand for protein, and unless the
expectant mother alters to a diet which provides more protein, she
may not get sufficient, whilst still eating too much carbohydrate.

The nutritional needs of a pregnant woman have been considered
in great detail by high-powered committees in many countries, and
the optimal, or best, daily allowance for a woman weighing about
55 kg (121 lb) has been worked out to be:

Calories	2500
Protein	65 g
Calcium	1000 mg
Iron	15 mg
Vitamin A	6000 u
Vitamin D	400 u
Vitamin B:	
Thiamine	1.0 mg
Riboflavine	1.5 mg
Nicotinic Acid	15.0 mg
Vitamin C (Ascorbic acid)	50.0 mg
Folic acid	0.3 mg

To the average expectant mother, the above table is so much
jargon, but it can easily be translated into foodstuffs. This is shown
in Table 11/1, and is summarized here: (1) *Dairy products:* The
expectant mother should drink 500 to 750 ml (1 to 1½ pints) of milk
a day, either raw or made up in drinks or used in cooking. If she
wants, she can substitute cheese for milk, 30 g (1 oz) being equivalent
to 250 ml (½ pint). (2) *Meat and eggs:* She should eat 60 to 120 g (2
to 4 oz) of meat, fish or poultry a day, and usually have an egg. (3)
Vegetables: She should eat green leafy vegetables, cooked for less
than 10 minutes in a minimum of water, at least three times a week,
and other vegetables as she wishes. (4) *Bread, cereals, sugar, sweets,
potatoes:* These provide the energy, but in excess these are the ones
which put on the weight. Some carbohydrate is needed, but as the

expectant mother has to pay attention to her weight, she should eat these sparingly. (5) *Fruits:* She should eat an orange or a grapefruit each day, and any additional fresh fruit she fancies.

Table 11/1
Nutritional Needs in Pregnancy

Food		Calories	Protein (g)
Dairy products	A daily total of 600–900 ml (1 to 1½ pints) of milk, either raw or used in cooking or in hot drinks. Cheese can be substituted, 30 g (1 oz) being equal to 300 ml (½ pint) of milk. Butter or margarine can be taken as required (say 60 g, or 2 oz).	600 480	32 –
Meat products	The meat product may be *lean* meat, poultry, fish or liver. A serving of 60–120 g (2–4 oz) a day will provide for the needs. More meat may, of course, be eaten if desired. It is best grilled, roasted or stewed, rather than fried.	250	20
Egg	One a day (or at least most days).	90	6
Bread and other cereals (including sugar as required)	Three to four slices, which is equal to 120 g (4 oz) is probably sufficient. A half-full teacup of breakfast cereal equals one slice of bread. Wholemeal bread is preferable to white flour bread. Sugar or jam, say 60 g or 2 oz.	320 240	10 –

Vegetables	*Potato:* One to two medium-sized potatoes (150–300 g, or 5–10 oz). The potato can be cooked in any way, but the most nutritious are those cooked in their skin. If desired, potatoes can be replaced by squash, pumpkin or turnips. In working out a diet, the bread and potato are changeable.	140	5
	Vegetables: Salads and other green or yellow leafy vegetables, peas, beans and lentils contain valuable vitamins if they are cooked properly. About 60–120 g (2–4 oz) should be eaten daily.	50	3
Fruit	The old adage 'an apple a day keeps the doctor away' applies in pregnancy. For variety, the apple can be replaced by citrus fruits (orange, grapefruit) or by tomato juice, which are all rich in Vitamin C.	·50	1
		——	—
		2260	77

How she divides up the foodstuffs, having what at which meal, must be her decision. How well, or badly, she cooks the food is the result of her upbringing. How efficiently she chooses and buys the proper foods is the result of her education. If a mother wishes her child to be a good housekeeper, she will have the opportunity over the years to teach her, and this teaching will be reinforced in the schools. To start the lessons, the expectant mother can remember most of what is needed about diet and nutrition in pregnancy if she recalls the following slogan: 'Buy all you can afford from the butcher, the greengrocer and at the dairy; spend only little at the confectioner, the grocer and the chemist'.

DOUCHING

Vaginal douching is a peculiarly American habit, founded on an exaggerated need for so-called 'personal hygiene'. The vagina is self-cleansing. Douches are usually unnecessary at any time, and particularly in pregnancy, when they have a slight danger. So do not douche!

DRUGS IN PREGNANCY

After the 'thalidomide' tragedy, doctors have been even more careful in prescribing drugs to pregnant women. It will be remembered that thalidomide was given in early pregnancy as a sedative or to alleviate nausea. Later it was found that it had prevented the development of the arm and leg buds of the fetus, so that the affected babies were born alive but without arms or legs.

No new drugs are now prescribed for pregnant women unless they have been investigated by the most exhaustive tests, and most doctors only give expectant mothers drugs which they *really* need. The mother herself, particularly in the first 12 weeks of pregnancy, should avoid taking any drug unless she has checked with her doctor, and then only if it is really required.

Today, the expectant mother can rest assured that none of the drugs commonly prescribed during pregnancy has any damaging action on her growing baby.

EMPLOYMENT

Provided that the expectant mother enjoys her work and that it does not subject her to too great a physical strain, the job may be continued throughout pregnancy. In many countries legislation has been enacted which gives paid maternity leave for the last 6 to 8 weeks of pregnancy. After delivery it is usual to be given paid leave from work for 4 to 6 weeks, so that the baby may be cared for, and the mother may adjust to her new duties.

EXERCISE

Pregnancy is a normal event and should be treated as such. Exercise should be encouraged if this is the usual habit of the patient, but if the expectant mother normally takes no exercise beyond housework, she need not change her habits. The average woman takes a reasonable amount of exercise, and can continue to take it in pregnancy. If she enjoys swimming, she may swim. If she plays tennis or golf, she may continue until the enlarging uterus prevents accurately placed strokes! If she enjoys walking or gardening, then she should continue to walk or garden. In general, she need not alter the pattern of exercise to which she is accustomed, just because she is pregnant.

FAINTING

Fainting attacks, palpitations and headaches occasionally occur in pregnancy, and are due to the alterations in the expectant mother's circulatory system produced by the pregnancy. Although annoying, they have no sinister significance, and in Victorian days a faint was the way the modest wife announced to her husband that 'a little stranger was on the way'!

FREQUENCY OF URINATION

Irritability of the bladder is quite common in early pregnancy, and occurs again in the last weeks when the baby's head presses into the pelvis. Nothing much can be done about it, except to pass urine more often. If urination is associated with pain and scalding, the expectant mother should consult her doctor.

HAEMORRHOIDS

Haemorrhoids, or piles, are not infrequently found in pregnancy. They are more common in multigravidae, and seem to occur in families. The usual complaints are of bleeding during a bowel motion, the presence of a tender lump noticed during the use of toilet paper, or pain. Constipation and straining to empty the bowels aggravate these complaints. The expectant mother can reduce the discomfort of haemorrhoids by avoiding constipation, and making sure that the stool is never hard. Her doctor will be able to prescribe ointments which relieve the pain and reduce the swelling of prolapsed piles.

HEARTBURN

Heartburn is an annoying and fairly common complaint, which is more frequent in late pregnancy. It is due to the passage of small amounts of stomach contents into the lower part of the food tube (or oesophagus), which leads from the mouth to the stomach. In pregnancy this occurs because the valve guarding the entrance to the stomach relaxes, and because the enlarging uterus pushes up against the stomach. It is often worse at night, when the burning sensation in the upper abdomen can be quite distressing. Despite its name, it can be seen that heartburn has nothing to do with the heart. The expectant mother can relieve heartburn by eating small meals more frequently, and by taking a glass of milk to bed with her, and sipping this if heartburn occurs. She would also be wise to sleep propped up on one or two extra pillows. If heartburn persists, her doctor will prescribe one of the many antacid tablets or liquids. The more modern ones, based on aluminium or magnesium, are preferable to those containing sodium (salt), such as sodium bicarbonate, as this increases the patient's intake of salt, which may not be advisable.

IMMUNIZATION

Apart from immunization or vaccination against smallpox, which should be avoided in the first half of pregnancy, immunization programmes can be carried out as required. Indeed, because of the apparently increased risk of poliomyelitis to pregnant women, the expectant mother should be immunized against this disease if she has not previously taken her Sabin vaccine. Since the vaccine is given by mouth, it is quite painless and devoid of side-effects. There is a belief, too, that pregnant women are more susceptible to chest complications of influenza, and many doctors recommend that pregnant women should receive anti-influenza injections if an epidemic is expected. I am doubtful of the truth of this, as so many strains of the influenza virus exist, that the injection may only protect the patient, if it does, against one. Moreover, the injections are painful. In case of doubt, the patient should consult her own doctor. It is possible that a safe, painless, effective anti-influenzal vaccine may be developed soon which can be sprayed into the nose. If this happens, the views I have expressed can be ignored.

LEG CRAMPS

Some expectant mothers develop leg cramps in late pregnancy. These occur mostly at night, and the cause is not known. Treatment is not very satisfactory, and there is some evidence that excessive milk intake may be the cause. This is why the total milk intake recommended was 750 ml (1½ pints). If the patient has leg cramps, a drink of milk from the allowance may help. However, the evidence that excessive milk is the cause of leg cramps is not very secure, as leg cramps occur in Asian women who do not habitually drink milk. Recently a doctor has suggested that the cramps will be less if the foot of the bed is raised 25 cm (10 inches).

MATERNAL PRENATAL INFLUENCES

A considerable literature has grown up about how maternal influences can affect the baby. This obstetric superstition has been propagated from antiquity, and sought to explain the birth of deformed or blemished infants. This tribal myth has been used by playwrights and novelists to tell dramatic stories, and is still widely believed. It has, of course, no substance. There is no evidence that maternal impressions can affect the baby in any way. The reasons are many: first, there is no nervous connection between the mother and her baby; second, the blood of the mother is quite separate from that of the baby; and third, the infant is completely formed by the 8th week of pregnancy, so that for the impression to have any effect it must occur before this time. In most cases, the 'shocking experience' which the mother 'knows' is the cause of her baby's birth defect occurred much later. The truth is that maternal impressions have no effect on the growth or development of the baby. The baby will not become a famous television actor if the expectant mother spends hours watching television. The infant will not be exceptionally gifted musically if the mother persistently listens to, or plays, music during pregnancy; nor will he be a famous sportsman if her husband insists that she watches all the ball games she can over the 40 weeks of pregnancy; nor will the sight of a one-eyed black cat crossing the road mean that her baby will be born one-eyed and black!

It is true that a few babies are born with congenital defects, but the number with a defect is less than three in every hundred. This means that 97 of every 100 babies born are perfectly formed, and of the three which have defects, most can be treated. But it is not true that the defects are due to prenatal influences. They are usually due to an inherited defect in one of the genes which make up the new individual. Occasionally, however, they are due to infection by the rubella virus occurring during pregnancy. This is the virus which causes German measles, and the problem is discussed further on page 264.

NAUSEA

About 50 per cent of pregnant women experience some degree of nausea, and a few vomit. This complaint occurs in the first 12 weeks of pregnancy, disappearing at the end of this time, but sometimes recurring in late pregnancy. The cause is almost certainly a sensitivity to the hormones of pregnancy, but the condition may be exaggerated if the expectant mother is over-anxious or emotionally stressed. Most often the nausea occurs in the morning, hence the name 'morning sickness', but it may occur at any time of the day. Nausea in the morning is more common than at other times of the day, because the stomach contains the overnight accumulation of gastric juices.

Most women are able to overcome the nausea by simple means. The constitution of the diet should be adjusted to exclude greasy, fatty foods, and fried foods should be avoided. Small carbohydrate-rich meals are taken at more frequent intervals, the first being brought to the wife by her husband as soon as possible after waking. This may consist of toast or biscuits, and tea. After this, small meals are eaten every 3 hours until bedtime. Some women find it better to avoid drinking at meals and to take the fluids, either as sweetened fruit drinks, weak tea or milk and soda-water, at other times.

An example of a suitable diet for the day is:

On waking   A slice of toast or two Cream Cracker biscuits, with a
             drink of weak tea.
8.00 a.m.   Light breakfast of cereal, or toast with honey or jam,
             and perhaps weak tea. If the expectant mother feels she
             can eat more, she adjusts the diet to her own needs.
10.00 a.m.   Toast with a glass of milk, tea or a fruit drink.
12.30 p.m.   Lunch. Soup with toast or Cream Crackers; rice or
             noodles with lightly boiled vegetables.
3.30 p.m.   Tea. Toast, jam, fruit juice, and perhaps plain cake.
6.30 p.m.   Dinner. Lean meat or chicken, green vegetables,
             potatoes, salad and rice pudding.
9.30 p.m.   A drink of tea, cocoa, warm milk, or milk and soda.
To bed   A drink and Cream Crackers to take if the expectant
             mother wakes up during the night.

This is only an example, and a great number of variations can be
chosen by the individual herself. If the nausea is troublesome, the
expectant mother should consult her doctor. Although many and
varied drugs have been prescribed in the past, doctors today are very
wary of new drugs in early pregnancy. However, two kinds of drugs
are safe and fairly effective; one is a barbiturate derivative, and the
other an antihistamine.

NOSE BLEEDS

Slight bleeding from the nose is not unusual in pregnancy. It is due to
the increased blood supply which occurs, and in most cases needs no
treatment. It does not mean that the expectant mother has a high
blood pressure.

PICA

For some reason, which the psychiatrists try to explain, bizarre
cravings for strange foods may occur in pregnancy. Unfortunately,
each group of psychiatrists has a different explanation, so the *fact* of
bizarre cravings remains, but the *reason* remains unknown. If the
craving is for substances other than foodstuffs, the craving is called
'pica'. The word comes from the Latin term for 'magpie', a bird which

collects strange articles. Severe craving is not very common, and true pica is rather rare. Most women who do have cravings want carbohydrates, either sweets or laundry starch, or large amounts of fruit. A few have cravings for more exotic things, such as pickles, caviare or avocados. The very few who have true pica may urgently crave to eat coal, clay or pencils. If the expectant mother develops strange cravings for foods in pregnancy, she must realize that she is not going mad, but that the cravings exist and need to be controlled.

PLACIDITY

To the annoyance of the intellectually alert expectant mother, she notes an increasing placidity and drowsiness as pregnancy advances. She no longer has the clarity of mind and precision of thought she had before pregnancy. Even small intellectual matters become a trial; to do anything is an effort and she fears she is becoming bovine. The cause is the increased circulation of the pregnancy hormone progesterone, and she can be reassured that the placidity will pass once the baby is born. Meanwhile, she will have to look inwards into the warmth of her womb, rather than attempting to equal Einstein!

SEX IN PREGNANCY

If the expectant mother's pregnancy is normal and she has no tendency to premature labour or repeated abortions, sexual intercourse may continue at a frequency which is normal for that couple. Some women find that they desire more frequent coitus in pregnancy; others find they are less stimulated. Coitus should be gentle, at all times, and in the second half of pregnancy the wife may find that penile entry from the rear, the wife lying in front of her husband, is more comfortable and satisfying. Alternatively, sexual desire may be satisfied by non-coital methods. The man may help his partner reach orgasm by manipulating her clitoral area with his fingers or by caressing it with his tongue (cunnilingus). These varieties of sexual techniques are both enjoyable and safe, except that, a man should never blow into a pregnant woman's vagina during cunnilingus. This is because air may enter a blood vessel causing a fatal air embolism.

Sexual activity, including coitus, can continue throughout pregnancy, right up to the time of confinement and can resume after childbirth as soon as the woman wishes and finds it enjoyable. There is no truth in the myth that sexual activity, including orgasm, in normal pregnant women can produce premature labour or abortion, nor will it lead to infection of the fetus if continued up to the expected time of delivery.

SHORTNESS OF BREATH

In late pregnancy a number of expectant mothers find that even moderate exertion causes shortness of breath. Provided their doctor has checked that their heart and lungs are normal, the shortness of breath, although inconvenient, is without danger.

SMOKING

The influence of cigarette smoking on pregnancy has been studied in the last few years. The evidence at present is that cigarette smoking, particularly if more than 10 cigarettes are smoked per day, has an adverse effect on pregnancy. There seems to be an increased risk that abortion will occur, and the birth weight of the baby is likely to be less than that of a baby born to a woman who does not smoke. Expectant mothers should avoid excessive smoking during pregnancy, although as far as the baby is concerned, fewer than 5 cigarettes a day can be smoked without any harm. However, smoking is a probable cause of lung cancer, and pregnancy might be a good time to stop smoking altogether.

SWEATING

In late pregnancy, many expectant mothers find that they sweat more easily and in hot, humid weather 'feel the heat intolerably'. Sometimes night sweats occur, the expectant mother waking up in a 'lather of sweat'. The excessive sweating is due to dilated blood vessels in the skin, which in turn dilate because of pregnancy. No specific treatment is available, and all that the expectant mother can do is to avoid excessive exertion, to take frequent rest periods, and have frequent cool showers. Because of the increased fluid lost by sweating, the expectant mother should increase her fluid intake.

SWELLING OF THE ANKLES AND LEGS (OEDEMA)

Retention of fluid in the tissues of the body is normal in pregnancy. The average expectant mother retains between 3 and 6 litres (6½ to 13 pints) of fluid, half of it in the last 10 weeks of pregnancy. Swelling of the ankles, the lowest part of the body, is therefore common. If it occurs in the evening, it is not serious, and all that the expectant mother needs to do is keep her feet up. Women who are overweight for their height by the 20th week of pregnancy, and overweight women who gain more than 0.5 kg (1.1 lb) per week after the 30th week, have almost a 50 per cent chance of developing evening oedema. In general this is unimportant, but if these women, and all others, develop swelling of the legs earlier in the day, it is a warning sign that 'toxaemia of pregnancy' may be developing, and the mother-to-be should hasten to see her doctor.

TRAVEL

Apart from the restriction by airlines on carrying women more than 32 weeks pregnant who have no certificate of fitness from their doctor, an expectant mother can travel wherever she likes during pregnancy. She may safely travel by aeroplane, by ship or by car – or at least as safely as other motorists will let her! The only problem may be that she may go into labour at her destination, and will have to find a new obstetrician.

URINARY TRACT INFECTION

About 5 per cent of women have a hidden infection of the urinary tract, which causes them no trouble until they become pregnant. In pregnancy, owing to the muscle-relaxing effects of progesterone, the collecting area in the kidney and the tube which connects the kidney to the bladder becomes larger. Urine tends to stagnate in these areas, and in the bladder. Women who have hidden urinary tract infection (called 'bacteriuria'), unless treated, have twice the chance of developing anaemia, a raised blood pressure, and of delivering a 'premature baby'. It is usual for doctors to examine the urine in early pregnancy for the presence of bacteriuria, and if this is found, to give treatment. This treatment will also prevent the onset of kidney infection, or pyelonephritis. The collecting area of the kidney is called the renal pelvis, or *pyelos* (a Greek word meaning a trough). If the urine becomes infected, the kidney pyelos and the kidney tissue itself may become inflamed – which is why this type of kidney infection is called pyelonephritis.

The symptoms of pyelonephritis are pain in the loins, fever and shivering, sweating, and painful urination. Should these symptoms occur in pregnancy, the expectant mother should call her doctor without delay, as treatment using sulfa drugs or antibiotics is very successful.

VAGINAL DISCHARGE

During pregnancy the normal secretions which keep the vagina moist are increased, and additional secretions derived from the glands of the cervix add to the quantity. About 30 per cent of expectant mothers are conscious of the increased vaginal discharge. If the quantity necessitates the wearing of a pad, the mother-to-be should consult her doctor, so that investigations may be undertaken to determine if the discharge is merely an exaggeration of the normal; if it is due to infection by the fungus, *Candida albicans*, which causes thrush; or if it is due to infection by a small parasite, the size of the point of a pin, called *Trichomonas vaginalis*. Usually infection with either of these causes an irritating vaginal discharge, but occasionally it does not. The doctor can only determine the actual cause of the vaginal discharge by examining a smear taken from the vagina with a cotton-wool swab. He looks at this under a microscope, and is then able to prescribe the appropriate treatment.

VARICOSE VEINS

Pregnancy provokes the appearance of varicose veins in the legs of women who are predisposed to them. The veins may appear at any time during pregnancy, but on the whole tend to enlarge and become more obvious in the later months. They may appear either as enlarged, worm-like tubes beneath the skin, or as spider varicosities around the ankles and behind the knees. The legs feel heavy, look ugly and may be painful or swollen. Most of the veins disappear once the baby is born, which is why doctors do not recommend surgical treatment in pregnancy. Some remain, however, to enlarge in subsequent pregnancies. Treatment is to keep the feet up as much as possible, and certainly to sit with the feet down as little as possible. As well as this, well-fitting supportive stockings, which are today indistinguishable from normal nylon stockings, should be put on each morning before the expectant mother puts her feet out of bed.

VITAMIN AND MINERAL SUPPLEMENTS

It is the habit of doctors, encouraged by the beautiful advertisements which appear in medical journals, to insist that all pregnant women receive tablets of vitamin and mineral 'supplements'. This habit is approved by convention, and the majority of women (at least in the U.S.A.) would feel that their doctor was being rather incompetent if he failed to prescribe a 'pregnancy pill'. The pregnant dietary supplementary pills often contain a multitude of minerals (for some of which it is admitted that no use has been found) and a variety of vitamins. These pills are swallowed with fair regularity by pregnant women, and I suspect in most cases the contained minerals and vitamins emerge from the other end unaltered, to join the vast concentration of the contents of swallowed pills and potions in the sewage. The question which has to be answered in the affluent countries, and particularly amongst the more affluent citizens in these countries, is: 'Are the pregnancy dietary supplements necessary?' Would not the money expended be better spent on some other natural foods? The answer must be a qualified 'Yes'! The great majority of women do not need pregnancy supplements provided they eat a reasonable diet. At the most they need to take each day a single pill containing iron. The 'submerged' 10 per cent of poor women in the affluent societies and the 90 per cent in the developing countries do need supplements, particularly of iron, but even more they need additional protein. These people are the very ones who all too often receive little antenatal care, usually get inadequate food, and most often receive no dietary supplementary pills in pregnancy. Their need is great; that of their affluent sisters is minimal.

The expectant mother should eat a balanced diet; she should obtain proper antenatal care; she should have the haemoglobin concentration of her blood tested, as described previously; and she should be given a prescription for a tablet containing an iron salt (and it does not matter which iron salt). She should take one of these tablets each day from about the 14th week of pregnancy, but if she happens to miss a couple of days, it does not matter much.

There has been some discussion recently about whether pregnant women should be given a particular vitamin called folic acid. It is called 'folic' acid because the vitamin was first found in the leaves of green vegetables, and *folium* is a leaf in Latin. This vitamin is needed for the growth of cells, and since little is stored in the body, a steady intake is required. In pregnancy the demand increases considerably, particularly in the last 10 weeks, and the level of folic acid in the mother's blood tends to fall. If the diet contains green or yellow leafy vegetables, lightly cooked using only a small amount of water, there is generally no need for additional folic acid tablets. But because the baby demands and takes so much folic acid from the mother, it may be wise to give supplements to the mother who is carrying twins. The dose she needs is very small, and the vitamin is only needed after the 30th week of pregnancy. The vitamin should only be taken after discussing the matter with the doctor.

What then is the situation regarding vitamin and mineral pills in pregnancy? Beyond taking a single iron tablet each day, and in special cases taking a folic acid tablet, the pregnant woman in an affluent society, who is not poor, does not require to take the vitamin and mineral pills so attractively displayed and bottled by enterprising pharmaceutical companies.

WEIGHT GAIN

It is quite obvious that women put on weight during pregnancy. The question to be answered is how much is permissible. Until very recently weight gain was restricted very considerably, as obstetricians believed that there was a close relationship between weight gain and the onset of 'toxaemia of pregnancy'. Whilst there is a relationship, it is now known that it is by no means as close as was previously thought. The rigid restriction on weight gain was especially propagated by American obstetricians, possibly because as a race Americans eat too much. At all events, women were bullied, frightened and indoctrinated into believing that a weight gain in pregnancy of more than 8 kg, or 18 lb, was dangerous, and in trying to restrict their weight gain to below this figure, many women had a miserable and anxious pregnancy. Today, it is known that this attitude was unnecessarily restrictive, and much more latitude can be allowed.

To appreciate how much weight gain is normal, it is helpful to analyse the various things which increase the expectant mother's weight in pregnancy. Obviously, the fetus, the placenta and the liquid in which the fetus lives all contribute. Equally obvious is the increased weight of the uterus and the breasts. Not quite so obvious is the fact that the increased volume of blood, which circulates in an expectant mother's arteries and veins, adds to the weight gain.

Two other factors are involved. The first is the increased deposition of fat in the mother's tissues. In part this is caused by the conversion of excess carbohydrate eaten in the diet, but in part is a normal event caused by the hormones of pregnancy. The amount of fat deposited varies very considerably, but averages 2,000 g or 4½ lb. It is believed that evolution of man led to this deposition of fat in pregnancy, so that the mother had extra energy stored which might later be needed for the care and feeding of her baby. Finally, and again because of the hormones of pregnancy, water is retained in the body. Again the amount varies, but about 4 litres, or 6¾ pints, is retained, half of it in the last 10 weeks of pregnancy.

It is possible to make a table showing how the various factors lead to weight gain in pregnancy:

Fetus, placenta and amniotic liquid	4400 g	(10 lb 0 oz)
Uterus and breasts	1100 g	(2 lb 7 oz)
Blood volume increase	1000 g	(2 lb 4 oz)
Fat deposited	up to 2000 g	(4 lb 7 oz)
Water retained	up to 4000 g	(8 lb 14 oz)
	12.5 kg	(28 lb 0 oz)

As can be seen, a total of 12.5 kg, or 28 lb, is a normal weight gain in pregnancy. Because of this, the doctors who restricted severely the patient's weight gain were being unnecessarily harsh.

The weight gain is not spread equally throughout pregnancy. After the 20th week, the fetus gains weight more rapidly, fat is deposited in greater amounts, and fluid is retained more readily. In fact, the expectation is that in the first 20 weeks a weight gain of 3.5 kg, or 8 lb, will occur, and in the last 20 weeks a weight gain of 9 kg, or 20 lb, can be considered normal. Of course, there are individual variations. The expectant mother who is underweight for her height may be encouraged to put on more weight, and the overweight mother will be firmly told not to put on so much weight.

More important than overall weight gain is the weekly gain in the last 20 weeks of pregnancy. A weight gain of more than 1 kg (2 lb) a week is suggestive of excess fat or fluid retention. This may be the first sign of 'toxaemia of pregnancy', so that the expectant mother should *avoid gaining more than 0.5 kg, or 1 lb, a week in the last 20 weeks of pregnancy.*

A final point: if an expectant mother gains more than 16 kg, or 35 lb, in pregnancy, she will find it almost impossible to lose the extra weight. Her clothes will not fit, her sylph-like figure will be a memory, and perhaps her husband will object. And that wouldn't do!

Chapter 12

The Three Stages of Labour

The process of childbirth is usually called 'labour'. The term is appropriate, for labour is a time of work. Considerable energy is expended in the contractions of the uterus. For this reason the pregnant woman is in ways like an athlete. If she has had proper training during pregnancy, so that she knows what to expect and what to do in labour; if she is in good physical condition; if her mental attitude to labour is good, the process of childbirth is relatively easy. One of the objectives of good antenatal care is to enable her to reach this peak of fitness at the time labour is due.

Before we consider the process of labour from the viewpoint of the expectant mother, it is helpful to consider what happens in labour. With the aid of diagrams, we will see how the baby is expelled from its heat-controlled capsule, to journey down the dark curved birth-canal, and to be pushed out into a world where it has to use many functions for which it had no need while in the uterus. It has to obtain its oxygen from the atmosphere, not from its mother's blood. It has to get rid of its own waste products. It can no longer depend upon its placenta to act as a liver and a kidney. It has to obtain food instead of depending on the transfer across the placenta of required foodstuffs from the mother's blood to its own blood. In all these functions, the newborn baby succeeds admirably. However, the more normal the process of childbirth, the easier it is for the baby to adjust to independent life.

THE LAST FEW DAYS OF PREGNANCY

In late pregnancy, just before the onset of labour, the baby has grown to an average weight of 3,300 g (7½ lb), and is 50 cm (20 in) long. It has occupied more and more space in the amniotic sac, and the amount of amniotic fluid has been reduced from a maximum volume of 1,000 ml (1¾ pints) at 36 weeks' gestation, to about 600 ml (1 pint) at 40 weeks' gestation, or 'term'. If it is a first pregnancy, the baby's head is likely to have settled into the mother's pelvis. The uterus is becoming increasingly sensitive to stimuli, and increasingly active. The cervix is soft, has shortened in length, and is likely to have begun to open a bit, usually about 1 to 2 finger-breadths. If a doctor performs a pelvic examination at this stage, he will feel the 'bag of waters', which is the inexact term used for the amniotic sac, and in it he can feel the baby's head. If he could see the baby, he would find in more than three-quarters of cases that its face was looking towards the mother's right or left hip bone (Fig. **12/1**).

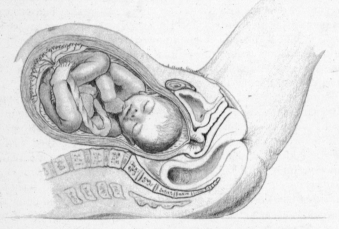

FIG. 12/1 The baby in late pregnancy. Its head is 'fixed' in the mother's pelvis and it 'looks' towards one hip bone. The cervix is soft but not yet drawn up

THE FIRST STAGE OF LABOUR

For reasons which are quite unknown, at a specific point in time labour starts. The uterine contractions initially are not very strong, and only occur at long intervals. However, with the passage of time, they become stronger and more frequent. This phase of labour does not distress the patient unduly, and is called the quiet phase. It lasts an average of 8 to 9 hours in a first labour, and 4 hours in subsequent labours.

With each contraction, the muscle fibres of the uterus shorten a tiny fraction, so that a pull is exerted on the cervix, which is the weakest part. This is because the muscle is thickest in the upper part of the uterus, and becomes less thick in the lower part. The cervix has only 10 per cent of muscle.

The pull on the cervix first shortens it until it no longer hangs down into the vagina like a cuff, but is drawn up flush. Doctors call this 'cervical effacement'. The pull then opens the cervix, and it slowly opens wider and wider. This the doctors call 'cervical dilatation', and patients may hear nurses or doctors saying that the cervix is so many finger-breadths, or so many centimetres dilated. The quiet phase of labour usually lasts until the cervix is 2 to 3 finger-breadths (or 4 to 5 centimetres) dilated. Three fingers, or 5 centimetres, means that the cervix is half-way to its complete opening, which doctors call 'full dilatation'.

During the quiet phase, the baby's head flexes more so that it tucks in its chin, and the head moves more deeply into the pelvis. This can be seen in the illustration. It will be noted that the 'bag of waters' is still intact (Fig. 12/2). The end of the quiet phase is heralded by a change in the character of the uterine contractions. They become stronger and more frequent, and the expectant mother may request drugs to reduce the discomfort. The cervix continues to dilate, and the baby is pushed further into the pelvis, where it may cause pressure on the bladder and back-passage (Fig. 12/3). As the dilatation of the cervix becomes nearly complete, the contractions of the uterus are quite strong, but the degree of discomfort felt by the patient will depend on the adequacy of her preparation for labour, and on her attitude to labour. When the cervix is fully dilated, the uterus and vagina together form a curved passage, along which the baby can pass aided by uterine contractions and the mother's additional use of her abdominal muscles.

The period of time from the onset of labour to the full dilatation of the cervix is called the *first stage of labour*. It lasts, on an average, 10 hours in a first labour, and 7 hours in a subsequent labour, although, of course, the duration of the first stage varies very considerably between different expectant mothers.

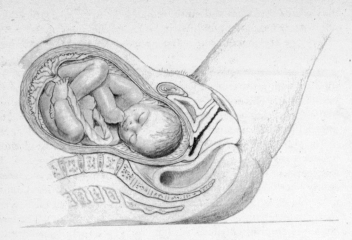

FIG. 12/2 The baby in early labour. Note how it has
tucked its chin well in. The cervix has been drawn up,
and the bag of waters is still intact

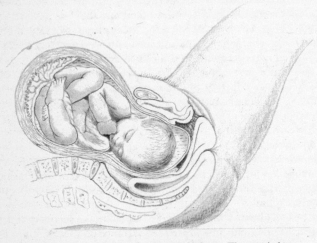

FIG. 12/3 Late in the first stage of labour. The cervix has
almost completely opened and the bag of waters bulges
in front of the head

THE SECOND STAGE OF LABOUR

The second stage of labour is the time when the mother-to-be has to help. In the first stage she helps most by relaxing during contractions, and by reading, talking, listening to the radio, or watching television. In the second stage she has work to do. She has to aid in the expulsion of the baby from the birth-canal, which is formed from the uterus and the vagina. The second stage usually lasts less than 1½ hours, extending in time from the full dilatation of the cervix to the birth of the baby. If the second stage lasts longer than 1½ hours, the attending doctor usually helps the birth by forceps (see Chapter 17). The beginning of the second stage is announced frequently by the bursting of the 'bag of waters', with a resulting gush of fluid from the vagina. The bursting of the 'bag of waters', called by doctors 'rupture of the membranes', may occur much earlier in labour, or occasionally not until the baby is ready to be born. Usually, however, it occurs at the very end of the first stage of labour.

At the same time the expectant mother gets the urge to push. This is caused by the pressure of the baby's head on the tissues in the middle of the pelvis. A message is sent to the brain, which makes the mother want to fix her diaphragm, and contract her abdominal muscles to push her baby out into the world. The baby is therefore pushed downwards, and because of the shape of the muscles which stretch across the pelvis, its head turns so that it comes to look backwards (Figs. 12/4 and 5). Evolution has caused this, for when man expanded his brain and developed a round skull, he made childbirth more difficult. The widest diameter at the entrance to the bony pelvis is the one stretching across it between the hip bones, and the baby adjusts so that the long diameter of its head (that from the forehead backwards) fits into this. In the lower part of the pelvis, the longest diameter is from before backwards, and the baby's head rotates to fit this so that its face now looks backwards towards the mother's back.

With each contraction of the uterus, and aided by the mother's 'pushing' efforts, the baby's head moves nearer the vulval cleft. Soon the top of its head can be seen by the doctor who will deliver the baby. The head advances a bit with each contraction, and retreats a bit between contractions, but overall the advance continues, more and more of the head becoming visible. The mother is working very hard during this time, her pulse rises, she sweats from the effort, and between contractions she rests, dozing and obtaining energy for the

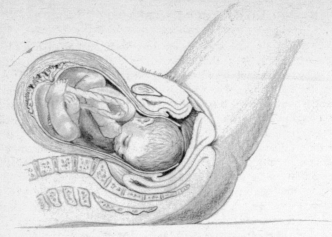

FIG. 12/4 The early part of the second stage of labour. The child's head is beginning to turn so that it faces towards its mother's back. The bag of waters has 'broken'. The mother feels pressure on her bladder and rectum, and she has the desire to push

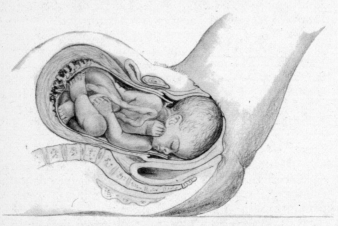

FIG. 12/5 Late second stage. Labour is nearly over. The baby's head appears at the vulva, and the shoulders are turning to fit into the bones of the pelvis. The face is turned completely towards the mother's back. The mother's perineum is being stretched

next effort. And despite this, it is said that women are the 'weaker sex'! Finally, the head stretches the vaginal entrance and the tissues between it and the back-passage (or anus). This area is called the perineum, and it becomes tightly stretched over the baby's head which bulges through it. This is quaintly called 'crowning of the head'. At this point the doctor may inject a local anaesthetic into the tissues of the vulva, if he has not done so already. This prevents the mother from the pain of stretching of the tissues, which many say feels as if their bottom was about to burst. It is also said that it resembles the feeling of trying to open the bowels after being consti-pated for a month! The next contraction pushes the baby down further, and the head sweeps over the vulval tissues, the forehead, the eyes, the nose, the mouth and the chin appearing successively (Fig. 12/6).

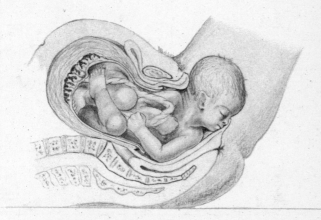

FIG. 12/6 The baby's head is being born, emerging from
the vagina and sweeping the perineum backwards

The delivery of the baby's head can be seen in the series of drawings (Fig. 12/7), and it can be noted that once the head is born, it turns back to face the mother's hips. This has been arranged by evolution so that the shoulders of the baby and the rest of its body can slip out of the birth-canal easily. The baby is born! The mother, no longer expectant, looks delightedly at her baby, and as its first cry echoes, she fondles it and then relaxes and sleeps momentarily.

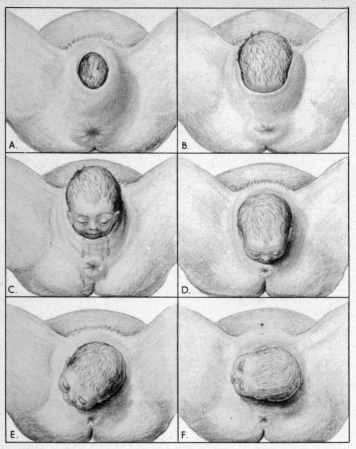

FIG. 12/7 The birth of the baby's head as seen by the doctor. Note how the perineum is stretched by the baby's head before it is born

THE THIRD STAGE OF LABOUR

Little more remains but to wait for the expulsion of the placenta, or afterbirth, so-called for obvious reasons. This has separated from its attachment to the wall of the uterus as the baby was born. The doctor either awaits its expulsion or, as is more usual today, aids its rapid removal by giving an injection of a drug called ergometrine, or one called syntometrine which makes the uterus contract firmly. This, of course, reduces the blood lost by the mother, which is desirable. The injection is given either as the baby's head is being born or as the baby's shoulders emerge.

Chapter 13

Childbirth Without Pain

In the year 1847 in the city of Edinburgh, in the dining-room of a house in Queen Street, three respectable physicians sat sniffing the contents of various bottles. The bottles contained mixtures of chemicals which were said to cause loss of consciousness. They had spent many evenings in this pursuit, sniffing and recording their observations. On a cold, wet evening in November, the group led by James Young Simpson gathered as usual. One of the mixtures that night was a rather pleasant, sweet-smelling fluid. After one large whiff each, the three men became strangely excited and gay; after two, they all became sleepy; and after a third large inhalation, they lay sprawled on the floor, only awaking after a few minutes. In this way the anaesthetic qualities of chloroform were discovered. It was clear to Dr Simpson that chloroform could help to relieve the pain of women in labour – for at that time no pain-relief of any kind was given, and as no patient received antenatal care, labours were often difficult, painful and dangerous. But when Simpson announced, in a paper published in the Monthly Journal of Medical Science, that chloroform could be used to relieve the pains of childbirth, he was criticized vehemently, attacked in print and from the pulpit by clergy and leaders of the public, as well as by many members of the medical profession. The use of chloroform was against God's Will, they cried, for was it not written that because Eve tempted Adam to eat the forbidden fruit, a curse was laid upon her that 'in sorrow would she bring forth her children'? If the pain and sorrow were reduced, it was irreligious. To this Simpson replied that in the Bible the first reported surgical operation had been performed under anaesthesia. The Lord God had caused 'a deep sleep to fall upon Adam; and he slept; and He took one of his ribs, and closed the flesh thereof'. Simpson was told by an American that to give chloroform was to interfere with nature, since the pains of childbirth were a natural function. Simpson agreed but asked, 'Is not walking also a natural function? And who would think of never setting aside or superseding this natural function. If you were travelling from Philadelphia to Baltimore, would you insist on walking the distance by foot simply because walking is man's natural method of locomotion?' An Irish woman visiting Scotland attacked him by saying, 'How unnatural it is for you doctors in Edinburgh to take away the pains of your patients when in labour'. His reply was, 'Madam, how unnatural it is for you to have swum over from Ireland to Scotland against wind and tides on a steamboat'.

Most of the objections were from the clergy; to each Simpson had an answer, and little by little his opponents were silenced, particularly as women appeared to approve of his attempt, in his own words, 'to alleviate human suffering, as well as preserve human life'. The cachet of approval was put upon his method when Queen Victoria was given inhalations of chloroform during the birth of her eighth child. Simpson was vindicated, and when he was later knighted, as Sir James Simpson, the opposition was in disorder. Yet to some extent, although they did not know it, they were partly right. Chloroform, although sweet-smelling, quick-acting and not irritating to breathe, is not a safe anaesthetic, because it may damage the liver. Consequently it is no longer used in obstetric practice.

No one would now deny that women should have the discomfort of childbirth relieved, and countless methods have been introduced in the past. Some were dangerous to the mother, some to the child; but today a reasonable approach has been made, and women need no longer fear the pain of childbirth. There are very real dangers though if the sedation is pushed too far, and the doctors have to find out the point at which adequate sedation and analgesia (that is, pain-relief without unconsciousness) can be given without risk to the mother or baby. It is unfair to promise a mother that all discomfort can be relieved, but it is equally callous for a doctor to allow his patient to suffer unduly, or to permit the nurses, who are so much closer to the patient during most of labour, to appear indifferent to her discomfort or perhaps even to relish it. Luckily only a few of these midwives remain, and today the training of a nurse-midwife includes instruction in analgesia.

Today three main methods of relieving the pain associated with childbirth are available. These methods should be discussed with the doctor during pregnancy so that the expectant mother can make her own choice. But it must be emphasized that she can change her mind and make another choice right up to and during her confinement. She must not feel that she is 'stuck' with a particular method.

The methods are, first, psychoprophylaxis or natural childbirth; second, analgesic supported childbirth and third, 'painless' childbirth following an epidural analgesic. So that a woman has the knowledge to make an informed choice of the method which she believes will suit her, these methods are now discussed.

PSYCHOPROPHYLAXIS

In many cultures pregnancy and childbirth are considered shameful matters, to be hidden from view and not discussed. As a consequence of this, many women have no idea what happens in childbirth, and how a large baby can be born through what appears to be a small hole. Strangely, even today, some pregnant women believe, until told otherwise, that the baby is born through the umbilicus. Because childbirth is not discussed, many woman pregnant for the first time only learn of its processes from equally-ill-informed friends and older women, who all too readily tell the expectant mother of the 'terrible time I had before the doctor cut out the baby', and of the pain, agony and danger of childbirth. According to the Russians who introduced psychoprophylaxis, these snippets of misinformation sink deep into the memory of the pregnant woman, and a 'conditioned reflex' occurs. Because of this reflex, every time the woman thinks of childbirth, a mental image of pain, suffering, danger of death and fear is conjured up, so that a woman enters labour anxious and tense. Psychoprophylaxis seeks to eliminate this 'conditioned reflex', and replace the image of fear, anxiety and tenseness by one in which childbirth is known to be a normal event. It also seeks to alter the brain's appreciation of pain, and convert it into a sensation of discomfort which can be relieved by muscular activity.

The psychoprophylactic method depends on the belief that 'conditioned reflexes' can be changed by training, because they are not built into the person's personality, and arise because of the person's response, or conditioning, to outside events.

It is known that pain is a relative thing. Pain is felt in a different way at different times. A hypnotized person, although awake, feels no pain; a soldier in the field, cold, deserted, hungry and wounded, may feel considerably more pain from his wound than he would if he were warm, rescued and being looked after by a sympathetic nurse. The pain of a dentist's drill varies depending on how much confidence the person has in her dentist, and how she herself feels. And, of course, each person has her own threshold above which pain is felt: the stoic woman feels little pain; the anxious, nervous person, given the same degree of pain, will feel a lot.

These facts are utilized in the psychoprophylactic method. The brain of every person is thought to have a special threshold below which no pain is felt. The normal, everyday, potentially painful stimuli which occur are not interpreted as pain because they fall below the threshold at which pain is felt. But the threshold can be reduced by conditions such as fear, emotional upset, shock, hunger and cold. In these conditions, stimuli which are normally not painful cross the lowered pain threshold and are felt as pain. Psychoprophylaxis seeks to raise the pain threshold by explanation of the processes of labour, and by the exercises which are taught seeks to change the interpretation by the patient's mind, of any painful sensations which get over the threshold. By changing pain to muscular activity, the patient actively participates in the childbirth.

Training takes place along two main lines. First, the fear of labour is reduced or eliminated by a series of talks in which the mother is told how conception occurs, how the fetus grows, what happens in childbirth, and how she can help by learning breathing techniques. Secondly, she is taught certain exercises, which are thought to improve her muscular control.

The breathing exercises, which are taught in the second half of pregnancy, are of three kinds. The first two are for use in the first stage of labour, and the third for helping to expel the baby from the mother's birth-canal in the second stage of labour.

The breathing exercises for the first stage of labour are to learn slow quiet breathing using the rib muscles, and not the diaphragm. The patient learns by demonstration and by reiteration that the onset of a contraction of her womb is a signal for her to start her learnt breathing pattern. In this way she learns that a contraction is a signal for breathing activity, rather than pain. In the late first stage, when the contractions are stronger, she learns that a breathing pattern of quick, shallow breathing interspersed with breath blown out at intervals helps considerably, especially if she combines the breathing with 'effleurage'. This is a light stroking movement of the fingers over the abdomen.

In the second stage of labour the pattern of breathing changes again. The expectant mother now takes deep breaths, which steady her diaphragm against the upper part of her uterus. This is followed by a contraction of her chest and upper abdominal muscles, which form a girdle around the uterus adding its pressure effects to those of the uterine contractions. In the first stage of labour, she should lie on one side or the other, whilst in the second stage she lies on her back, reclining upon pillows beneath her head and shoulders.

As well as breathing exercises, many supporters of psycho-prophylaxis believe that certain exercises encourage muscular control. For a muscular contraction to occur, the message, or stimulus, must travel from the brain to the muscle, and when one muscle contracts, others have to relax. Muscles which act in this way are called voluntary muscles, as they are under the control of the mind. (Not all muscles are voluntary; some like those of the uterus and the heart, are involuntary and contract independently of the person's wishes.) To accomplish the delivery of her baby through her vulva in the second stage of labour with the greatest ease, the mother has to contract her abdominal muscles in time with the uterine contractions, and simultaneously relax the muscles which support her vagina and perineum. The exercises learnt in 'relaxation classes' help her to do this.

Throughout the training period, the mother learns that the breathing exercises and exercises for 'neuro-muscular' control will help her during labour, but she is told that if she finds she requires pain-killing drugs, these will be given readily, and she must not feel a sense of failure about needing them. It has been found that the best results are obtained if the patient is confident in her knowledge of the processes of labour, if she constantly receives support and encouragement from those attending her, and if she is told from time to time of her progress.

Women who have chosen the psychoprophylactic method find that the discomfort of childbirth is minimized if the attending nursing and medical staff treat the patient as an intelligent participant in her own confinement, and if she has with her in the delivery room the man who fathered her child. The support of a loved person, who has also learned about the processes of childbirth, is particularly important as it gives the woman a warm personal link in the relatively cold clinical atmosphere found in most maternity units and hospitals. Moreover the joy of sharing in the birth of their child enhances the pleasure bond of their relationship.

It is difficult to determine the number of women who choose 'natural childbirth', but it appears that between 15 and 20 per cent of women would choose the method if they were encouraged by their medical attendants. Unfortunately, some doctors think that women choosing the method are freaks or cranks, and others resist having the man who fathered the child present during labour and childbirth.

Of women who choose psychoprophylaxis, about 45 per cent require no sedation or analgesics, 45 per cent require some analgesic support, and 10 per cent change to one of the other methods available.

ANALGESIC SUPPORTED CHILDBIRTH

Whilst most women in the developing nations receive little or no analgesics during their confinements and because of cultural attitudes have no wish for their husband to be present, the majority of women in the developed nations are given (or, more rarely, choose) the method of analgesic supported childbirth. An analgesic is a drug which reduces or eliminates pain without clouding the consciousness of the person to any significant extent. The principle behind the method is that women in labour should have the pain of labour reduced by being given sedatives or analgesics at appropriate intervals, but the dose of the drugs should be regulated to avoid damaging the fetus.

In the quiet phase of the first stage of labour, the uterine contractions are relatively painless and few women ask for analgesics, although an apprehensive woman may welcome some form of sedation. In the past, barbiturates were widely used but recently some concern has been expressed that the drugs may depress the baby's breathing and the newer sedatives and, more usually, tranquillizers are being given. Many different tranquillizers have been given but, currently, promazine (Sparine) and diazepam (Valium) are used most frequently. The former drug is given by injection into a muscle when labour is established, and gives the woman a warm woozy feeling. Diazepam can be given as an injection or by mouth.

Once the quiet phase of labour merges into the active phase, the uterine contractions become stronger and more painful and most women want an analgesic which will reduce the painful sensations. In pride of place is pethidine (called meperidine in the U.S.A.). Pethidine is given by injection into a muscle, usually in the thigh or the upper arm. Within 20 minutes of the injection, the pain is reduced, often considerably, and the woman relaxes and feels drowsy between contractions. The effect of an injection of pethidine lasts from two to five hours, so that several injections may be needed in the course of labour.

Towards the end of the first stage of labour and in the second stage, the mother may need further help to reduce the discomfort. Two analgesics are available (which in higher concentration lead to the complete loss of consciousness and therefore are really anaesthetics). If either is chosen, the woman holds a mask over her face and breathes deeply during an uterine contraction. The drug in the gas mixture dulls the pain, and once the contraction has ceased, the mother puts the mask on one side. The two anaesthetic mixtures are 'gas and oxygen' and 'Trilene'. There is little to choose between them. 'Gas' (really nitrous oxide) is mixed in a special machine with oxygen, so that there is never less than 30 per cent of oxygen in the mixture. The patient breathes this mixture through a tube and face-mask. 'Trilene' is a sweet-smelling, blue liquid, which vapourizes into a gas when air is passed over it. Trilene is placed in a small box-like inhaler, and this is connected by a rubber tube to a face-mask. When the patient breathes in through the tube, air passes over the Trilene and some vapour is taken up. As a contraction starts, the mother breathes in, and inhales Trilene vapour which dulls her pain. Between contractions she puts the mask to one side. Not every woman can use Trilene.

Many women, particularly those delivering a second or subsequent baby, find that the pain relief from pethidine supplemented by inhalational analgesics is all that they need, but some women require more. The only person who can determine the amount of pain felt is the person herself, so that the woman in labour has the right to ask for additional sedation and receive it.

Pain is likely to be more severe in a woman delivering her first baby, as its head presses down and stretches the vaginal entrance. A local anaesthetic injected into the tissues will relieve this pain, so that the 'bursting feeling' is eliminated. The doctor may give the injection into the stretched tissues between the vaginal entrance and the anus. This is called a perineal nerve block. An alternative and better method is for the doctor to give an injection to numb the nerves which supply the vulva as they pass through the pelvis. To do this, the doctor puts a finger in the woman's vagina, and gently pushes to one side until he reaches a triangular shaped bone which is a part of the pelvis. He then pushes a small needle, which is attached to a syringe, along his finger and injects the local anaesthetic around the triangular bony promontory. He repeats this on the other side of the woman's pelvis. Quite quickly all painful sensations in the vulva and lower vagina are eliminated, so that the baby's birth is relatively painless, although the contractions of the uterus are still felt.

About 50 to 60 per cent of women choose analgesic supported childbirth (or are given the method without any choice); but in many Western nations more women are seeking to have 'painless childbirth' using an epidural analgesic.

'PAINLESS CHILDBIRTH'

Unfortunately painless childbirth, using an epidural analgesic, is a rather complex method. In the first place, the epidural injection can only be made when labour enters the active phase, or the contractions may cease. This means that during the quiet phase of the first stage of labour some sedation or analgesic may be required. Secondly, the injection can only be made by a trained person, usually an anaesthetist who has a special interest in obstetric anaesthesia. Thirdly, a woman who has had an epidural anaesthetic requires to be observed meticulously as the drug may cause vomiting and, sometimes, a fall in blood pressure. Fourth, because the woman has no sensation of pain, she finds it difficult to aid her baby's birth by using her abdominal muscles and pushing when she has a uterine contraction. This means that the second stage of labour may last longer than in women choosing the other methods, and forceps delivery of the baby is more frequent. Provided that the woman is attended by a skilled doctor this is of no importance, but many women are delivered by nurse-midwives who are not trained, or permitted to use obstetric forceps.

For all these reasons epidural analgesia is only available for a minority of women. But if a woman chooses the method, generally she can find a doctor who uses the method and who can deliver her in a hospital which has the facilities available. So that the expectant

mother can make an informed choice she should understand where
the injection is made and how it works.

Epidural anaesthesia

The backbone is made up of separate vertebrae, and protects the
spinal cord, which extends as far down as the pelvis through a hole in
each vertebra. The spinal cord is made up of millions of nerve fibres,
and is linked to all parts of the body. Impulses are constantly passing
from all parts of the body to the brain along the spinal cord, and out
again from the brain to all parts of the body. A substantial number of
the nerves relay to the brain sensations received by the various parts
of the body, such as feelings of cold, heat or pain. The nerves relaying
these sensations are called sensory nerve fibres, and they pass along

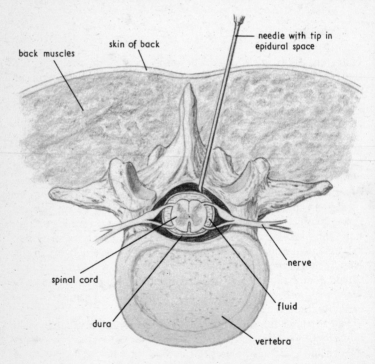

FIG. 13/1 Epidural anaethesia

different routes from the nerve fibres which bring messages from the brain to the muscles and other structures. Since many of these fibres make the muscles contract, or move, they are called motor fibres. If it were possible to anaesthetize, or numb, the sensory fibres from the uterus without also anaesthetizing the motor fibres to the uterus, labour could be made painless. Luckily this can be done safely, provided the anaesthetist is an expert.

The spinal cord is surrounded by a glistening envelope (called the dura) for all of its length, and the envelope contains a fluid. Between the envelope and the bony hole in the vertebrae is a space, through which nerves pass from the spinal cord on their way to and from the structures of the body (Fig. 13/1). The anaesthetist inserts a thin needle through the muscles of the mother's back, and with great care gets the tip to lie in the space between the dura and the bone – this is the epidural space. He pushes a fine polythene tube through the needle so that it is in the space, and then withdraws the needle, leaving the polythene tube in the space. He can now give a local anaesthetic into the epidural space, and, if needs be, keep 'topping' it up when the anaesthetic effect begins to wear off. You can see that epidural anaesthesia has the advantage that a woman is relieved of most of the pain associated with childbirth, but has the joy of helping in the birth of her baby, of seeing it being born, of hearing its first cry and of cuddling it as soon as it is born.

In this chapter, I have tried to stress, that a woman has the right to be informed about the methods available to relieve the pain associated with childbirth, to discuss them with her chosen medical attendant, and to choose which method she prefers. Whichever method she chooses, it is the duty of those helping her during child-birth to inform her of the progress of her labour, to obtain her co-operation and to treat her as a participant in a wonderful process.

We have advanced a long way from the time when the Biblical curse on Eve that 'in sorrow would she bring forth her children', dominated men's minds.

Chapter 14

What to Expect in Labour

The mechanical processes which lead to the birth of the baby need to be understood by the expectant mother, so that she may have insight into what happens and what is expected of her. But she also needs to know what happens to her and what she is to do.

LATE PREGNANCY AND PRELABOUR

In the last weeks of pregnancy, the baby is settling into its final position preparatory to birth. In the majority of first pregnancies the baby's head has settled into the pelvis and is exerting pressure on the pelvis, the rectum and the bladder. Varicose veins become more obvious as the blood returning from the legs is dammed back; backache is more common; frequency of urination usual. The expectant mother, too, is becoming impatient. She wants to see and fondle the baby she has nurtured all these weeks. Sleep is less sound, and on hot nights sweating may be a problem. It is quite proper for the expectant mother to ask her doctor for sleeping tablets to help 'tide' her over these last few weeks; but most women adjust to the disturbed nights, and rest during the day to make up for it.

False labour

In these weeks, the uterus is increasingly sensitive, and the painless contractions which have been felt in the preceding weeks become more frequent. Painful contractions may also occur, usually at night and at irregular intervals. This is 'false labour', but it may be mistaken for the onset of true labour, and many an expectant mother has been admitted to hospital, only to be discharged home the next day. The difference between false and true labour is that the contractions in false labour are irregular in duration, occur at irregular intervals, and rather than increasing in intensity, or strength, as time passes, diminish in intensity after a few hours and then disappear altogether. Often they occur at night, and are usually felt in the lower abdomen and back. This is in contrast to true labour, in which there is an increasing frequency and intensity of contractions, which develop an almost predictable regularity as time progresses. But no mother should be ashamed of having gone into hospital in false labour, as sometimes the two types are most difficult to differentiate.

What to take into hospital

By this time the expectant mother will have prepared the things which she will require in hospital, and will often have a bag packed in readiness. What she needs depends to some extent on her own desires and local custom. In general the bag should contain the following:

Nightdress or pyjamas (2 or 3 sets). Many women prefer pyjamas, and wear the top only. In many ways pyjamas are more convenient than nightdresses, particularly if the mother is going to breast-feed. A few hospitals, regrettably, insist that the patient wear a hospital gown. This is generally ugly. The practice is disappearing, and the sooner it goes, the better.

Brassières. Two nursing brassières are usually required.

Bed jacket

Dressing gown. This is essential as 'early ambulation' is now normal, and patients are usually up and about within 24 to 48 hours of childbirth.

Bedroom slippers

Sanitary belt. Sanitary pads are usually supplied by the hospital, but some hospitals ask the patient to supply her own, and to bring them in before labour so that they may be sterilized.

Handkerchiefs or tissues

Toothpaste, toothbrush, toilet soap, washing flannel, nail brush, hairbrush, comb, hand mirror, cosmetics, perfume, talcum powder. Beauty may be in the eye of the beholder, and the new mother has every right to feel and be beautiful. But artifacts help in our society, and why not?

Writing paper, envelopes, stamps and a pen. It is surprising how many letters need to be written once the baby is born.

Books. The lying-in period is a time of rest, interspersed with moments of activity. Books fill in the time, although portable television sets are replacing them.

Baby clothes. A set for dressing the baby on discharge from hospital. Hospitals usually supply nightgowns and napkins (diapers) for the hospital period.

THE ONSET OF LABOUR

The onset of true labour is announced by one or more of the following three signs:

(1) The onset of regular, rhythmic uterine contractions, which may be painful.

(2) The passage of a small amount of blood-tinged, sticky mucus from the vagina (the 'show').

(3) The 'gushing' of liquid from the vagina. This is due to rupture of the membranes which form the amniotic sac.

Regular painful contractions

If false labour has been experienced in the last weeks of pregnancy, the patient may be able to detect a change in the character of the contractions when true labour starts. If no false labour has been experienced, the patient will be able to determine if this is indeed true labour from the character of the contractions. The contractions of true labour initially last about 30 seconds, and occur at regular intervals of about 15 to 20 minutes. During the contraction, the uterus can be felt to become hard, and some degree of pain is felt, either only in the small of the back, or, as labour progresses, radiating from the flanks into the abdomen. In fact, as a rule the less backache there is, the more efficient is the labour. The pain begins as a small 'twinge', it increases to a peak, and diminishes to fade away entirely. In the opinion of many women, it is like a severe menstrual cramp.

As labour progresses, the duration of the contraction extends from 30 seconds to 90 seconds; the interval between contractions diminishes from 20 minutes to 3 or 5 minutes, and the intensity of the contraction increases, so that the expectant mother may ask for pain-reducing drugs.

In general, the patient should go into hospital when the contractions are regular and are recurring at about 10 minute intervals, but of course this is only 'in general', and individuals may feel the need to go into hospital earlier or later.

The 'show'

The discharge of blood-stained mucus precedes or accompanies the onset of painful contractions as often as it follows them. What has happened is that the 'plug' of mucus which has filled the cervical canal from early pregnancy is dislodged as the uterine contractions draw up (or 'efface') the cervix and begin to dilate it at the onset of labour. The discharge of the blood-stained mucus is called the 'show', and labour generally starts within 24 hours of its appearance.

Rupture of the membranes

In a few cases, labour is heralded by a sudden gush of liquid from the vagina. This occurs because the membranes of the amniotic sac, which lines the uterus and in which the baby has grown, suddenly rupture. This event may occur before term, or it may occur at term. In either event, the patient should go to the hospital without delay, so that she may be examined, as occasionally problems arise which need to be checked as soon as possible. In general, labour starts within a few hours of spontaneous rupture of the membranes. If labour has not started within 12 to 24 hours and the pregnancy is near term, the doctor will give an infusion of a drug called oxytocin, into an arm vein of the expectant mother, to hasten the onset of labour.

ADMISSION TO HOSPITAL

From time to time newspaper stories appear of women who failed to reach hospital in time, and the baby was born in the car, in a taxi, or perhaps on the front steps of the hospital. These occurrences are rare, and most expectant mothers get into hospital in good time.

For doctors and nurses a hospital is a familiar workplace; for many patients it is a strange and frightening place, where unbending people order the patient to do unpredictable things, and where everyone seems too busy to talk to her and to explain what is being done and why. This authoritarian, inhuman approach is fast going, and hospitals are becoming places in which *people* work to help other people. As childbirth is an essentially normal event, this humanist approach is even more important in a maternity hospital, and happily it is becoming much more common. One way in which the expectant mother can reduce her anxiety is to visit the hospital during pregnancy. Many hospital authorities co-operate in arranging these visits, when the patient can see the labour ward, or delivery floor, and the type of room, or ward, in which she will stay.

More is needed. Hospital authorities, at all levels, need to remember that a maternity ward must be run for the benefit of an informed woman who wishes to participate in the birth of her baby. Unfortunately too many hospitals still 'depersonalize' the expectant mother from the moment of her admission. She is interviewed, apparently irrelevant questions are asked (for example, what is your husband's occupation), her pubic area is shaved, she may be given an enema and she is then put in an ugly, unglamorous hospital 'gown'. Most of this is unnecessary, as you will read.

Hospitals must review their procedures and re-organize their physical arrangements, to meet the expectations of the 'about-to-deliver' couple. The hospital should provide a comfortable, well-decorated lounge, which has coffee and toilet facilities for 'expectant fathers', in which the couple can walk about or sit if they wish, talking to other couples in the early part of labour. Hospitals should ensure that the rooms on the delivery floor are single rooms and are made as 'unclinical' as is compatible with hygiene and safety. The staff should be certain that no woman in labour is left alone at any time. If the woman wishes, the father of her child (or some other close relative) should be able to remain with her throughout the labour, including times when she is being examined.

Once her baby has been born, the child's father should be able to visit her whenever she wishes, and to remain with her as long as she wishes.

In addition, 'rooming-in' should be permitted without question if the mother desires it (p. 245). During the time she is in hospital, information and counselling on parenting, how to cope with the infant in the first weeks at home, child-development and family planning should be provided for her and the child's father. If hospitals do not provide such services at present, women's groups should exert pressure to make sure that they do as soon as is practicable.

What happens at present is that on admission, in early labour, the woman is examined by a doctor on the hospital staff or a nurse, who then informs the patient's own doctor, depending on the custom and staff pattern of the particular hospital. The first thing which is done is to determine if labour is really under way, and how far advanced it is. This information is obtained from the patient's description of what has happened in the preceding few hours, aided if necessary by an abdominal examination of the position of the baby in the uterus. If labour is not far advanced, it is usual for the patient to change into a hospital gown and to get into bed, so that she may be 'prepared' for delivery. In the past this preparation was fairly complex: the patient had a hot bath, was given an enema, and the pubic and vulval hair was shaved. Today, the hot bath is replaced by a warm shower, if the patient feels she needs one. The enema is omitted, or replaced by the use of a small pill which is inserted into the back-passage, and induces bowel motion with much less discomfort and distress than did the enema. The 'complete' shave is reduced to shaving the area of the perineum, the hair on the pubis merely being clipped short. The old method of a complete shave was uncomfortable (nurses are not very skilful with a safety razor), undignified, the patient feeling that she looked like a 'plucked chicken', and not really necessary unless an abdominal operation was anticipated. It should also be questioned if a woman needs to wear a hospital gown. It is usually ugly, leaves the woman's back and bottom bare and depersonalizes her into a 'patient'. I can see no reason why a woman should not wear her own nightwear which is pleasant to look at and which makes the woman feel glamorous.

When these preliminaries are over, the resident doctor usually reviews the patient's antenatal record if this is available, and checks that she is not suffering from any infectious disease such as a cold. He then examines a specimen of urine and takes the patient's blood pressure. Next he re-examines the abdomen to make sure that the baby is lying normally, and that its head or its breech is fitting into the expectant mother's pelvis. He may also wish to perform a pelvic examination so that he can make a full evaluation of the progress of labour. This examination is in no way different from the pelvic examination performed in pregnancy, except that increased precautions are taken to avoid infection. Whilst the doctor is cleaning his hands, the patient is placed on a sterile cloth and may put on leggings. The doctor cleans the vulval area with an antiseptic solution, and pours some obstetric antiseptic cream into the vagina. This not only prevents infection, but also renders the examination easier. During these examinations the doctor will be able to answer any questions which the patient may have.

THE FIRST STAGE OF LABOUR

The first stage of labour is the time during which the cervix must be drawn up and opened fully so that the birth-canal is established. It is a time when the expectant mother can actively do little to aid the delivery of her baby. It is a period of waiting intelligently, with the knowledge of the preparations for the birth of her child which are occurring within her body.

Since it is a period of waiting, more and more hospitals and obstetricians are coming to realize that during the first stage the patient requires to be in an atmosphere which is as home-like as possible, and only when the end of this stage is approaching does she need to be taken to the more antiseptic hospital-like surroundings of the delivery room. To meet the needs of this new philosophy, hospitals are building, or converting other accommodation into first stage areas, which contain individual rooms and a commonroom, decorated pleasantly, furnished with comfortable chairs, and perhaps with a television set so that the patient may occupy her time more happily, often together with the baby's father.

As has been noted, the patient who has insight into the processes of labour, and who has perhaps been to psychoprophylactic classes in pregnancy, is much better equipped to cope with the first stage of labour. At some time it is likely that the contractions will become uncomfortably strong. When this occurs, the expectant mother usually wishes to go to bed, and may request pain-reducing drugs, which are readily available. She will also be confined to bed if the membranes have ruptured or if any other complication has been detected. In the first stage the patient should not lie on her back on a hard bed. She should either recline propped up on pillows supported so that she can lie at an angle of 45 degrees to the horizontal or lie on her side, as in this way she improves the flow of blood through the uterus, and provides more oxygen for her baby.

During the first stage of labour, she will not be permitted to eat any solid food, for the good reason that in labour food remains in the

stomach and is not digested; and she may not be permitted to drink
any fluids. Some doctors do permit their patients to drink tea, water
or sweet drinks; others feel that all fluid should be given as an
infusion into an arm vein.

THE SECOND STAGE

This is the stage of expulsion of the baby from the warm womb into
the outside world. This is the period when the active aid of the mother
is required to help her baby be born. It is a time of some discomfort,
which is reduced by modern anaesthetic methods or by the injection
of local anaesthetic into the tissues at the entrance of the vagina.

The help of the mother is needed. With each uterine contraction
she takes in a big breath, filling her lungs with air. She then holds her
breath, which makes her diaphragm rigid, and by contracting her
lower chest and abdominal muscles, she pushes down, adding a
further expulsive effort. Often she finds that she can get a better
'push' if she lifts her head and clasps her legs, drawing them up onto
her abdomen (Fig. **14/1**). During a contraction she works hard, between contractions she relaxes completely. To dull the pain of the
contraction, she may breathe 'gas and oxygen' from a machine, or
another gas called 'Trilene', or have an epidural anaesthetic. The
practice differs in different hospitals.

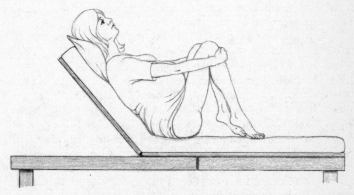

FIG. 14/1 The ideal position for delivery

At last the baby's head appears, stretching the tissues of the perineum. Rather than allowing the perineum to tear jaggedly, as may happen, the doctor often makes a deliberate small cut with scissors. This is called an 'episiotomy'. It is easier to stitch, is much less painful if stitched properly (in fact using one technique it is virtually painless), and heals far better.

A final push 'crowns' the baby's head and the doctor now helps in delivering the baby. The expectant mother only pushes when she is asked to do so, instead panting quietly as the baby is slowly and gently born. The birth of the baby from 'crowning of the head' takes about 2 or 3 minutes, and many doctors give an injection at this time to expel the placenta more rapidly. But not all agree that this is necessary.

The baby is born, and lies between the mother's legs whilst its nose and throat are cleared of mucus. The cord which has been its lifeline for 40 weeks ceases to beat; it is tied and cut. The baby takes a breath and its first cry is heard by the mother, who is lying back relaxed. The doctor makes sure that the baby is normal – and over 97 per cent are – and then hands the baby to the mother, so that she may fondle and cuddle it whilst the afterbirth is being expelled.

Indeed, some doctors – and I am one of them – encourage the patient to witness the birth of her baby. If the expectant mother is propped up on pillows, she can see the baby being born once the head has been crowned, and can hold its waving hands whilst the buttocks are still emerging from her body.

Labour should be as pleasant and enjoyable a process as possible and both doctor and nurses should try to make the mother as comfortable as possible by creating a quiet, happy environment. This idea has been extended by the French obstetrician, Dr Leboyer, who believes that the passage of the baby into the world and its adaptation to life outside the uterus should be gentle, or problems will arise later. Some of his views are perhaps exaggerated, but the principles he holds are good. The environment of the delivery room should be as 'homely' as is compatible with the need for cleanliness and good observation of the mother during labour. The light in the delivery room should not be more than that needed for the medical attendants to be able to see what they are doing and to ensure the safety of the baby's birth. The attendants should be supportive, communicative and helpful. They should let you see and cuddle your baby; after all you have waited 40 weeks for this exciting moment! Dr Leboyer believes that a baby should not cry at birth and should be put in warm water until it adjusts to the different environment. There is much dispute about this view, as the cry a baby makes at birth is necessary for it to fill its lungs with oxygen for the first time, and I believe it better for the baby to be cuddled by its mother – so that it has the warmth and contact of her body, rather than the impersonal warmth of a bath. Nevertheless, the influence of Dr Leboyer is beneficial if it induces obstetricians to think more of the human aspect of childbirth and less of the mechanical processes of parturition.

THE THIRD STAGE

The third and final stage of labour is the time during which the placenta is expelled. It rarely lasts for more than 20 minutes, and is painless. Usually, today, the doctor assists the expulsion of the placenta by pressure upwards on the abdomen just above the pubic bone, and by gently pulling on the cut cord at the same time. A small amount of bleeding is usual during the third stage, but it is less than 300 ml (½ pint) in most cases, particularly if the injection mentioned earlier has been given. The injection makes the uterus contract firmly, and the blood vessels which have supplied the placenta are squeezed tightly in the lattice of muscle fibres.

Labour is over. The episiotomy is stitched. The proper repair of a torn perineum, or of an episiotomy, is most important, as the discomfort can make the new mother's first few days uncomfortable and the idea of a 'damaged' part of her genital area can disturb her body image. It is a good idea to ask for a mirror so that you can look at your perineum when the stitches have been taken out (if that needs to be done), so that you can see how normal it is.

The mother, no longer expectant but fulfilled, is washed and powdered. She relaxes and sometimes sleeps whilst the nurses check that the uterus is contracted, and about one hour after delivery she returns to her room in the lying-in ward. She is emotionally happy. She has done a unique and wonderful thing.

THE FATHER IN LABOUR

What of the father? It was his spermatozoon which fertilized the egg; it is he who has contributed half of the genes to the child. What is his place in labour? This depends greatly on custom and culture. In some tribal societies the man undergoes a mock labour, is pampered and cossetted during the time his wife, either alone or attended by a single female, delivers her child. In other societies, the man is excluded from the vicinity of the place where the woman has her baby, and is expected to ignore the whole episode, holding that it never happened.

In modern Western society, there is a trend to involve the father in the process of childbirth. He, as well as the mother, reads about the process of growth of the child in the uterus; he learns about the course of labour; together they are involved in the sequence of events leading up to childbirth. This approach has much to commend it. It culminates in the presence of the father during childbirth. In the first stage of labour he remains with his wife, so that in the unfamiliar surroundings of the hospital, she has someone whom she knows, loves and with whom she can share her experiences. An expectant mother should never be left alone in labour. This ideal is often difficult to achieve, and the presence of the father can be invaluable. In the second stage of labour, he sits by the head of the delivery bed, attending to his wife, encouraging her, being involved with her. Together they witness the birth of the baby, and together their emotional bonds are strengthened. In using this method for some years, I have observed its value repeatedly; and the look of joy on the faces of father and mother as together they help in the delivery of their child is wonderful.

The question which must be answered is, 'Who decides that the father shall attend his wife's confinement?' The answer is simple, unequivocal: the wife. If the expectant mother wants her husband to be present, and *only* if she wants him, may he attend. Certainly it may be necessary to ask him to leave if some operative procedure is required or some untoward event occurs, but if this has been discussed during pregnancy, no difficulty should arise.

LABOUR – A WOMAN'S CHOICE

Until very recently women usually went into labour at a specific, but usually unpredictable, time when the pregnancy had lasted about 40 weeks. Labour started and continued for a variable number of hours, interference only taking place if the baby's life seemed threatened or, in rare cases, if the life of the expectant mother was at risk. This 'hands off' philosophy meant that about one woman in ten had a labour which lasted for more than 24 hours, and some women laboured for days. This attitude has changed. Today it is unusual for a woman to continue in true labour for more than 24 hours without help being given to deliver her of her baby, and many doctors intervene if a woman has been in true labour for more than 12 hours. What I have written does not apply to women in 'false labour', so some women continue to feel that they have been in labour for days, usually because no one has bothered to explain what was happening.

The change to earlier 'interference' has been beneficial in that expectant mothers have been spared hours of pain and it has reduced the threat to the baby which occurs if labour is prolonged. It has also had the effect of permitting a different attitude, by doctors, to labour.

Today, a woman can choose one of three ways for her labour to be conducted. These ways are first, 'natural childbirth'; second, traditional childbirth and third, elective childbirth. Of course, the choice may have to be altered if something occurs in late pregnancy or during the labour which threatens the life of the baby.

Natural childbirth

In this method the woman expects to go into labour spontaneously, to have her man with her during labour, to receive few or no drugs and to be delivered without the aid of instruments, although she may require an episiotomy. This method, in which psychoprophylaxis is often used, is splendid for those women who prefer it and who are attended by sympathetic, helpful, communicative medical attendants. Of course, if the labour lasts for more than 18 to 24 hours, the doctor may decide to intervene, but usually only does so after discussion with the expectant mother.

Traditional childbirth

The woman goes into labour spontaneously, and is given drugs, as needed. In the active part of the first stage and in the second stage, she may choose an inhalational analgesic, or request an epidural anaesthetic. If labour is progressing more slowly than expected, she may be given an intravenous drip into an arm vein. This drip contains a drug called Syntocinon which has the effect of stimulating the uterus to contract more strongly, so that the duration of labour is reduced.

Traditionally, the progress of the labour is followed and notes are made by the nursing staff. The nurses make sure that the expectant mother is not becoming dehydrated and check her pulse rate, her temperature and her blood pressure at intervals. They also examine her abdomen to see how deeply the baby's head is settling into the mother's pelvis, and to check on the frequency and strength of the uterine contractions. (These examinations are also made in women who have chosen natural childbirth).

Recently a change in management has occurred which I believe to be an improvement. The nurses make the same observations, but instead of writing notes, they mark them on a special chart, called a partogram, which gives a visual display of the progress of labour. By studying a large number of partograms, doctors have been able to determine more accurately how labour normally progresses. They have found, for example, that the cervix normally dilates, or opens, at a fairly steady rate, once labour is established and they can anticipate how much dilated it is expected to be after any chosen number of hours of labour. They have recommended that if the dilatation of the cervix is lagging two or more hours behind what it was expected to be, labour should be encouraged by setting up an intravenous drip containing Syntocinon. If this method is chosen, as it is increasingly, a woman in labour needs to be examined vaginally every 2 hours as well as abdominally so that the degree to which the cervix is dilated can be estimated accurately. The value of using partograms is that the duration of labour is reduced but the doctor only intervenes to set up the drip if progress is slow. Since delivery is often accelerated it is also called accelerated labour.

Elective accelerated childbirth

Elective childbirth is derived from the accelerated form of traditional childbirth. In this method the woman and her doctor decide beforehand on what day childbirth will take place. Of course, the choice of the day is only finally confirmed when everything is ready. This means, in general, that the pregnancy is near term, that the baby's head has settled snugly into the woman's pelvis and that the cervix is soft, shortened and at least 2 centimetres dilated.

On the elected day, the woman comes into hospital early in the morning. The doctor examines her to confirm his findings and then breaks the bag of waters with a special instrument. This procedure is called an amniotomy. At the same time he sets up an intravenous drip containing Syntocinon which stimulates the uterus to contract. Syntocinon is run at a rate which is increased until the uterine contractions occur regularly and strongly at about 3 minute intervals and each lasts about 90 seconds. The rate at which the drip flows is adjusted by a nurse who has to be in attendance constantly so that the dangers of too fast a drip are avoided. If the drip runs in too fast it may make the uterine contractions too strong and too frequent so that the baby fails to get enough oxygen from the mother's blood, and its life is in danger. Many hospitals now use a machine called an automatic infusion pump, which automatically regulates the rate of the drip, increasing or slowing the rate if the contractions are too infrequent or too frequent.

Because of the possible risk to the baby from the intravenous drip its heart rate is monitored by a special machine called a fetal heart monitor. The changes in the rate of the baby's heart are electronically converted into a pictorial graph on the machine and give a good indication of whether or not it is getting sufficient oxygen.

Once labour is properly established, an epidural anaesthetic is started, so the woman feels no pain. Labour continues in this way and most women can be expected to give birth within 12 hours. If this does not occur the doctor usually recommends that a caesarean section should be performed, or he may permit the woman to sleep and repeat the drip on the next day.

You can see that the advantage of elective accelerated childbirth is that you know the day on which your baby will be born, and can plan accordingly; you know that you will only be in labour for 12 hours at the longest and that your baby will be born by the evening. You can also be pretty sure that your doctor will be present to deliver your baby because he or she can arrange his work load better, and can keep himself free of other activities on the day he electively induces your labour and augments the uterine contractions with the intravenous drip.

The disadvantages are that the method requires a good deal of electronic equipment and constant observation by a nurse which makes labour a mechanical, impersonal process. A further disadvantage is that a woman, who chooses this method for the delivery of her baby, should be aware that although the duration of labour is reduced and she knows that she will deliver her baby on a certain day, the chances of her having a caesarean section are doubled, to between 7 and 12 per cent of all elective accelerated inductions, and that a larger number of babies become jaundiced in the first week of life.

It is also essential that the woman and her doctor are sure that the pregnancy has reached its full duration and that the baby is not premature. As I have written earlier, the best way of making sure is for a woman to be examined in the first 10 weeks of pregnancy. But if she has not, there are other ways of finding out if the baby is mature or not. These are rather complicated and may involve putting a needle into the fluid surrounding the baby and taking a sample. The needle is pushed into the amniotic sac through the mother's abdomen, and the fluid is tested for certain chemical substances which indicate that the baby is mature.

What I have tried to suggest is that today there are different approaches to labour, but the final choice is yours, provided of course that nothing occurs which makes it necessary for the doctor to intervene to rescue your baby from a hostile environment. You are having a baby: you should be able to choose how you want to have it after discussion with your doctor.

THE BABY AFTER BIRTH

The mother gives one further push, her husband sits beside her whispering to her, encouraging her. Her doctor gently and skilfully steers the baby's head through her vulva, so that it is born. Mucus streams from its nose and mouth; its mouth moves in sucking motions; and it may open its eyes. A further contraction occurs, the mother gently pushes and the baby slips out, still guided by the doctor, to lie on the bed between the mother's legs. It is born. It blinks it eyes; it jerks its arms and legs, clasping and extending its fingers. The umbilical cord, which has been its lifeline for so long, still beats. The nurse sucks its mouth clear of mucus with a rubber tube attached to a suction bulb. The baby takes in a convulsive gasp, and cries for all to hear.

The baby, which has grown from a single cell only visible under the microscope, has now developed into a living being made up of millions upon millions of cells. Some are formed into complex organs; some into bone; some into skin; some into the blood which carries the life-giving oxygen around the body. Its colour becomes pinker and pinker; the umbilical cord stops beating. It is cut. The baby is an independent, perverse, beautiful, irritating, intelligent, dependent, stupid, helpful individual. Which characteristics it will develop depends to a large extent upon its inheritance, but to no small extent upon the upbringing it will receive from its mother and father. The attitudes it will adopt will largely be theirs.

What does it look like, this newborn infant, as it lies crying between its mother's legs, or cuddled within her arms? It will be about 50 cm, or 20 in, long and will weigh anything from 2,500 g (5½ lb) to 4,500 g (10 lb) – with an average of 3,300 g (7 lb 4 oz). Its birthweight depends on several factors, such as the physique of its parents, its race, whether or not its mother was ill in pregnancy, and the socio-economic level of its parents. But between these weights, the baby will be normal and healthy, and cause no anxiety.

Its head is rounded, the bones firm, although still separated to leave a diamond-shaped soft space above the forehead and a Y-shaped edge at the back of the head. The baby's brain will grow in the first years of life, and the separation of the bones enables the skull to expand easily. Its head is likely to be covered with fine hair, but some babies are almost bald. You cannot tell from this how its hair will grow later, nor whether it will be prematurely bald! Its ears stand out firmly. Its nose is developed. Its eyes open and blink, but are a slate-grey colour. The real colour of its eyes comes later. Its mouth moves as it makes sucking noises or cries. Its body is rounded; its skin smooth. The lanugo hair which covered it in the uterus has gone, except on its shoulders. Its arms and legs are normal, and the fingers and toes have nails which project beyond their tips. It moves its arms and legs, and if a loud sound is made near it, jerks them convulsively. Its genitals are normal. If a boy, the penis hangs limply, the foreskin projecting beyond its tip, and the testicles are in the scrotum. If a girl, the labia majora are well developed and in contact, so that the vulva is concealed.

It lies peacefully, breathing gently, moving its limbs from time to time. It is this miracle of life which the mother has fed in her womb for the 40 weeks, and has now expelled during the hours of labour (Fig. 14/2).

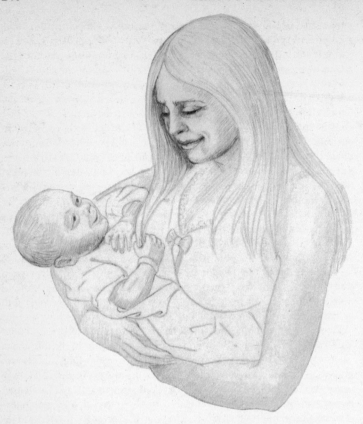

FIG. 14/2 The new-born baby held in its mother's arms

EXAMINATION OF THE BABY

Over 97 per cent of newborn babies are perfect, but in the remaining
3 per cent a defect may be found. The majority of the defects can be
treated successfully, often by surgery, provided that they are
detected in the first days of life. The doctor will examine the baby
systematically and carefully, once its breathing is established. He will
examine its head, and look into its mouth to make sure that it has no
cleft palate. Because of the pressure on the head of the baby during

its passage along the birth-canal, the scalp is often swollen and misshapen, particularly over its posterior part. The swelling is due to congestion of the skin and seeping of fluid into the scalp tissues. It is called a 'caput', and disappears completely within three days. The doctor will then test the movement of the baby's arms and legs, and will pay special attention to its hips, as there is a congenital condition which causes dislocation of the hips. If this is detected and treated by special splinting in the first three months of life, it is completely curable. He will listen to its chest, and examine its abdomen. In particular, he will look at its genitals to make sure that its testicles are normal if it is a boy, and that its vagina is properly formed if it is a girl. Some of the congenital defects cannot be detected by examination – one of these is a strange, and rare, defect called phenylketonuria. If this is not detected early in life, accumulation of a certain substance in the body can lead to mental retardation of the child. Only 1 in 10,000 babies has the defect, but it is now considered that all babies should be tested in the first week of life. The test is quite simple. A sample of the baby's urine is placed on a specially treated piece of paper, which stains if the baby has the defect. Treatment is to give a diet which does not contain phenylalanine, the offending substance.

THE FIRST BATH

It was traditional that soon after birth the baby was weighed (everyone wants to know its weight!) and then bathed. The white, greasy vernix was washed off with soap and water, and the baby powdered and dressed, to be admired by all. It is now known that this method of bathing the baby removed all the protective grease from its skin, and permitted the germs in the air, or blown from its mother's mouth and nose, to settle on the skin, to grow and cause infections. Today, in general, babies are not bathed. Their skin is cleaned with a cleansing agent which is also antiseptic, called pHisohex, but not all the vernix is removed, a fine, invisible layer remaining. Since hospitals have used this method, the incidence of skin infection in babies has dropped very considerably.

CIRCUMCISION

The Jews circumcise their boys on the 8th day of life to fulfil
Abraham's covenant with God; the Muslims circumcise their boys at
puberty as a symbol of reaching manhood; Aboriginal tribes in the
Australian desert circumcise their boys, partly ceremonially as an
initiation to manhood, partly for hygiene as the desert sand can
irritate the foreskin. Circumcision of males has a long religious
tradition; but in modern times, in the U.S.A. and Australia particularly, it has become a routine performance, not for religious reasons,
but because it is the custom. It is said that mothers demand it, doctors
profit by it, and babies cannot complain about it. The reasons given
are that removal of the foreskin makes the penis cleaner, prevents
masturbation, makes it less sensitive so that ejaculation is delayed in
coitus, prevents cancer of the cervix in women, and prevents cancer
of the penis in men. The evidence for all these arguments, except the
last, is very shaky. The normal foreskin is adherent to the glans of the
penis until the infant is a year old. After this time, it can be drawn
back, and if the boy is taught to do this, he can keep his foreskin clean.
It will not fix his mind on sex. Nor does the absence of a foreskin
prevent masturbation, which anyhow is a normal activity. Circumcision does not improve a man's sexual performance, nor does it
decrease it: it has no effect. There is no evidence, at all, that secretions which may be found under the foreskin cause cancer of the
cervix in women, although many researchers have tried to prove this.
The only men who develop cancer of the foreskin are those who are
unhygienic. If as children they had been taught to draw back the
foreskin and to clean it, cancer would not have occurred.

None of the so-called medical reasons for circumcision is valid, and
there is strong evidence that the foreskin *protects* the glans of the
penis, which is a delicate, sensitive structure. Circumcised babies may
develop tiny ulcers around the 'eye' of the glans, and in a few cases
have developed a tightness of the opening, which causes pain on
urination. Although these are minor happenings, they suggest that
the foreskin has a protective function, especially in infancy.

The decision whether the baby shall be circumcised is, of course,
that of the parents, but they should consider the evidence before they
decide, and not decide just because 'everyone has it done, and he will
feel different from his friends if he hasn't been circumcised'. That is
not a reason at all.

Chapter 15

Lying-in and Going Home

The puerperium is the time during which the genital organs, particularly the uterus, slowly return to their non-pregnant state, and when all the other changes which occurred in pregnancy disappear. This period lasts about 8 weeks.

Traditionally the first part of the puerperium was a time of 'lying-in'. It was a time when the woman was kept away from others (particularly men) because she was losing a bloody substance from her vagina and was therefore 'unclean'. It was not realized at that time that the bloody substance, called lochia, was a mixture of blood and the break-down products of tissues discharged as the uterus slowly became smaller and more like a non-pregnant uterus. The tradition of segregation during the lying-in period has largely gone, but many of the surrounding influences, such as the belief that the woman was unclean, have persisted until quite recently.

Up to the last decade, women in the first weeks of the puerperium have been treated as ignorant, idle, ill women who required careful discipline so that they did not damage themselves, and who were expected to fit into hospital routine, however ridiculous, with humbleness and without question. The medical staff 'knew' that if the patient got up before the seventh day after childbirth, prolapse of the uterus would result. So the patient was confined to bed, she found difficulty in passing urine and became constipated. When she did get out of bed, her muscles were so weak that her first steps were faltering. These changes confirmed in the medical attendants' eyes that a puerperal woman was a 'sick woman'. They knew this despite the evidence that in many lands women started work very soon after childbirth without ill effect. Women are often emotional after childbirth which is, after all, a most moving experience, and the mood changes again confirmed the opinion that the patient was ill. For three decades, the baby was separated from the mother and placed in a nursery to be observed by the father like watching fish in an aquarium, and to be brought out to the mother for feeding, who was treated like a battery hen.

Today a new and more sensible approach dominates the care of the puerperal woman. This new philosophy recognizes that the puerperal woman is an intelligent, healthy individual, who has just achieved a most memorable event: she has given birth to a live, healthy baby. She is a person who is subject to emotional moods, for childbirth is a heady thing. She will have to adjust to the demands which the infant will make of her life. This can be difficult, but is less so if she is treated with helpful understanding in the early days of the puerperium, and has received adequate instruction in the 'right approach to parentcraft' during pregnancy.

She is a person who is anxious to see, to touch and to care for her child with the helpful co-operation of the nursing staff. Of course, there may be problems, but most of these can be readily overcome.

The new approach to the puerperium makes three main points. First, although more rest is needed in the early days, the patient should be able to get up and walk about as soon as she wishes. Secondly, in general it is far better from many points of view for the baby to 'room-in' with the mother. Thirdly, mother and baby can go home not on a fixed day, but when conditions are most suitable for them.

Rest

Immediately after the drama of delivery and the excitement of receiving her husband's congratulations, the patient is full of emotional well-being and rather tired. Most women sleep for a while, a few asking for a sedative as they are too excited to sleep. When the mother wakes, she will certainly want to see and hold her baby, and from this time it may well join her in her room. She can get out of bed when she likes, but many women prefer to stay in bed for the first 24 hours, and luxuriate in rest! After this time she should get up, and walk about. It improves the tone of her muscles, it increases the blood flow through her tissues, and it enhances the drainage of the lochia. Moreover, women who practise early ambulation feel much fitter. Swabbing rounds and bed-pans (which are revolting but necessary things) are no longer required. The new mother still requires rest, but she can get this by having a siesta of two hours between lunch-time and visiting time. In many hospitals visiting hours are becoming much more generous as they should be, and children are allowed to visit their mother and newly born brother or sister.

Rooming-in

This term implies that for all, or most of the day, the child remains in its cot beside the mother's bed. Of course, if either the mother or child are not fit, perhaps after an operation or because the baby is premature, rooming-in cannot be practised. But most mothers prefer to have the baby with them, instead of seeing it through the nursery window, and touching it only at feeding time. Rooming-in enables the mother to become adjusted to the child, to become accustomed to its behaviour, and to interpret its needs at a time when experienced help is available to reassure her. Rooming-in has the additional advantage that by treating mother and child as a single 'set' or 'unit', cross-infection between babies, always a bug-bear in maternity hospitals, is reduced to a minimum. 'Rooming-in' also seems to make breast-feeding easier. This is so important a subject that it deserves, and gets, a chapter to itself (see Chapter 18).

Getting to know your baby

Unfortunately many hospitals seem to be organized more for the benefit of the staff than for the mothers and the babies. Hospital routines become fixed and are followed without thought for the real needs of the mother. Such routines can be destructive to the period of adjustment every woman has to go through as she gets to know her baby.

Rooming-in helps a good deal and even more important is the help given by informed, unhurried, communicative staff. It may surprise you that many women find that at first they do not feel an overwhelming love for their newborn baby. They have been taught that once the baby is born, they will find that they have a sudden burst of mother-love, only to be disappointed, when the baby has been born, that it is not there. The baby is neither as exceptionally beautiful nor as cuddly as the new mother had expected. The lack of a surge of mother-love can induce guilt, but a woman should know that this is normal. Mother-love does not happen instantaneously. It takes time to get to know your baby, and you will find quite quickly that you have fallen in love with it. The development of mother-love is helped by rooming-in and particularly by cuddling, yet in some hospitals neither are encouraged. Cuddling, which means body contact, is a strong force in helping you create the bonds of love which unite you with your baby. Touch, body contact, is equally important to your baby; because it gives it the feeling of warmth and security it needs. The cuddled baby is the contented baby. You cannot cuddle your baby too much. You will not spoil it, whatever the old wives say.

Going home

The day of discharge should vary to suit the particular mother and her baby. If the mother is normal, as is likely, she should be able to go home whenever she feels fit, once lactation is established, confident that she can cope with the baby. During her stay in hospital, she will have learned to bath the baby, and will have acquired the confidence that it is not as fragile as she had thought. She will have learned to interpret its cry, and to know which cry means 'I'm wet, change me', which 'I'm hungry, feed me', and which 'I'm full of wind, burp me'! She will have learned how much the baby depends on her, and yet how much it has its own character.

It is wise to remember that babies feel atmosphere. Quite often the change from the noisy hospital to the quiet home is noticed but not understood by the baby. Because of this, in the first two days at home it is irritable and fractious. The mother may think that her milk 'isn't doing it any good', but this is not the reason, and is no occasion for changing to a formula milk. What the baby wants is to feel secure. This it does when it is held close to its mother and cuddled. The prescription for fractious babies in the first few days at home is frequent cuddling.

THE LOCHIA

The three most obvious indications that the mother is no longer expectant are that her stomach is at last flat, or at least flatter than it was, that she has a baby to feed and care for, and that she is discharging lochia. The lochia is the bloody discharge from the uterus which is now shrinking back (or involuting) to its normal size. During pregnancy the uterus was the capsule within which the fetus lived and grew. It protected the fetus from the outside environment; it provided for its nourishment through the placenta; and, finally, by its muscular contractions it expelled the baby into the world. Now these functions are over, the uterus undergoes involution. Immediately after birth it weighs 1,000 g (2⅕ lb) and can be felt as a firm, globular bulge reaching up to the umbilicus. By the 14th day after childbirth, it will have shrunk to 350 g (11 oz), and can no longer be felt in the abdomen. By the 60th day (8 weeks) after childbirth, it is back to normal size. Involution is brought about by a shrivelling-up of the muscle fibres and the absorption of their substance, partly into the blood stream and partly into the lochia. The lochia is made up of blood from the site where the placenta was attached, and the crumbling of the lining of the uterus which had developed so greatly in pregnancy. In the first 5 days after childbirth, the lochia mostly consists of blood, and is consequently red in colour. For the next 5 to 10 days, it is reddish-brown as the blood loss lessens and more of the uterine lining is expelled. By the 12th day, it has become pale, either yellowish or white; and the discharge persists, varying in amount, for up to six weeks. However, in most cases the discharge has ceased by the end of the third week. The duration of the red lochia varies very considerably, and occasionally it continues for 10 or more days, or episodes of red lochia may recur in the following weeks. They often follow urination, particularly when the mother is not breast-feeding her baby. If the red lochia persists for longer than three weeks, if it becomes as profuse as the amount lost on the first day of a menstrual period, or if clots are passed, the doctor should be consulted.

AFTER-PAINS

After delivery, the uterus does not stop contracting. The contractions continue painlessly for the most part, but in some women, particularly multigravidae, painful contractions persist in the first few days of the puerperium, and may require analgesics. They are especially likely to occur during breast-feeding.

BOWELS

In the past constipation was a problem, but today with early ambulation it is less so. Should a patient become constipated and feel uncomfortable, she should ask for treatment. Usually a gentle laxative, such as Senokot, or a rectal suppository, such as bisacodyl, is given.

URINATION

In the first 24 hours after childbirth, the mother sometimes finds it difficult to pass urine because of the stretching during delivery of the vaginal tissues and the tissues around the bladder. Early ambulation helps, and in fact most women have no trouble.

DIET

The old music hall song 'A little bit of what you fancy does you good' applies in the puerperium. Most women want a meal, certainly a cup of tea, after delivery; and in the puerperium a good wholesome diet, rich in protein and vitamins, with not too much carbohydrate, is needed. Most nutritionists recommend that the puerperal woman who breast-feeds should get at least 2,500 calories a day. The diet of a puerperal mother should be as generous as that she took during pregnancy, with an additional 500 ml (1 pint) of milk a day (some of which may be used in cooking).

ABDOMINAL BINDERS

Formerly it was believed that an abdominal binder was necessary to prevent prolapse and to help the uterus to involute. It is now known that a binder neither prevents a prolapse nor encourages involution, and is not necessary on medical grounds, although a girdle may be required. Some multigravidae feel that the uterus 'flops about' and are more confident and comfortable if they wear a girdle. The choice should be that of the patient, but she should know that the reason for her choice is not medical but psychological.

THIRD DAY BLUES

On about the third day of the puerperium, the excitement of the new baby has diminished a bit. The mother has found that she has an independent, demanding infant to cope with, milk may be filling her breasts which may be tender, and the emotional sensitivity noted earlier may produce a reaction. Depression, mood changes or fits of crying occur for no reason. Everything is going well, but suddenly the patient bursts into a sobbing fit, and after the episode feels better. She knows that she is being silly, but can do nothing to stop it. The thing to remember is that 'third day blues' (which may occur on the fourth or fifth day) are not uncommon, and need sympathetic understanding from the husband and the medical attendants.

EXERCISES

With early ambulation and an intelligent mother, the routine exercises recommended in the past are probably unnecessary. However, many doctors still believe in exercises, and some women require them. Each woman must make up her own mind. The exercises shown in the following diagrams have been used with success in The Women's Hospital, Crown Street, Sydney (Fig. **15/1**).

FIG. 15/1 Postnatal exercises. The following exercises are to restore your muscle tone, and your figure after childbirth. The exercises should be done daily, each one at least five times, for a period of three months

Exercise 1
To tighten abdominal muscles
Lying on back, one pillow under head. Knees raised up. Place hands on tummy, tighten muscles, relax, and repeat five times. Make sure this is done correctly, the movement is inward. If your chest moves during the exercise the movement is incorrect

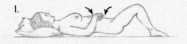

Exercise 2

To close separated abdominal muscles

Both hands on tummy, one hand placed over the other, hold the muscles down and against the resistance of your hands, lift head and shoulders off pillow, trying to rise to a sitting position. Repeat five times

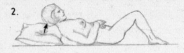

Exercise 3

To tighten the pelvic floor

Press the hollow of the back into the mattress, pull tummy muscles inward, tighten up inside as though preventing the bladder from working

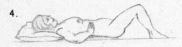

Exercise 4

To restore your waistline

Place hands on waist and tighten as though fastening a very tight skirt. Relax, and repeat five times

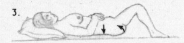

Exercise 5

For circulation and leg strengthening

Lying on back with legs straight.

(a) Move feet up and down
(b) Move feet round in circles
(c) Feet straight up, toes curled over
(d) Tighten the kneecap and tense leg muscles
(e) Ankles crossed, press thighs together, tighten up inside

Exercise 6
Kneeling
(a) Kneeling on hands and knees, first arch and then hollow the back, keep tummy muscles tight.
(b) Then move head and hip to the right. Relax and then move head and hip to the left

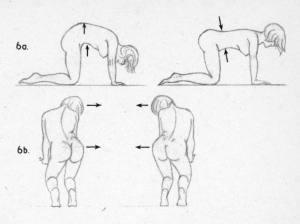

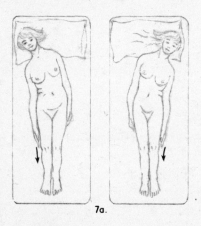

Exercise 7
Stretching exercises
Lying on back.
(a) Tummy muscles tighten, stretch arms down to each side alternately as though trying to grasp ankles.
Relax, and repeat five times
Lying on side.
(b) Lying on the left side, tighten tummy muscles, stretch top arm and top leg down so that body is in one long line.
Relax, and repeat the same exercise lying on the right side.
Relax, and repeat five times

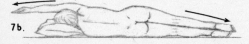

Exercise 8
Sitting up
Hands above head, tummy muscles tightened, tighten internally, stretch
forward and touch toes. Relax, and repeat five times

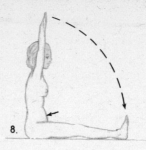

Exercise 9
Standing
When allowed to stand
Stand tall, tummy muscles
pulled inward, tighten up inside

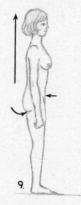

Exercise 10
Lying face down
Spend at least 20 minutes lying face down, one pillow under the face, one
pillow under the tummy, tightening the muscles

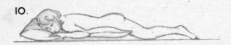

FIG. 15/1 (continued) Advanced postnatal exercises. These exercises require greater muscular energy, two are 'isometric', and all can be done when you feel ready

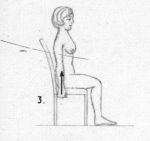

Exercise 1
Lying on back on bed, abdominal muscles tightened, arms folded across chest, raise head and shoulders and legs slowly. Slowly lower

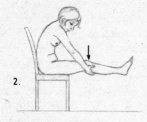

Exercise 2
Sitting on chair, legs extended, abdominal muscles tightened, place hands below knees and press legs down into the hands. Hold this position to the count of six

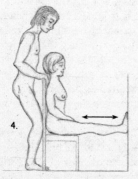

Exercise 3
Sitting on chair, place hands under the seat of the chair, feet firmly on floor and tighten all muscles. Imagine lifting self and chair towards the ceiling. Hold to count of six

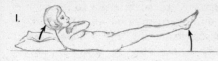

Exercise 4
Sitting on chair, feet on wall, push away from wall with abdominal muscles braced

VISITORS

In the matter of visitors, attitudes are changing. At one stage only the husband might visit, and this had a venerable tradition. In the seventeenth century, a great French obstetrician referring to the habit of holding a party on the third day of the puerperium when the child was baptised, wrote, 'Though there is scarce any of the company, which do not drink her health, yet by the noise they make in her ears, she loses it'.

Today it is realized that this attitude is unnecessarily restrictive. The husband should be allowed to visit at any time of the day, and it is nonsense to say that this interferes with hospital routine; the hospital is there for the patient, and not the patient for the hospital. Other visitors should be permitted at specific times each day, but should inquire first if they may visit. Each woman feels differently about visitors: some women want very few, preferring to be with their husbands; others want to keep in touch with their friends. But the friends should realize that the demands of a young baby, and the odd schedule of early waking found in hospitals, may make the mother very tired. For this reason, visits should be cut short. The visitor can always see the mother when she goes home, and nowadays this is tending to be sooner after childbirth.

ADJUSTING TO BEING A PARENT: THE 'CRISIS' OF PARENTHOOD

Unfortunately in most maternity units or hospitals, the mother is not encouraged to ask the questions which trouble her, and has little opportunity to make any real contact with a changing, busy nursing staff (who often give conflicting advice) and a busy, often uncommunicative doctor. Because of the routine of many hospitals, which excludes rooming-in and restricts the time her husband or some other close relative can visit her, she has difficulty in learning to know her baby and to understand the altered relationship she will have with her husband on her return home.

After her return home, five to ten days after childbirth, she may become increasingly isolated, particularly if it is her first child and if her relatives live at some distance. Because of costs of land, houses and high rents, most young couples have to live in the newer suburban areas of the cities, where public transport is inadequate, and shopping, mainly in supermarkets, can only be done if the woman has a car. The isolation is intensified as she realizes that she has to cope with mothering a new and unpredictable baby, whose needs fill her time by day and often by night. Even those visitors who come to see her, give her conflicting advice, and if she seeks medical help she often has to wait for an hour or more for a five minute consultation. Her isolation and the feeling of strain in trying to cope are intensified if her husband is unco-operative, and leaves most or all of the household tasks to his already over-burdened wife. No one has told her, neither during her upbringing nor during pregnancy, that mothering is not an instinct but has to be learned. No one has bothered to explain that she will have to adjust to her new role: that of being a mother, responsible for a 'small, utterly dependent creature', as one mother wrote to me. She had expected motherhood to be instantaneously joyous, but she found that the joy was often less than the tears and feelings of inadequacy. When extended families were usual, one or more people were immediately there to help to reassure and to comfort the anxious new mother. In our Western urbanized society, the nuclear family, mother, father and children living in suburbia, distant from relatives, imposes increasing strains on new mothers, so that exhaustion is common.

At unpredictable hours the baby asks to be fed, needs to be changed and cries. Crying may be a demand for food, for changing, for mothering and/or for cuddling, which gives the baby the tactile stimulation so needed for its development. But it is difficult to distinguish, at least in the first weeks, between a hunger cry, a discomfort cry and a cry for mothering.

Faced with the problems of learning how to mother her infant, often lacking knowledge and understanding of the baby's needs; more important, lacking support, the new mother begins to feel that her baby's demands are excessive, and that she is never going to be able to satisfy them. Many babies cry a great deal more than the mother expected, many sleep far less than expected, particularly at night. Because of this the new mother lacks sleep, and becomes increasingly exhausted. In her exhaustion she wonders if she will ever be able to be a good mother and why it is that she lacks the ability other women appear to have to cope with the small, selfish, continually demanding infant. She feels a failure and begins to be resentful towards the small infant who has disrupted her life so effectively, and may be damaging her relationship with her husband, even if he is particularly understanding.

She resents that she has been brought up to be a housewife *and* a mother, but now has not time to keep the house as clean and tidy as she would wish, and care for her intrusive child at the same time. This compounds her sense of failure. Her resentment towards her child may be replaced by temporary hostility. As one woman wrote 'you try to do everything to please the little leech, but it sobs and seems to reject everything you do, yet it dominates your life'. The new mother may feel helpless and believe that her failure to cope is a reflection on her. This may be followed by brief feelings of violence towards the baby and depression.

The baby, in turn, seems to notice the hostile environment. It vomits after feeds, it cries even more, it may have diarrhoea. All these suggest to the already harassed mother that she is not caring for it properly despite all her efforts. Her depression can worsen and she has periods of crying, periods of exhaustion, periods of irritability and even of irrationality.

Any sexual feeling she may have is dampened by the depression, and this in turn aggravates her anxiety as she worries about her husband's feelings towards her. If she is breast-feeding she wonders if it is weakening her and whether her milk is 'suiting' the baby. She may change to bottle-feeding only to find that the bottle-fed baby continues to make the same demands. Her anxiety and depression worsen and can last for weeks. She is in the 'crisis of parenthood'.

How do you cope with the 'crisis'? How can the problems of adjusting to parenthood be reduced?

Coping with the 'crisis'

It will help you if you remember that the period of adjustment is short, and that each day you and your baby learn to know each other better. In the first weeks you may find you have to feed your baby every two hours, but you can be sure that by six weeks it will have found its feeding pattern. If your baby cries 'too much' at first, you can be sure that it will cry less as time goes on. And a baby which cries, because it wants to be cuddled and to see and hear what is going on about it, instead of being left alone in a cot, is likely to be a more interested, intelligent child. You can go on doing the things you have to do and still cuddle your baby if you buy a baby-sling. Most peasant women carry their babies all the time and still do hard work in the home or in the fields. Why not do what they do, put your baby in a 'mei-tai', either on your back, or, if the baby is very young, across your front? The baby will like it and you will not feel so impatient if you are able to do what you have to do. If your baby cries a lot at night, wanting food or company, bring it into your bed and let it sleep with you, warm against your breathing body. You will not lie on it or smother it. Babies wriggle and move, so that if you started to lie on it, it would wake you within moments. If, at times, you feel guilty because you think that you hate your baby for demanding so much from you, do not worry. You do not really hate your baby and the hostile emotion was only a brief reaction to your tiredness.

In any 'crisis' it helps to have a sympathetic person with whom you can share your problem. If you and your husband have a close relationship, he will help care for the baby and will relieve you of some of the chores in the house. He will cuddle the baby, change the nappies and be generally supportive, so that you can rest more. He will know that during the period of adjustment the baby controls your lives, and he will understand and help. Also, if you have a near relative who can help you care for the baby, or who can relieve you so that you can get out of the house for a while, ask her. But if you have not, join one of the community helping organizations which exist. These are the Nursing Mothers Associations and Parent Education Centres in Australia, The La Leche League in Britain and the U.S., and Play Group Associations. This supportive help can make all the difference. Make sure you find out the addresses and telephone numbers of one of the organizations, before you leave hospital and that you join it. The organizations provide 24-hour telephone counselling and home visiting when needed.

Reducing the problems of adjusting to parenthood

The way to do this begins long before the baby is born. When I was researching this part of the book I wrote asking women if they had difficulties in adjusting to parenthood. The women were members of the Childbirth Education Association or the Nursing Mothers Association of Australia. The response was tremendous, and the suggestions which follow were made by them.

● In schools and at home, education for parenthood should be part of the curriculum for both boys and girls. The course should include discussions of the emotional and psychological changes which occur during pregnancy and after, as well as the physical changes which occur, so that women can build up confidence in themselves as mothers, and so that men can learn that as fathers they have an important role in helping their wives during the period of adjustment to parenthood.

● In the pre-natal months expectant mothers and expectant fathers should have the opportunity to learn about adjusting to parenthood so that both are involved in the process, and both understand that supportive help is needed, especially by the new mother.

● Mothers must remember that they are not superwomen and so must their husbands! It is almost impossible to care for home, husband and baby as efficiently as a woman would like. You can not be a full-time housewife and a full-time mother; one function has to be neglected during the period of adjustment to some extent at least, and that must be the role of housewife.

● Mothers must remind themselves that their feelings of inadequacy are shared by large numbers of other mothers and they are neither alone nor abnormal.

● Women must exert pressure to make sure that there are centres in hospitals and in the community where they can meet other mothers, share experiences, obtain confidence, and where they can meet experienced, helpful counsellors. In the future it is to be hoped that in every community there will be a Resource Centre or a Family Health Service which will supplement the work of existing organizations.

● Women should work to see that in each community a baby-sitting service and an emergency home help service is provided for mothers, at a reasonable cost.

If women go on using their influence, we may obtain what Caroline Pearce of Adelaide sees as needed to supplement the other suggestions. She says that the corner shop should be 'restored to its rightful place as a convenience', and as a social contact point. She believes that home deliveries of household goods should be encouraged. She asks that town planners help to reduce physical isolation by locating shops sensibly, by designing them well, and by making them accessible to mothers with babies and small children.

She writes: 'In our society, women need help and support so that they may develop healthy relationships with their children, who may in turn be capable of healthy and meaningful relationships with others'.

THE POSTNATAL CHECK-UP

It is usual for the doctor to request that the puerperal mother return to see him between 6 and 8 weeks after confinement. This postnatal check-up is of considerable importance, as it enables the doctor to make sure that all is well, and it gives the mother the opportunity to discuss any problems which may still cause her anxiety. Many doctors want to see the baby as well as the mother.

The examination is quite painless, and the extent of the investigations which need to be made depends on whether the pregnancy and labour were normal or complicated. If they were normal, the doctor will merely palpate the mother's abdomen, examine the cervix with a speculum, and perhaps take a further cervical smear. He will also do a pelvic examination so that he can determine if the uterus has involuted properly. If the mother has any complaints, he will deal with these.

In recent years, the postnatal visit has provided the opportunity to discuss with the doctor the subjects of birth control for herself and immunization programmes for her baby. These two matters are today probably the most important aspects of the postnatal visit.

SEXUAL INTERCOURSE AFTER CHILDBIRTH

Although it is usual to await the postnatal examination before sexual intercourse is resumed, this is not necessary. Provided that coitus does not cause pain, it may be resumed once the lochia has ceased. Whether or not sexual intercourse is resumed is a matter for the couple to discuss, the woman making the final decision.

A number of women who have been 'torn' during childbirth or who have had an episiotomy, find that intercourse is painful. Often the husband needs to spend more time arousing the wife sexually by kissing, hugging and by mutual pleasuring so that she is fully relaxed and her vagina is wet before they start having sexual intercourse. Sometimes, however, coitus continues to be painful. If this occurs you should see your doctor and explain exactly how and where it hurts so that help can be given you. You should not be ashamed to see the doctor; you are not 'wasting his time'.

THE RETURN OF MENSTRUATION AFTER CHILDBIRTH

If the mother is breast-feeding, menstruation does not usually return for about 24 weeks, or 6 months. Ten per cent of women menstruate by 10 weeks after childbirth, 20 per cent by 20 weeks, and 60 per cent by 30 weeks. Ovulation is unusual before the 20th week after childbirth, but about 2 per cent of lactating women do ovulate before this time. However, pregnancy rarely occurs in the first 20 weeks of the puerperium. Even if the menstrual periods start, breast-feeding can be continued as the quality of the milk is not altered during menstruation.

In modern Western society, about 70 per cent of mothers do not breast-feed. These women are at much greater risk of pregnancy, as in over 80 per cent menstruation and ovulation have begun by the 10th week after the birth of the child.

Chapter 16

The Rhesus Factor and Other Matters

THE RHESUS PROBLEM

Until 1940 the reason why a number of babies were born-dead, swollen with fluid and looking like small Buddhas, puzzled many obstetricians. They were also puzzled by the fact that some babies, who were apparently normal at birth, became severely jaundiced and died within a few days. The explanation of these two phenomena suddenly became clear. In 1940 two scientists had noted that the red blood cells of certain women had a strange substance, called an antigen, attached to their surface. If these red blood cells were injected, as in a blood transfusion, into the blood stream of another person, they would provoke the formation of substances called antibodies in that person's blood stream. But this reaction only occurred if the person receiving the blood transfusion did not have any red cells of her own which had the same antigen on their surface. If she had such cells, no reaction occurred.

Once the antibodies were formed, they attached themselves to the antigen sites on the injected, or foreign, red blood cells; and, in a complicated way clumped (or agglutinated) them. The red blood cells agglutinated in this way first became swollen, then burst and were destroyed. (In a way, this is similar to what happens when a heart is transplanted into another person, and is then 'rejected' by that person.) During their experiments with the antigen, the doctors had prepared a serum by injecting the red cells of Rhesus monkeys into guinea pigs, and had found that all Rhesus monkeys had the antigen attached to their red blood cells. Because of this, they called the antigen the Rhesus antigen, or the Rhesus factor. They then decided to study how many Americans had the Rhesus factor attached to their red blood cells. After much investigation, they found that 85 per cent of Americans had the Rhesus factor attached to their

red blood cells, and 15 per cent had no Rhesus factor on their red
blood cells. Those with the factor they called Rhesus positive; those
without it Rhesus negative. Further investigations of other races
showed some differences. For example, Europeans had the same
proportion of Rhesus negative people; but in North India, the incidence of Rhesus negative people was only 10 per cent; and in South
India less than 5 per cent; whilst Rhesus negative people were almost
never found amongst Chinese. This strange difference of numbers of
Rhesus negative people in different races is not understood.

More importantly from the point of view of our discussion, other
investigators remembered the unexplained deaths of the jaundiced
babies, and inquired what was the Rhesus group of their mothers. In
every case the mother had been Rhesus negative and the father had
been Rhesus positive. And in every case the mother had previously
received a blood transfusion, or had one or more previous pregnancies.

A woman marries a man not because of his blood group, but
because he is attractive to her, or has qualities which appeal to her. In
short, because she is in love with him. Since 85 per cent of people are
Rhesus positive and 15 per cent Rhesus negative, the odds are that in
10 per cent of marriages the wife may be Rhesus negative and the
husband Rhesus positive. At some stage, quite naturally, they decide
to have a baby. Because it inherits half of its genes from its father, it
may be Rhesus positive or it may be Rhesus negative. If it is Rhesus
negative, no problem arises; but if it is Rhesus positive, problems
may occur with a later pregnancy, although the first baby will not be
affected. During the pregnancy, the Rhesus positive baby grows
happily in its mother's womb, but off and on in late pregnancy tiny
numbers of its Rhesus positive red blood cells may seep across the
placenta and enter the mother's blood stream, where they are
destroyed. At delivery, however, much larger amounts of fetal blood
get into the mother's blood stream. The amount may be too great to
be destroyed immediately, and the surviving cells are recognized as
being foreign invaders, which have Rhesus positive badges on them!
The mother's defence system goes into action and special commando
cells, called immuno-competent cells, manufacture the destroying
substance (or antibody) which attaches itself to the foreign Rhesus
positive cells, coats their surface, clumps them and literally blows
them apart.

The mother's defence system, once stimulated, remains ever on the alert should any further Rhesus positive cells enter her body.

The couple decide to have a further child. Again it inherits half its genes from its father, and again it may be Rhesus positive. If it is, a strange thing now happens. The anti-Rh antibody, which the mother's immuno-competent cells have continued to manufacture, circulates through her blood stream, and because of its peculiar shape is able to pass through the placenta and enter the blood stream of the fetus. This does not happen in very early pregnancy, but becomes more and more likely as pregnancy advances. In the blood stream it meets the baby's normal Rhesus positive red blood cells, and coats them so that they burst. The burst red cells release a substance called bilirubin, which accumulates in the baby's blood and some of it is excreted into the amniotic sac in the baby's urine. As its red blood cells are destroyed, the baby becomes progressively so anaemic that it is bloated, Buddha-like and dies. If fewer red blood cells are destroyed, the baby remains alive but is born anaemic and jaundiced from the accumulation of bilirubin in its blood.

Once these facts had been discovered, it was possible to find out first, if the Rhesus negative mother had been stimulated to manufacture antibodies, by doing a test on her blood; and secondly, to determine how badly the baby was likely to be affected, by taking a sample of the amniotic fluid and estimating the amount of bilirubin in it. This test on the amniotic fluid was done first at about 28 weeks, and repeated once or twice more. The object of all these tests was to find out when it was more dangerous for the baby to be inside the uterus than to be born. Once born, its damaged blood could be replaced in an 'exchange transfusion' by Rhesus negative blood, which the antibodies could not attack since the red cells had no antigen on their surface. The transfused blood kept the baby alive whilst such antibodies as remained slowly decayed over the following weeks. Some babies needed further 'topping-up' transfusions, but by six weeks of life, they were all well. None of the antibodies the mother had transferred to them remained, and their Rhesus problem was over. Using these methods of care, most Rhesus affected babies now survive, but a few still die in the uterus. A New Zealand doctor thought that some of these could be saved if they could be given a transfusion whilst still in the womb, to help them survive there until they were slightly more mature and able to survive outside. He suggested that very badly affected babies, who were not yet Buddha-like but were still less than 34 weeks mature, should be treated in this way. It is a complicated procedure to perform an 'intra-uterine transfusion', but one-third of the babies treated in this way survive.

Today a treatment is available which will almost eliminate the problem, at least for those Rhesus negative women who have not started to manufacture antibodies. Scientists in Britain and the U.S.A. have discovered that Rhesus negative women can be protected by giving them an injection of a special antibody, made in the blood of Rhesus negative volunteers. The injection is only useful if given to a Rhesus negative mother who has not yet made any antibodies against Rhesus positive blood. The scientists believe that the special antibody works by coating and destroying any fetal Rhesus positive red blood cells which have entered the mother's blood stream during labour. The injection is painless, and is effective if given up to 72 hours after birth.

Provided the mother has been tested in pregnancy so that it is known whether she is Rhesus negative, and a sample of the cord blood of the baby is tested and found to be Rhesus positive, the special injection can be obtained and injected into the mother. This will protect her completely against the 'Rhesus problem'.

A number of doctors with different skills – immunologists, haematologists, obstetricians and paediatricians – have combined their activities to obtain this result. It is an example of team-work in medicine for the benefit of women.

GERMAN MEASLES (RUBELLA)

The careful observations by Dr Gregg in Sydney in 1941 first brought to our attention the dangers of German measles in the first half of pregnancy. German measles (rubella) is caused by a virus which can cross the placenta and infect the baby. It is a peculiar virus, as it prefers to grow in tissue which is just forming. Before the 10th week of pregnancy it has a wonderful opportunity, for the heart, the ears, and the skull of the fetus are forming at this time. If the virus gets into the tissue, the heart may be damaged, the hearing impaired, the eyes may develop cataracts, and the skull may not expand. Because of these serious complications affecting more than half of the babies, many doctors believe that a therapeutic abortion should be performed if a woman develops rubella in the first 12 weeks of pregnancy.

Some pregnant women come into contact with a case of rubella, either in their own family or in a neighbour's. Until very recently it was the custom to give them an injection of 'gamma globulin', which was painful, but which was said to protect the fetus from the virus. It is now known that the injections of 'gamma globulin' are of no value in protecting the babies.

It would be sad if nothing more could be said, but it can. A test has now been developed which will tell if a patient has had rubella, and once you have had rubella, you are protected for all time. A specimen of the person's blood is taken and the test made. In Australia, the U.S.A. and probably in most other countries, it has been found that more than 85 per cent of women have rubella before they reach the age of 16. The other 15 per cent have not had rubella, but a vaccine is available which will give these women a mild attack of rubella. They will not know that they have had rubella, but they will be protected.

Testing to tell if a woman has had rubella is rather complicated and expensive, and because of this the vaccine now being offered to all schoolgirls when they reach the age of 14. But since many women do not know if they have had rubella, it is expected that they will be tested if they wish. The most suitable time for testing to see if a woman has had rubella is when she decides to marry, or just before she decides to have a baby. If her test is positive, she knows that her baby is in no danger of being damaged by the rubella virus. If she decides that she will have the injection, she must take precautions to avoid becoming pregnant for two months after the injection. After that time she will have become protected against rubella, and there is no chance of her baby being damaged by the rubella virus.

GENERAL DISEASE AND PREGNANCY

Two conditions, in particular, require extra care during pregnancy. These are diabetes and heart disease. Any woman who is a diabetic or has heart disease should see her doctor as early as possible in pregnancy. The amount of insulin the diabetic requires during pregnancy fluctuates, and proper control of the diabetes can only be obtained by regular blood tests for sugar. In diabetes it is usual for the mother to be admitted to hospital at about the 32nd week, and to be delivered in the 37th week, but each case requires individual attention. Regular antenatal visits at short intervals are essential, and often the patient's doctor will seek the help of a physician who is interested in the disease. In diabetes, the help and co-operation of the expectant mother is essential if she is to have a live baby.

The patient with heart disease usually has no trouble in pregnancy, but in the more severe forms may require to go into hospital at about the 30th week for bed-rest. As is the case in diabetes, regular, frequent visits to her doctor throughout pregnancy are essential. She must also avoid putting on too much weight, which means that she must eat a balanced diet, avoiding excess carbohydrates, sweets and sugar. She must also avoid becoming anaemic, and her doctor will undoubtedly test her blood for anaemia and prescribe iron tablets. She must not omit to take these.

BREECH BABIES

In the middle of pregnancy, because the fetus is small and the amniotic sac relatively large, the baby tends to move around a good deal. At this time about 40 per cent of babies present with their bottom nearest the mother's pelvis. These are called breech presentations. By the 28th week, the percentage has dropped to 15 per cent; by the 34th week to 6 per cent; and by the 40th week less than 4 per cent of babies still present by the breech. The reason is that as pregnancy advances, there is more room for the legs in the upper part of the uterus, and the baby gets into the most comfortable position! Most of the babies which remain as breech presentations have their legs straight, the feet under the chin (Fig. 16/1).

In the past breech babies often died during delivery, but today with skilled attention, teamwork by the obstetrician, the anaesthetist and the nurses, these problems have been overcome. However, if the expectant mother still has a breech presentation when the pregnancy has reached 34 weeks' gestation, the doctor may try to 'turn it'. This is a simple manipulation, and is not painful, so the expectant mother does not need an anaesthetic. He is very gentle as he attempts to do the 'external version', and if the baby does not turn easily, he does not persist (Fig. 16/2). Before the manipulation, the mother should be sure that her bowels and bladder are empty, and that she is relaxed. If the doctor fails to turn the baby, he will probably ask the mother to have an X-ray to make sure that the pelvic bones and the cavity of the pelvis have a normal shape. A few obstetricians who fail to turn the

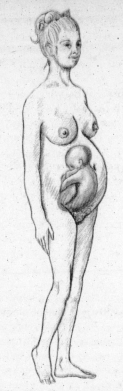

FIG. 16/1 The breech baby

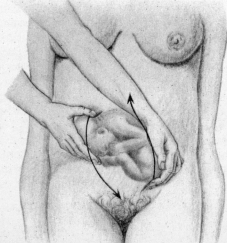

FIG. 16/2 Turning a
breech baby

baby without anaesthetising the expectant mother make a further attempt after giving her a general anaesthetic. When this is done, the woman may feel some slight abdominal discomfort and tenderness for a few days but, generally, the procedure is not followed by much pain.

Most breech babies are born easily, after a labour which is no longer or more difficult than if the baby was 'head-down', or more correctly was a cephalic, or vertex, presentation. But in certain cases, particularly if the baby is very large, a caesarean section will be performed.

The mother whose baby remains as a breech need have no anxiety, and when her baby is born she will see that its head has a beautiful round shape. When the baby lies as a cephalic presentation, its head is often temporarily distorted for a few hours after birth. It is of no consequence to the baby, and the shape becomes normal very rapidly.

MULTIPLE PREGNANCY

It is quite normal for most mammals to have a multiple pregnancy or litter. The human female usually only has a single baby in each pregnancy, but one pregnancy in 90 is a twin pregnancy; one pregnancy in 90×90 is a triplet pregnancy; and quadruplets occur once in $90 \times 90 \times 90$ pregnancies. There are two ways in which a multiple pregnancy can occur: either two, or more, eggs are released from the ovary at one time, and are fertilized by two different spermatozoa; or the single fertilized egg cell may completely divide at the stage of the blastocyst, and then *two* individuals develop, but have a single placenta. The first kind of twins are fraternal twins, who are no closer to each other in characteristics than any brother and sister. The second kind are identical twins, and are mirror images of each other. The fraternal twins make up 75 per cent of all twin pregnancies; identical twins only 25 per cent.

Twins are more frequent in African and Asian countries, and this is due to the higher proportion of fraternal twins, as identical twins occur equally often whatever the race or age of the mother. Amongst Caucasians, or Europeans, fraternal twins occur more frequently in families with a history of twins, in older women, amongst women who have had several children previously, and after injection of drugs which induce ovulation.

Each twin is always lighter than a singleton baby at the same stage of pregnancy, although, of course, the combined weight of the twins is greater than that of the singleton. Because of this, twins tend to be underweight at birth. As well, the size of the twins can vary very considerably. The difference between them is greater when they are identical twins, as one of them is greedy and takes the greater part of the nourishment which arrives through the placenta. Inside the womb, the twins lie side by side. In late pregnancy, it has been shown that in 45 per cent of cases both lie with the head over the mother's pelvis; in 25 per cent the leading twin has its head down, and the other twin is a breech; in 10 per cent the breech leads the head; and in 10 per cent both are breeches (Fig. **16/3**).

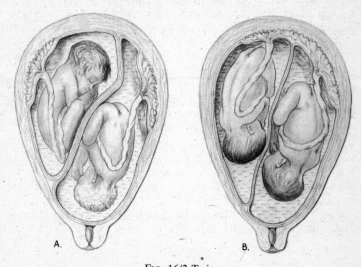

A.   B.

FIG. 16/3 Twins
(a) Fraternal twins from the chance fertilization of two ova
(b) Identical twins, from the fertilization of a single ovum and its later division into two identical embryos

The doctor may suspect twins when he finds that the uterus is larger than he anticipated calculating from the date of the last period (see Fig. **8/3**). There are other causes for the undue enlargement of the womb, but twins is the most common cause. It is possible he will be able to feel both babies, but this is unusual before the 28th week of pregnancy, by which time the expectant mother may herself suspect that she has twins. If the doctor is uncertain, he will arrange for an X-ray picture, which will show the two babies and their positions in the uterus. X-rays are usually avoided before the 24th week of pregnancy to reduce the risk of radiation to the babies.

A multiple pregnancy is a little more risky than a single pregnancy, but provided the expectant mother attends regularly for antenatal care, the risk is small. 'Toxaemia of pregnancy' occurs more frequently, as does anaemia. Many doctors prevent anaemia by giving the expectant mother iron tablets with a tiny amount of folic acid added, from about the 30th week of pregnancy. In late pregnancy, twins usually impose more discomfort on the expectant mother, than does a single infant. Her abdomen feels heavier, she has more backache, and swelling of her ankles and legs is quite common. It has also been found that twin pregnancies tend to end prematurely, and about one-quarter of twin babies are delivered by the 36th week. This premature rate can be reduced considerably with good antenatal care, and if the mother rests for a good deal of the day from the 32nd week on. She should certainly give up work, if she can afford to, by the 28th week.

Contrary to popular belief, labour in a twin pregnancy is no longer than in a single pregnancy, but the delivery of one or both of the twins is often aided by the doctor. There is often an interval of about 10 minutes between the birth of the twins, but no doctor today would allow an interval as long as the 65 days which was reported some years ago.

Finally, an old myth should be demolished. Twins are not less fertile than singletons when in their turn they marry.

AGE AND OBSTETRIC PERFORMANCE

Examination of the records from very large numbers of pregnancies in many countries has been made to see if age has any effect, good or otherwise, on obstetric performance. There has been surprising agreement that the least complications in pregnancy and during childbirth are found if the mother has been well-nourished from childhood, has some knowledge of what happens in pregnancy, is more than 155 cms (61 ins) tall, not over-weight nor emaciated, and aged between 18 and 30! Of course, this does not mean that younger or old mothers, fat or excessively thin mothers, or short women do not perform well. They do, but there is apparently a greater chance that complications will arise.

The teenage mother

There has been concern, particularly in the U.S.A., Britain and Australia, about the increasing number of teenage mothers, particularly those under the age of 17 who are unmarried. In Eastern countries, it is normal for marriage to take place soon after puberty, and for consummation of the marriage to occur either then or, as with Hindus, two to three years later, so that teenage pregnancies are not unusual. There is nothing to suggest that the teenage mother is in any way disadvantaged in pregnancy, provided that she seeks antenatal care as early as possible. In a study of teenage mothers which we have conducted in Sydney, we found that if the girl received antenatal check-ups, she had a slightly greater chance of developing 'toxaemia of pregnancy' than her older sisters, and was a bit more likely to become anaemic. The duration of labour was not increased; in fact labour seemed easier, and the average birthweight of her baby was not different from that of her older sisters, nor was there any increased risk that her baby would be born dead or die soon after birth. If the girl did not attend the antenatal clinic until late in pregnancy, as happened with many of the unmarried teenage mothers, we found that there was twice the chance that she would develop 'toxaemia of pregnancy' or become anaemic; and although the duration and conduct of labour was not altered, she had double the risk of losing her baby.

The importance of these observations is that every teenage girl who becomes pregnant, whether she is married or not, should seek antenatal care as early as possible. She need not be worried that the doctors and nurses will condemn her for getting pregnant – they will not; and they will be happy that she has had the sense to come along so that her pregnancy and labour may be made as easy as possible. Often the unmarried girl has many problems to face, and most maternity hospitals have a staff of qualified social workers who can advise and reassure her, can give her confidence, and talk to her with kindness and wisdom.

The older primigravida

About 5 per cent of women, usually of the higher socio-economic groups, delay becoming pregnant until they are more than 30 years old. Such a patient is called an 'older primigravida', rather than the previous term 'elderly primigravida', which is somewhat insulting to the expectant mother! The older primigravida may develop more complications in pregnancy than her younger sister, and because of this she should obtain antenatal care as early as possible in pregnancy so that any complications can be diagnosed and treated quickly.

The older primigravida has three times the risk of developing 'toxaemia of pregnancy', and a slightly greater chance of having a breech baby or a twin pregnancy than her younger sister. As 'toxaemia' can be controlled by bed-rest and drugs, this is of no great danger provided she is receiving competent antenatal care. Labour in the older primigravida tends to last rather longer than amongst her younger primigravid sisters, and her baby's birth needs to be helped by forceps or caesarean section more frequently. Even so, only about 10 per cent of these patients require caesarean section, whilst 35 per cent are delivered by forceps.

The grande multigravida

This term was first used in Dublin to describe those women who have had at least four previous pregnancies. These mothers are more likely to have complications in pregnancy and labour than women who have had fewer children, and the risk is greater if the mother is aged 35 or more. Unfortunately, this is the patient who most frequently neglects to obtain antenatal care. If she does seek antenatal care, the chance of a complication occurring in pregnancy or labour is greatly reduced. She is more likely to develop bleeding in pregnancy, and 'toxaemia of pregnancy' is a little more frequent. Although she may deliver a bigger baby, labour is usually quite rapid. However, she has a risk of bleeding after delivery until action is taken.

These findings emphasize the importance of regular antenatal visits, and delivery in a well-equipped hospital under the care of a well-trained doctor.

Chapter 17

Pregnancy Complications

In more than 70 per cent of pregnancies the antenatal period and the confinement are completely normal. In the remaining 30 per cent of pregnancies conditions may appear which require treatment so that a live, healthy baby is delivered by a healthy mother. The detection of the conditions whilst they are still mild is one of the purposes of good antenatal care. It is for this reason that the expectant mother was recommended to make regular visits to her doctor as described in Chapter 10. It can safely be said that the conditions only prove serious if the expectant mother fails to attend her doctor at the first sign of abnormality.

What are the signs which should lead an expectant mother to contact her doctor immediately, so that she may visit him or he may visit her at her house?

They can be listed as follows:

1. Bleeding in the first half of pregnancy, with or without cramping abdominal pains.
2. Severe abdominal pains in the first weeks of pregnancy.
3. Bleeding with or without abdominal pain in the second half of pregnancy.
4. Swelling of the fingers or face, particularly if accompanied by headaches or blurring of vision.
5. A gush of water from the vagina in the second half of pregnancy.

BLEEDING IN THE FIRST HALF OF PREGNANCY

The usual cause of bleeding in the first half of pregnancy is that the expectant mother is threatening to abort. About one pregnancy in seven ends as a 'spontaneous' abortion, which is the correct term for the lay euphemism of 'miscarriage'. All that the word abortion means is that the embryo or fetus is expelled from the uterus; it does not mean that the expectant mother has gone to an abortionist – that is called an 'induced' or 'criminal' abortion. In at least three-quarters of cases, the reason for a spontaneous abortion is that the fetus was not properly formed, and Nature is getting rid of it. In a few cases an abortion may follow a severe fever, such as pneumonia, and in even fewer cases the doctor may find an abnormality of the uterus or a weakness of the cervix. In the past a retroverted uterus (one which is 'bent back'), excessive coitus, fatigue, 'undue exertion', or a 'severe shock' were blamed for the occurrence of an abortion. It is now known that none of these causes an abortion.

The first sign of an impending, or threatened, abortion is usually bleeding. This may merely be some slight irregular 'spotting' of blood, followed after a few hours or days by a moderate discharge of blood from the vagina, which may resemble a menstrual period.

In other cases the bleeding is heavier at the start, and may be accompanied by some slight cramping pains, resembling period pains. Despite the anxiety caused to the expectant mother by the appearance of these symptoms, it is reassuring that more than 80 per cent of cases of threatened abortion settle down, and the pregnancy continues. If this happens, the baby will certainly be quite normal.

The expectant mother should inform her doctor at once if she bleeds in early pregnancy. He may suggest that she goes to bed for a few days, and that coitus is avoided for a couple of weeks. If she is anxious, as she may well be, he will probably prescribe a sedative to calm her down. The sedative also reduces the sensitivity of the uterus and calms it down. For many years a variety of vitamins and hormones were given to patients with threatened abortion. A favourite was progesterone, or one of the chemical substitutes for the natural drug. A great number of women received expensive injections or took expensive tablets of the progesterone-like drugs. There is now clear, certain evidence that neither progesterone, nor its chemical substitutes, is of any value in the treatment of threatened abortion, apart from a psychological value. There are cheaper and more effective ways of providing the expectant mother with the psychological support, and a wise, honourable New York obstetrician once recommended 'T.L.C. frequently every day'. T.L.C. stands for tender, loving care!

In 20 per cent of cases of threatened abortion, the bleeding increases and abdominal cramps become severe. The abortion is now probably inevitably going to occur. Many women who abort do not notice the threatened and inevitable stages, as they succeed each other too quickly. These patients complain of sudden bleeding and painful cramps, and on going to the toilet, expel 'something' from the vagina. The doctor should be called at once, and everything which has been discharged from the vagina should be kept for his inspection. If this is done, it makes his task much easier. On his arrival, the doctor usually gives the patient a pain-relieving drug, and then performs a pelvic examination. This will tell him if all of the fetus and the placenta have been expelled, or if some remains inside the uterus. If it does, the doctor will certainly wish the patient to go to hospital so that he may 'clean out', or curette, the cavity of the womb.

Statistics show that if a patient has seven pregnancies in her lifetime, one is likely to end as an abortion. The fact that a patient has had an abortion in one pregnancy does not mean that it will happen again. If she has an abortion, there is an 80 per cent chance that the next pregnancy will produce a live, normal, healthy baby; if she has two abortions in succession, the chance of the next pregnancy producing a live, healthy baby is 75 per cent; and even after three abortions, one after the other, she still has a 70 per cent chance of producing a live, healthy baby with her next pregnancy.

In fact, however disappointed an expectant mother may be, she should not be anxious if a pregnancy ends as an abortion; her next pregnancy has every chance of being normal.

Most threatened abortions occur in the first 12 weeks of pregnancy, but a few women complain of vaginal bleeding between the 12th and 20th week of pregnancy. It is much less common for a woman to abort during this period, but it does occur. These women are sometimes found to have an abnormality of the shape of the uterus which can be detected by an X-ray picture taken (after injecting some oil into the uterus) when the woman has recovered from the abortion.

About 20 per cent of women who have a late abortion, especially if it is not their first late abortion, are found to have a weakness of the cervix (the neck of the womb). Women with this condition, which is called cervical incompetence, usually only know that all is not proceeding normally when the 'waters break' unexpectedly and without apparent reason. This means that the fluid filled bag (the amniotic sac) which encloses the fetus, breaks above the cervix and 'water' leaks, or pours out, through the vagina. This is followed by some bleeding and by uterine contractions which expel the fetus.

Normally, the cervical canal is quite firm and remains closed although the uterus is enlarging as the fetus grows. In women with cervical incompetence the cervix begins to open more and more after about the 12th week of pregnancy. As it opens, the bag of waters is pushed through the opening and, unless the condition is detected and treated, it eventually bursts. When this happens an abortion is nearly impossible to stop.

If the doctor is aware that this may happen, usually because it happened before, he can prevent the bag bursting by putting a stitch around the cervix and pulling it tight; rather like pulling the string around the mouth of a purse. The operation is relatively simple and about three-quarters of women who have cervical incompetence and have the operation can expect to have a live baby. But the condition is rare. In other words, only a very few women have this weakness of the cervix, and the operation is therefore not often needed.

Recurrent, or habitual abortion does require investigation, and if a woman has the misfortune to have three or more abortions in succession, she would be wise to consult her doctor. He will make several investigations, which include a full physical examination and a pelvic examination. As well he usually makes some laboratory tests to make sure that the woman has no undetected disease, and often takes an X-ray picture of the uterus after injecting an oily substance into it.

ABDOMINAL PAIN IN EARLY PREGNANCY

An expectant mother who develops severe abdominal pain, fainting and slight bleeding in early pregnancy should at once consult her doctor, as she may have an ectopic pregnancy. In this condition the fertilized egg plants itself in the lining of the oviduct. This lining is thin, and is surrounded by a thin muscle wall. As the embryo grows, its placenta eats into the muscle wall, which eventually bursts. Ectopic pregnancy is not too common, occurring in 1 in 150 pregnancies. The treatment is surgery to remove the damaged portion of the oviduct. Of course, as every woman has two oviducts, she can become pregnant again after an ectopic pregnancy.

BLEEDING IN THE SECOND HALF OF PREGNANCY

Bleeding from the birth-canal occurs in the second half of pregnancy in about three per cent of women. Usually they are women who have previously delivered children, and primigravidae uncommonly develop this complication. If an expectant mother bleeds sufficiently to soil a sanitary pad, or to make a large stain on her clothes or her bed sheets, she should call her doctor at once. He may visit her in her house, or he may insist that she go into hospital immediately where he will examine her.

Bleeding in the second half of pregnancy is called 'antepartum haemorrhage'. Apart from the few cases due to local conditions of the cervix, there are two main causes, which were first distinguished in 1775 by Dr Edward Rigby in Norwich. At that time maternity care was conducted by untrained midwives, and they only attended the woman when she was in labour. If labour failed to progress, or was abnormal, the midwives called in the doctor. Because of the current ideas of modesty at that time, he usually had to make his diagnosis without a pelvic examination, or if he performed one, he did it under a sheet! Considering the difficulties, Rigby made a remarkably clear distinction between bleeding that was *inevitable* because the placenta was filling the lower part of the uterus in front of the baby, and the bleeding which occurred *accidentally* because a portion of the placenta separated from its bed on the wall of the uterus.

Today the two types, the inevitable bleeding due to a placenta praevia, and the accidental bleeding of abruptio placentae, still require to be distinguished as treatment is different. The position of the placenta in the uterus can be found by modern equipment, either using ultrasound (see p. 142), or by recording the activity of a special safe radio-isotope injected into an arm vein. The substance mixes with the blood, and as the placenta has a good blood supply, its activity is most marked over that part of the uterus in which the placenta lies. The activity is measured with a Geiger counter, and the number of 'bleeps' recorded on a chart (Fig. 17/1). Ultrasound sends high frequency sound waves through the body. When these waves meet a tissue some are absorbed, some are reflected and some pass through. What happens depends on composition of the tissues. The reflected waves can be converted into light waves and these will make a picture. The picture appears on the ultrasound machine and is photo-

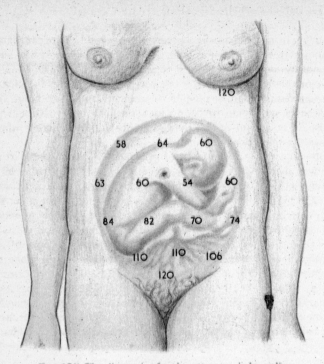

FIG. 17/1 The diagnosis of a placenta praevia by radio-
isotopes. The placenta lay under the area of the highest
count of 'bleeps'. This was proved at caesarean section, a
live boy being born

graphed. This enables the doctor, if he has been trained, to detect the
position of the placenta in the uterus. An expectant mother who is
diagnosed as having a placenta praevia remains in hospital until the
pregnancy has reached the end of the 37th week. This is called
'expectant treatment', and is used so that the baby may grow in the
uterus rather than having to cope with life in a premature nursery. At
the 37th week, a decision is made by the doctor whether it is safer for
the expectant mother to be delivered normally or by caesarean
section. Four patients in every 10 can deliver normally, and 6 in every
10 who have a placenta praevia require to be delivered by caesarean
section.

Abruptio placentae, the other main condition which causes bleeding in the second half of pregnancy, is of two kinds. In most cases the amount of separation of the placenta is slight, and the pregnancy can safely continue. In a few cases – no more than one-quarter of all – the amount that the placenta separates is greater. In these cases the expectant mother may lose a good deal of blood. Because of this, the doctor gives blood transfusions and brings on labour by breaking the bag of waters. Unfortunately, in the severe forms very few babies survive. However, as the condition usually only occurs in women who have previously had several children, the loss of the child may not cause so much grief as would the loss of a first baby.

SWELLING OF THE FINGERS OR FACE

In the second half of pregnancy, for reasons which are unknown, a condition may arise which is called 'toxaemia of pregnancy'. The name is a bad one for there is no toxin, but it has the advantage of being a shorthand reference to three symptoms or signs. These are oedema of the fingers, face or legs; a rise in blood pressure; and the appearance of protein in the urine. Although some swelling of the legs towards evening is normal in pregnancy, swelling of the legs present in the morning, or of the hands or face at any time, is a danger sign. Oedema can be detected by observing if the shoes are uncomfortable, or if the wedding ring is tight. It can also be anticipated by checking if a rapid gain in weight has occurred, and it may be remembered that a weight gain of more than 1 kg (2 lb) per week in the second half of pregnancy is a warning of impending 'toxaemia'. A more serious warning is blurring of vision or severe headaches, particularly if associated with oedema.

'Toxaemia of pregnancy' affects about 12 per cent of primigravidae and 6 per cent of multigravidae, but if detected early and treated properly is without danger to mother or child. After childbirth, it disappears rapidly, leaving no trace behind. But if it is neglected, serious complications such as convulsions or 'fits', and the death of the baby can result. This condition is called 'eclampsia'. The expectant mother can understand, therefore, the insistence made by the doctor for regular antenatal visits, when the blood pressure is estimated, the weight gain noted, oedema looked for, and the urine examined. She can also appreciate why she must follow her doctor's instructions implicitly should a rise in blood pressure or other signs of 'toxaemia of pregnancy' occur. The instructions may be simple, such as restricting the diet, particularly the amount of salt added to the food she eats, and by making sure that she rests more, as this improves the quantity of blood flowing to her placenta. Sometimes the doctor may ask her to be admitted to hospital, even when she feels she is quite well. In hospital she will be given sedative drugs, and the doctors and nurses will observe very closely her blood pressure, her weight gain, or one hopes loss, her 'fluid balance' (that is, the amount of fluids drunk against the quantity of urine passed), and the growth of the baby. The aim of the medical attendants is to control the 'toxaemia of pregnancy', so that the baby may grow and eventually be born unharmed.

A 'GUSH' OF WATER FROM THE VAGINA

A 'gush' of water from the vagina after the 28th week of pregnancy usually indicates that the bag of membranes, or amniotic sac, has burst. This is called 'rupture of the membranes' by doctors. As will be recalled, the baby grows in the amniotic sac which is filled with amniotic fluid, and the gush of water is the escape of the fluid. If rupture of the membranes occurs, the patient should at once go to hospital. In hospital treatment will depend on how far advanced the pregnancy is. Should this be less than 35 weeks, in all probability the doctor will give sedative drugs in the hope that labour will not start; but if the pregnancy has advanced beyond 35 weeks, he will generally give a drug which stimulates the uterus to contract. The reason is that after the 35th week, the baby is sufficiently mature to survive outside, and there is a slight risk that it may become infected if left in the uterus.

CONGENITAL MALFORMATIONS

If 1,000 women become pregnant and the pregnancy is diagnosed early, 150 may expect to abort (or miscarry) spontaneously in the first 20 weeks. Careful examination of the aborted fetuses shows that nearly half have been expelled by nature because the chromosomes were not the proper number or were deformed in some way.

A few women carrying babies with abnormal chromosomes, or with some other inherited congenital defect (which is usually one of metabolic function, the baby lacking the ability to make some special enzyme) fail to abort spontaneously. The pregnancy continues but a congenitally deformed baby is born. The most common congenital defect due to abnormal chromosomes is Down's Syndrome. This affects one baby in every 1,500 born to women under the age of 30, but the incidence rises to one baby in 300 if the expectant mother is over the age of 35. Down's Syndrome used to be called mongolism, and the child affected by Down's Syndrome is mentally retarded. Scientists have found that two forms of chromosome abnormality can cause Down's Syndrome, and if the baby has one of them there is a high chance that a subsequent baby will also be affected.

Today, a mother who has previously had an affected baby or who is over the age of 35 can find out early in her pregnancy whether or not her baby will have Down's Syndrome. At about the 15th week of pregnancy a narrow needle is inserted into the uterus, through the woman's abdominal wall under local anaesthesia, and a sample of amniotic fluid is removed. The fluid contains cells shed by the fetus. The cells can be grown in specially equipped laboratories and chromosomal examinations can be made. The growth or culture of the cells and the study takes about 20 days. If the expectant mother is found to have a baby affected by Down's Syndrome she can choose to have the baby or can decide to have an abortion induced, using prostaglandins, as I discussed in Chapter 7.

Other congenital abnormalities occur which are not due to abnormal chromosomes. At present we do not know why they do occur. One important group are those due to abnormalities of the spine or skull. These abnormalities affect about 4 babies in every 1,000 born. But, oddly, the incidence varies in different countries – in some the rate is 10 in every 1,000, in others it is only 2 in every 1,000. A woman who has had a baby with a spina bifida (the spinal column defect) or an anencephalic baby (the skull defect) has twice the chance of having another affected baby compared with other women.

Two methods enable doctors to find out if the next baby will be affected. The first is to take an amniotic fluid sample, as I have described, and to measure a substance called alpha fetoprotein. If the amount found is high the baby will have the defect. The second method is to take an ultrasound picture of the baby, which often shows the defect. If the tests are made before the 20th week of pregnancy and a defective baby is found, the expectant mother can choose to have an abortion which is induced using prostaglandins.

OBSTETRIC OPERATIONS

Women are often most anxious because their friends – if you can call them friends – or neighbours have given them lurid descriptions of the operations they had in their pregnancy. Not only are these descriptions lurid, they are misleading.

Induction of labour

For several reasons, such as 'toxaemia of pregnancy', haemorrhage in pregnancy, Rhesus problems, or pregnancy which has become prolonged to more than 42 weeks, the obstetrician may decide that it is best to induce labour. The usual way in which this is done is to rupture or 'cut' the bag of waters just inside the cervix. The procedure is quite painless, although rather inelegant. The expectant mother is put on an obstetric bed with her feet in stirrups (Fig. 17/2). The vulva is cleaned, antiseptic lubricant is poured into the vagina, and the doctor makes a pelvic examination. In this, he feels the cervix and notes whether it is soft or not, and how wide open it is. If it is 'suitable', that is soft and at least one finger dilated, he will go ahead and rupture the membranes. This is done with a small instrument, which tears a hole in the bag so that the water runs out. The procedure is called 'surgical induction of labour'. The mother can feel the warm amniotic fluid running down her vagina.

Labour usually starts quite quickly, and the doctor may encourage it to start by setting up a drip into an arm vein of the mother, and carefully running in a drug (oxytocin), which stimulates the uterus to contract. He may decide to give the oxytocin as tablets, which the mother puts in her cheek pouch and allows to dissolve, although this method is not quite as satisfactory as the intravenous drip. With either method, over 95 per cent of women have delivered their baby within 24 hours of the induction.

Recently some doctors have begun to use the substance, prostaglandin, in place of oxytocin, but there seems little advantage in the change, and most obstetricians continue to prefer oxytocin to 'speed up' the start of labour after induction.

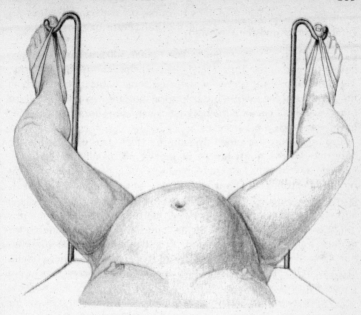

FIG. 17/2 The position in which the mother is placed for
certain obstetric manipulations

Another change which has become fashionable is for doctors to
perform surgical induction on most of their pregnant patients. I have
written about this on p. 236. The woman and the doctor agree that
labour will be induced near or at the end of pregnancy on a special
day provided that the cervix is 'suitable' and the baby's head is
'engaged' in the pelvis. If the doctor has a number of pregnant
women he induces labour by surgical induction on all of them on that
day, and starts an intravenous drip containing oxytocin at once. The
idea is that all his patients will have their babies during the afternoon
or the evening of the same day, which is convenient for the woman
and the doctor, who can rearrange his schedule. If you support this
attitude you can choose a doctor who uses this method. But for the
safety of the baby it is essential to know that it is not premature and
that it has grown sufficiently in the uterus to have the best chance of
being healthy after birth. There are now tests which can be made to
find out if the fetus is mature or not.

Fetal maturity and the L-S ratio

By convention a baby weighing less than 2,500 g at birth, or born before the end of the 36th week is said to be premature or 'preterm'. The definition is not very exact because some babies grow slowly in the womb, and are mature but below the 'normal' birthweight, whilst others are small because the pregnancy has been shortened and they have been born prematurely.

The first group are called dysmature babies. This implies that the baby has lacked nourishment in the womb, usually because the mother developed 'toxaemia' or had some other disease. This reduced the transfer of nourishment across the placenta so the baby's growth was retarded. These babies are mature as far as their ability to adjust to life is concerned, provided that they receive proper care.

The second group of low birthweight babies are genuinely premature. For one reason or another, pregnancy does not last 40 weeks but is curtailed, labour starting before the 37th week. These babies are less well able to adjust to life, as their vital processes have not become properly mature.

As doctors induce labour in more and more normal women for convenience, it is important to be sure before doing so that the baby is mature. Information that the baby is premature is also important when the doctor has to induce labour or do a caesarean section before the end of pregnancy because the baby is 'at risk' of dying in the mother's uterus (see p. 280). It is very important for you and your doctor to know the maturity of your baby and in this you and the laboratory can help.

The easiest way of knowing how much your pregnancy has advanced is for you to have kept a calendar of the dates of your menstrual periods, and to have visited your doctor between the 6th and the 10th week of pregnancy. A pelvic examination at this time enables the doctor to estimate the duration of the pregnancy accurately by detecting the size of the uterus. Later in pregnancy he can refer back to this information. If your periods are irregular or if you have failed to keep a menstrual calendar and if you have not visited your doctor in the first 10 weeks of your pregnancy, the doctor may have to use laboratory tests to determine the baby's maturity should he decide to induce labour.

The tests are made on a sample of the amniotic fluid in which the fetus lives. Under local anaesthesia a narrow needle is pushed through your abdominal skin and muscles and into the uterus. The doctor takes care to avoid pushing the needle through the placenta and often has an ultrasound picture made first to find out where the placenta is. When the needle enters the amniotic sac, a sample of about 10 ml of fluid is taken and sent to the laboratory, where chemical substances in the sample are estimated. These substances are secreted into the amniotic fluid by the fetus and give evidence of its maturity. The laboratory can measure many substances but two have proved the most helpful. The first test is to measure a substance called creatinine, which indicates whether the fetal kidney is sufficiently mature to cope with life outside the uterus.

The second test is even more useful. In this test two substances produced in the fetal lungs are measured. They are called lecithin and sphingomyelin. As the baby's lungs become mature, more lecithin is secreted and its quantity rises in the amniotic fluid. When there is twice as much lecithin as sphingomyelin in the sample, the baby's lungs are sufficiently mature for it to have little or no trouble in breathing after birth. But if the quantity of lecithin compared with that of sphingomyelin is less than twice as much (in other words if the lecithin:sphingomyelin ratio is less than 2), the baby has an increased chance of getting a lung disorder called hyaline membrane disease which can make its survival uncertain.

You can understand from this that if you choose to have your baby by the 'elective induction' of labour you may need to have the amniotic fluid test (called amniocentesis) made to estimate your baby's maturity before the surgical induction.

Caesarean section

The operation of caesarean section has nothing to do with Julius Caesar. The word derives from the Latin *caedere*, to cut, for that is what is done. If for some reason the baby cannot be born through the birth-canal, an incision is made in the lower part of the abdominal wall and through the lower part of the uterus. The child is removed through the incisions, which are then carefully repaired with stitches. The mother is anaesthetised throughout the whole operation, and wakes up to hear her baby crying. In the past 30 years, the incidence of caesarean section has increased considerably. Much of this increase is justified; but some inexcusable, either because the patient demands the operation, or the doctor takes the 'easy way out'. In

Australia and Britain, the incidence is about 4 to 8 per cent; in the U.S.A. it seems to be about 6 to 12 per cent.

Part of the reason for the higher rate in the U.S.A. is that there most obstetricians believe that once a caesarean section has been performed on a patient, all subsequent deliveries should be by caesarean section. A few take a different view, and believe that many women who have previously been delivered by caesarean section can be delivered vaginally as safely and with less discomfort in a subsequent pregnancy. This opinion is shared by obstetricians in Australia, Britain and most other countries. In a very careful study in Britain, it was found that 45 per cent of women who had previously had a caesarean section were delivered vaginally with safety in a subsequent pregnancy, and similar proportions have been obtained in Australia and Malaysia.

So 'once a caesarean, always a caesarean' is no longer valid, and an expectant mother whose first baby was delivered by caesarean section has a 50:50 chance of delivering her next baby vaginally. The only stipulation upon which all obstetricians agree is that a patient who has previously had a caesarean section must be looked after by a specialist obstetrician, and have her baby in a properly equipped hospital.

Forceps deliveries

In July 1569 – 400 years ago – a family of Huguenot refugees called Chamberlen fled from France and arrived in England. One son, Peter was about 6 years old, and two more sons were to be born subsequently in England, one of them also being called Peter. Although this may not have led to confusion within the family, it has led to the confusion of medical historians, for both Peters became doctors, and one of them invented a secret instrument for the help of women in labour. The elder Peter had a dramatic rise to fame, attended Queen Anne for her confinements, and it is thought that he was the inventor. The Chamberlens kept their secret most successfully, and it is said that when asked to help in a difficult labour, one of them would arrive at the bedside, sit in front of the patient, and have a sheet stretched from the abdomen of the patient and tied round his neck. In the obscurity of the sheet, he would draw a bundle from the pocket of his coat, and manipulations were seen to move the sheet; but the secret instrument was never glimpsed. It was in fact the first obstetric forceps. Chamberlen's forceps were like a pair of outsize sugar tongs, made of metal and covered with leather. He introduced them into the vagina, applied them to the side of the baby's head, and pulled. Sometimes he was successful in delivering the baby, other times not. But successful or not, the family kept the secret for over 100 years, son succeeding father. In about 1670, the grandnephew of the first Peter was in charge, and was tempted to sell his instrument. Hugh Chamberlen offered it for sale for £1,000, a very considerable sum of money in those days. He was invited to go to Paris and demonstrate the value of his instrument. The patient chosen was a dwarf, who had severe rickets, and who had been in labour for days. Chamberlen demanded that he be given a private room, and that no one should observe him at work. He struggled for three hours but failed to deliver the patient, as might be expected. His offer of sale was rejected, but six months later he was in Paris trying again. Finally in 1728, the male line became extinct, and 30 years later the secret instrument was sold and its design made public.

Since that time many changes in the design of the obstetric forceps have made it a precision-tooled, correctly constructed instrument. Over the years, too, the indications in which the forceps are needed, and for which they can be used with safety, have been identified.

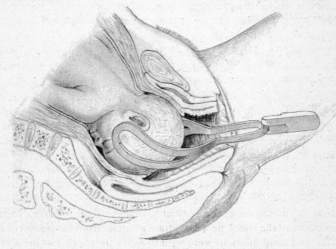

FIG. 17/3 The obstetric forceps. The mother has received a local anaesthetic, and the forceps fit snugly along the sides of the baby's head, like sugar tongs fit along a lump of sugar

Doctors who propose to practise obstetrics learn how to handle the instrument, or more correctly the instruments, for today each blade of the forceps is separate. Each blade is inserted into the vagina separately, so that it lies over the side of the baby's head, and once both are in position, the handles of the blades are crossed and joined together at a lock (Fig. 17/3). In this way the least possible damage is done to the mother or to the baby.

The percentage of mothers on whom forceps are used to effect delivery of the baby varies. In Asia about 1 per cent, in Britain about 6 per cent and in Australia about 12 per cent of the mothers are delivered by forceps; whilst in the U.S.A. the rate exceeds 30 per cent. This is because women in labour in America are very heavily sedated, and often are given an anaesthetic so that they are unable to help in pushing the baby into the world. It is a matter of custom, but even in the U.S.A. most obstetricians are realizing that the more natural childbirth is made, the better it is for mother and for baby.

If forceps are required, the mother can be assured that the operation will be quite painless. Either a local anaesthetic is given, or else an injection is administered into her spine, called an epidural anaesthetic. The forceps are only inserted into her vagina when the anaesthetic has taken effect. The baby may be born with red marks along the sides of its face corresponding to the shape of the forceps blades. The mother can rest assured that the marks will disappear rapidly.

'Taking the baby with instruments' is still regarded as a serious step by many expectant mothers. Years ago it was, but today with skilled doctors and well-made precision instruments, forceps deliveries are safe. By far the majority of forceps deliveries are made to help the head of the baby over the mother's perineum. This is called a low forceps delivery. In a few cases the baby's head may fail to advance in the second stage of labour, despite strong contractions and good 'pushes' by the mother. If the second stage lasts for more than one and a half hours, the doctor usually introduces the forceps and delivers the baby. This is termed a 'mid-forceps delivery', and it requires far more skill and experience than the low forceps delivery, which is really quite easy. It is usual for the doctor to make a deliberate cut in the perineum with a pair of scissors before delivering the baby. This prevents the tissues from tearing, and it is termed an 'episiotomy'. After the birth of the baby and the placenta, the episiotomy is stitched (see page 232). If the stitching is done properly, it is no more than slightly painful and uncomfortable for two days or so, and with one method of stitching it is virtually painless.

In the last 20 years, an instrument has been suggested which might replace many forceps deliveries. Actually it was originally invented 120 years ago by a famous Scottish obstetrician, Sir James Simpson, who also first used anaesthesia in childbirth. The instrument consists of a flat cap, about 7.5 cm (3 in) in diameter. This is connected to a vacuum apparatus. The cup is pushed against the head of the baby, and a vacuum created, so that it is held firmly against the scalp by the atmospheric pressure. The doctor then pulls on the tubing which connects the cup to the vacuum bottle, and the baby is delivered (Fig. **17/4**). The apparatus, called a ventouse, is simple to use, and is said to have the advantage that less is introduced into the vagina than when forceps are used. Because of this, damage to the mother's tissues is less likely to occur.

It does not really seem to make much difference in most cases whether forceps or a ventouse is used to deliver a baby which is delayed on its journey into the world.

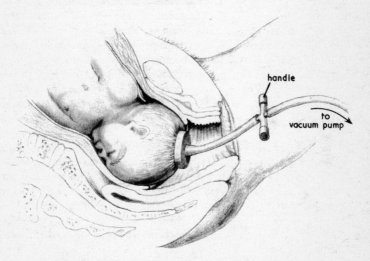

FIG. 17/4 The 'vacuum extractor'. In place of forceps, a small suction cup may be applied to the baby's head, a vacuum created and the baby delivered by pulling on the cup

Retained placenta

You will remember that normally the placenta (or afterbirth) is expelled within a few minutes of the birth of your baby, especially when the doctor has given you an injection of ergometrine as the baby was being born. Occasionally, perhaps once or twice in every 100 deliveries, the afterbirth is retained in the uterus. Often it will be expelled after a 15 minute interval but, in some cases, particularly if bleeding occurs, the doctor may decide to remove it. You are given an anaesthetic and the doctor introduces his hand, very gently, into your womb and eases the placenta from its attachments. The procedure is quite safe, painless and in no way affects your progress in the lying-in period, or your ability to have another child.

PERINATAL DEATH (STILLBIRTHS AND INFANT DEATHS)

Of 100 pregnancies which reach the half-way mark of 20 weeks, only 2 will result in the birth of a dead baby (a stillbirth) or in the death of the baby in the first month of life. The reasons why babies die in this way are rather complex and I discuss them in my book *People Populating* in some detail. In over 30 per cent the cause is unknown, although most of the babies are born either prematurely or weighing less than expected for the time of birth. About 15 per cent of the deaths do occur because of an antepartum haemorrhage (see p. 277); and a similar number are malformed babies. Nearly 6 per cent occur because of 'toxaemia of pregnancy' and about the same number because of disease in the mother.

The loss of a baby at this time is deeply distressing to the mother and to her husband, but the deaths of these babies (called perinatal deaths) have been reduced remarkably in the past 40 years. Forty years ago, 60 babies in every 1,000 born were stillborn or died in the first month of life. Today fewer than 20 in every 1,000 born are lost in this way.

The usual, and quite normal reaction to a perinatal death is one of emptiness, restlessness and physical exhaustion: in short a sense of bereavement. Many women believe, quite wrongly, that the baby has died because of something they did, or did not do during their pregnancy. Some women feel a sense of failure: that by losing the baby they have failed their family or themselves.

A woman who loses her baby in this way need feel no shame or anxiety about her grief: it is as strong as that following the death of an older child or spouse. She needs someone knowledgeable to talk to, usually her doctor. In the words of an editorial in the *British Medical Journal* 'a willing ear tolerant of confusion and anger is probably more important than tonics or sedatives'. A woman who has had the misfortune to give birth to a stillborn baby or whose baby dies in the first month of life has the right to expect that her doctor will try to explain to her clearly and simply the cause of the death, if it is known, and to tell her what she can expect in her next pregnancy. Both the doctor and the other medical attendants should show sympathy but not condescension to the mother; should answer her questions fully and unemotionally, and should offer her support, as should her husband and relatives, until her sense of bereavement diminishes. In this way she can overcome a troublesome, unhappy period.

To put perinatal deaths into perspective, remember that of every 100 pregnancies which reach the 20th week, 98 will end with the birth of a live baby which will survive.

HIGH RISK PREGNANCIES

Since the whole purpose of good antenatal care and careful observation during labour is to make sure that you have a live and healthy baby, and are as healthy, or healthier, after your pregnancy than you were before it, doctors have become increasingly aware that in some pregnancies a greater risk of losing the baby is present. These pregnancies include those in which bleeding occurred in the second half of pregnancy; 'toxaemia of pregnancy' developed; women aged 30 or more who became pregnant for the first time; women who previously had given birth to a stillborn or deformed child; women whose pregnancy had been prolonged for more than 42 weeks; women who had diabetes, high blood pressure or kidney disease; and women with a Rhesus problem. If a mother-to-be has, or develops any of these conditions, or other rarer ones, her baby is at greater risk of dying before birth, of being born prematurely or of dying during labour.

Today it is possible to 'monitor' the well-being of the fetus in pregnancy of such women by measuring a hormone, oestriol, in their urine during the last weeks of pregnancy or by using the ultrasound machine to check that the baby is growing normally in the womb. If persistently low levels of urinary oestriol are found over a period of days, or if ultrasound suggests that the baby is not growing, the doctor may decide to induce labour, by breaking the bag of waters, or performing a caesarean section.

If a woman with a 'high risk' pregnancy is permitted to go into labour, either spontaneously or after induction of labour, her baby is at greater risk during labour than that of a 'normal or low risk' woman.

Increasingly such women are confined in maternity units which have an array of electronic equipment, a special nursery for small babies and highly trained staff who are ready to rescue the baby, by delivering it quickly, should problems arise unexpectedly. The electronic equipment which has been developed helps the doctor in reaching a decision and also detects early which baby may be in jeopardy.

Two pieces of equipment are most useful. The first, which I mentioned in Chapter 14, is the fetal heart monitor. This apparatus electronically measures the fetal heart rate and determines the strength and frequency of the uterine contractions. The information is translated into a visual continuously moving graph. By studying the patterns on the graph, the medical attendants can make sure that the baby is well and that the uterine contractions are occurring at the correct strength and the best intervals for the baby to get all the oxygen it needs. If the doctor detects an abnormal pattern, he may decide to deliver the baby at once, depending on the stage labour has reached, or he may use the second piece of equipment. This machine measures the acidity of the baby's blood. A small sample of blood is taken from the baby's scalp as it presses into the mother's vagina. This blood is then put into the machine and its acidity is measured with great accuracy. If the scalp blood of the baby is very acid, the baby is in danger of dying, and the doctor can rescue it from the danger. If it is not acid then the baby is safe.

The machines are expensive, complicated and require careful maintenance. For this reason they are only available in bigger maternity units, which also have intensive infant care units attached to them. In the next few years, a woman with 'high risk' pregnancy will expect to be confined in these larger units, so that her baby has the best chance of surviving; and, in fact, the chances are very good.

Chapter 18

Breasts and Breast-feeding

A difference between man and woman which remains obvious despite similar hairstyles and almost identical clothes, is that woman has well-developed breasts. Although the main function of the mammary gland is to provide nourishment for the infant, in vast areas of the world this function has become secondary. The primary function appears to be that the hemispherical swelling of the breast is a potent attraction to males. The ideal of breast beauty varies considerably amongst different races. For example, the Polynesians admire small conical breasts; the Hottentots and North American Indians appear to prefer elongated, melon-shaped, drooping mammary glands; the Chinese women tend to be flat-chested; whilst most European or American men prefer their women to possess large, 'uplifted', hemispherical breasts. The women of the Western world try to please their men as far as they can, and when nature does not provide the appropriate shape and 'uplift', resort to mechanical aids is made, such as brassières, 'falsies', bust-developing creams, exercises and other appliances. The breast cult of modern man is a recent development, for in the Middle Ages it was considered that: 'The breast of a beautiful woman should be rather broad, and as white as snow or clear as crystal. The breasts must be small, round as a pear or an apple of paradise, and soft as silk to the touch. Large breasts and long hanging breasts are considered ugly.'

Breasts, then, have a functional purpose for milk production to feed the newborn infant, and an erotic function to attract the male. In different cultures and at different times, one or other has predominated.

THE DEVELOPMENT OF THE BREAST

The infantile breast in both sexes consists of a nipple which projects from a pink surrounding area called the *areola*. Around the 10th or 11th year the areola bulges, and the nipple projects from the centre. The development of the male breast ceases at this point, but the female breast develops further as the sex hormones (oestrogen and progesterone) are secreted by the ovaries (Fig. **18/1**). The milk ducts which grow inwards from the nipple, divide into smaller ducts and divide again to form tiny milk-secreting areas called *alveoli*. At the same time fat is deposited around the ducts, so that the breast becomes increasingly protuberant and conical-shaped. After puberty, the development is more rapid, and by the mid-teens the breasts have assumed their adult form, being rounded and firm. In fact, however, they are rarely as round and as firm as our fantasies would have us believe. When a young woman stands up, her breasts hang down slightly, the upper surface is slightly concave and the lower surface slightly convex, joining the skin of the chest at an acute angle. Pregnancy leads to a considerable growth of the ducts and the alveoli, and if the mother breast-feeds her baby, the development is even greater. But in the majority of women the breasts return to their non-pregnant size and shape once lactation has ceased.

The adult breast is of variable size, the size having no relationship to the ability to breast-feed. Small breasts can produce as much milk as large breasts. Anatomically the breast is divided into 15 to 25 sections, called lobes, which are separated from each other by fibrous tissue radiating from the nipple, so that the lobes are rather like the sections of an orange. Each lobe has its own duct system, which ends in a dilated area under the areola and extending into the nipple. This forms a tiny milk reservoir when lactation is established. From this a small duct opens onto the surface of the nipple. There are therefore 15 to 25 openings on the nipple. Going backwards, the main duct divides into smaller ducts, and like the branches of a tree, these ducts divide into still smaller ducts each of which ends in, and drains, a collection of 10 to 100 milk-secreting areas (Fig. **18/2**). The entire duct system is embedded in a pad of fat, and it is this which gives the breast its shape. The duct system of each lobe therefore resembles a tree, the alveoli being the leaves, the small ducts the branches, and the main duct the trunk.

During each menstrual cycle, changes occur in the breasts, the ducts developing and the alveoli budding in the second half of the cycle. At the same time fluid oozes into the fatty tissue of the breasts, so that they become firmer and heavier. In some women they may

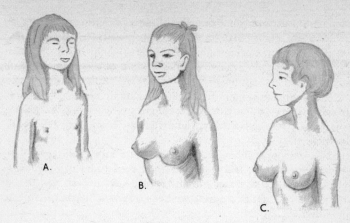

FIG. 18/1 The development of the female breast
(a) Prepubertal. (b) Late adolescence. (c) Maturity

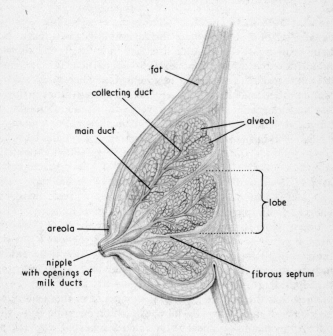

FIG. 18/2 The structure of the breast

become tender and cause discomfort, which is most marked in the week before menstruation. This is not abnormal, but merely an exaggeration of the normal, and treatment will help. In a few women, the swelling and tenderness persists instead of diminishing during menstruation and disappearing in the first half of the next menstrual cycle. The breasts remain tender and the gland tissue can be felt as irregular lumps. If this occurs, the woman must consult her doctor so that he may investigate fully, and give her treatment to relieve her discomfort.

As the woman becomes older, the breasts tend to get larger and the fibrous tissue bands tend to stretch, so the breasts droop more. After the menopause, the ducts and alveoli become smaller, and the fat starts to go, so that in old age the breasts become smaller, wrinkled and floppy.

IS A BRASSIÈRE REQUIRED?

Modern Western woman is conditioned to wear a brassière. The support has the advantage that it displays the breast more prominently, emphasising its sexual symbolism, and that it prevents premature stretching of the fibrous supports. However, the need for the 'bra' has been exaggerated, and it is probably only really necessary when the breast has become fully mature and hemispherical, during pregnancy and lactation, and if the breasts are very large. It is doubtful if a 'bra' is needed on medical grounds in the teenage years, or by a mature woman who has normal-sized, firm breasts. If a woman feels more comfortable and attractive in a 'bra', then she should wear one; if she is more comfortable and attractive without a 'bra', then she can happily do without. There is little sense though in mothers insisting that their young teenaged daughters require a 'bra': there is no danger of 'drooping', and little to which to give uplift.

In pregnancy, particularly in late pregnancy and during the time a woman breast-feeds her baby, it is advisable to wear a brassière, preferably all the time, both day and night. This is because the increased weight of the breasts at these times may cause stretching of the supporting tissues. The size of the brassière chosen will need to be increased as the breasts grow in pregnancy, and particularly after childbirth. It may be worthwhile buying 'nursing brassières', which have front openings over each nipple and changeable, washable pads to absorb any milk which may leak.

SMALL BREASTS

Because of the strong sexual symbolism of the female breast in Western society, many young adults are concerned if their mammary development fails to equal that of their friends, or more important their favourite film or television star. If the breasts have failed to develop at all, a doctor should be consulted; but if the breasts have developed to some extent and the menstruation has started, there is little that can be done to increase their size. Many women, beguiled by astute advertising, make use of costly oestrogen creams, rubbed assiduously into the breasts. If menstrual function is normal, enough oestrogen is being made by the girl herself and the extra oestrogen will do nothing. Anyhow, oestrogen only causes growth of the ducts of the breasts. What the small-breasted girl lacks is the pad of fat. Nothing, except a better diet, will deposit fat in the breasts. Of course, if the girl has a stooping posture, correction of this and exercises to strengthen the pectoral muscle which lies under the breasts will give them the appearance of being larger by 'throwing' them outwards.

A number of women who have large amounts of money but small amounts of breast tissue seek the attention of plastic surgeons who, for a fee, are prepared to introduce disc-shaped moulds of a plastic material (usually silicone) between the breasts and the pectoral muscles. Obviously, this will make the breasts look larger, although it will not improve their function in any way. Since the material is behind the breasts pushing them forward, their feel is unchanged. The operation may do a good deal to make an insecure woman feel more feminine and attractive, and provided the surgeon is skilled it can be most successful. An alternative method, in which a plastic substance is injected should be avoided, as cancer has followed this technique in some cases.

BIG BREASTS

The size of the breasts tends to increase as a woman reaches the age of 35, particularly if she has been pregnant. Most of this enlargement is due to deposition of fat, and although the Western culture approves of large breasts in a young woman, they are not so desirable in later years because instead of being high and firm, they are pendulous and floppy. Exercises are of little help, and although plastic surgery can be performed, it generally only restores the breast temporarily, the enlargement and drooping recurring after a time. And surely a well-designed, well-fitting brassière is preferable to surgery, which will probably only be temporarily successful? However, if the enlargement is gross, surgery may be required.

EXTRA BREASTS

In other mammals more than one breast on each side is normal. In the human, too, a breast (or at least a nipple) can develop anywhere along the breast line, which extends from the armpit to the pubic bone (Fig. 18/3). The most usual site for the extra breast is in the armpit. The extra breast, which has a nipple, appears as a 'tail' of the normal breast. In a few women nipples are found at other places along the breast line. No treatment is required.

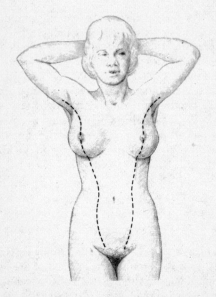

FIG. 18/3 Accessory breasts along the breast line

LUMPS IN THE BREAST

Most women fear that if a lump in their breast is found it may be a cancer. As cancer of the breast is the most common form of cancer in women, occurring twice as often as cancer of the uterus, it is a problem. In fact 5 women in every 100 may expect to develop cancer of the breast in their lifetime. But if breast cancer is detected early it is curable; detected late it is virtually incurable (see p. 350).

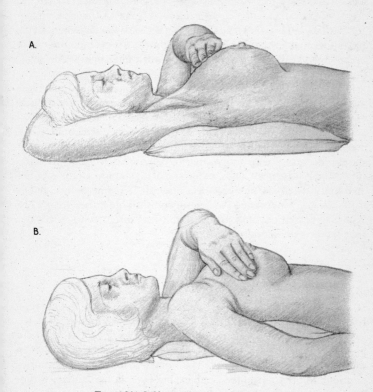

FIG. 18/4 Self-examination of the breasts

Although breast cancer is the most common form of cancer in women, benign lumps of the breast are much more common than cancer. But skill is needed to distinguish between the two kinds of lumps. This is why a woman should examine her breasts regularly, and visit her doctor every year so that he may check that she has not missed a breast cancer. Self-examination of the breasts is not difficult. It should be performed after the menstrual period is over in the younger woman, and once a month in women who have reached the menopause. The woman lies down comfortably, and with the tips of the fingers of the opposite hand palpates each breast in turn, systematically starting at the outer upper part and palpating each section of the breast until she has examined it all. The inner half of the breast is examined with the arm raised (Fig. 18/4A), and the outer half with the arm down at the side (Fig. 18/4B). If the patient palpates a small lump, she should go to her doctor at once. It may not be a cancer, but usually it is necessary to perform a small operation so that the lump can be removed and examined under a microscope.

Instead of finding a single lump, a number of women find that their breasts increase in size and become irregularly 'lumpy' in the week or so before menstruation. The lumpiness usually diminishes when menstruation starts, but persists in a few women, becoming more marked premenstrually each cycle. If you have this condition you should see your doctor so that he can palpate your breasts to make sure there is no cancer. The condition of irregular lumpiness is called mammary dysplasia or fibrocystic disease. It is not cancer, but is troublesome. Most women feel more comfortable if they wear a bra both during the day and at night, and it is often, but not always, relieved by taking oral contraceptives.

LACTATION

It is a disturbing fact that fewer and fewer women today breast-feed their babies. In one survey in Cardiff recently, it was found that by the seventh day of the puerperium, only 33 per cent of mothers were giving breast milk to their infants. These findings can be duplicated in many other Western countries. The women in less affluent countries continue to breast-feed their babies, but even in these lands bottle-feeding is gaining ground. Breast-feeding has several very real advantages. Firstly, the milk is sterile, balanced and appropriate to the human baby, just as cat's milk is appropriate for the kitten, bitch's milk is appropriate for the puppy, and cow's milk is appropriate for the calf. Human milk has slightly less protein and casein than cow's milk. The casein is the substance which makes curd. The curd of cow's milk is dense and difficult to digest, in contrast to the light, fluffy curd of human milk. Human milk contains more milk sugar (lactose) than cow's milk, more vitamins and more balanced minerals. In fact 'formula milks' made for bottle-feeding have to be modified from cow's milk by the manufacturers in many complicated ways to make them as much like human milk as possible. Furthermore, 'formula milk' requires care in mixing and in storing to keep it sterile and safe for the baby. Secondly, the act of breast-feeding brings the infant and its mother into a close physical relationship, and the stimulation of the nipple by sucking is pleasant (indeed it has some relationship to sexual stimulation). Not only this, but suckling leads to the release of a hormone from the hypothalamus in the brain, which increases the rapidity and efficiency of involution (or shrinking to normal) of the uterus. Thirdly, and rather facetiously, medical students are taught that the cat cannot get at breast milk and it comes in beautiful containers!

With all the advantages, one would think that all mothers would breast-feed unless there was a medical reason for them to avoid this, yet only one-third do.

The reasons for this distaste for breast-feeding have been studied, but no clear explanation has been found. One factor is that the rigid routine of hospitals, in which the baby is kept in the nursery and only brought to the mother at fixed hours, leads to difficulty in milk production because of restricted suckling. Because of this, and because the baby is obviously hungry, extra feeds using formula milk are given. By this stage, after battling with a fractious infant, a stern nurse and a feeling of failure, the mother's emotions further suppress her own milk production and the baby is put 'on the bottle' completely. In hospitals where babies room-in with their mothers and are fed 'on demand', breast-feeding problems are fewer and more mothers breast-feed. But if the mother has had difficulty with a previous baby leading to failure to breast-feed, the memory may deter her from trying to breast-feed the new infant, and she opts for bottle-feeding at once. Another possible reason for the reduced wish to feed may be linked to parental upbringing of the mother when she was a child. Despite the current display of the breast, despite its sexual symbolism, many mothers instil the belief into their daughters that the breast is a forbidden zone, to be hidden and never exposed. In a study of English mothers, two psychologists reported that 'modesty and a feeling of distaste' formed a major reason for their preference for formula-feeding, and in the U.S.A. another group reported that the mothers they studied were 'repelled' by the idea of giving their breasts to their infants. They were excessively embarrassed at the idea or were too 'modest' to nurse. In other studies of women of higher social groups, reasons for not wanting to feed were that feeding would 'interfere with the mother's social life'; bottle-feeding was so much easier; and breast-feeding would spoil the shape of the mother's breasts. These are selfish reasons, but are nevertheless felt.

If any advice can be given, it should be that for good reasons, breast-feeding is best feeding; but if the mother decides against breast-feeding for whatever reason, the baby will thrive provided the formula milk chosen is a reputable one, and the mother knows how to manage it.

PREPARING FOR BREAST-FEEDING

Nearly all women who want to breast-feed can do this successfully. In pregnancy you should prepare your breasts for lactation; whilst in hospital you need to have sympathetic motivated health-care professionals; doctors and nurses, to encourage you. When you get home it helps to have a friend to call if you have problems, or better still, join one of the nursing mothers' organizations who have informed, helpful counsellors on telephone stand-by at all times.

Preparing your breasts for easy lactation is quite simple. From about the 30th week of pregnancy put your hands around the outer part of your breasts and gently, but firmly, squeeze the breast tissue towards your nipples (Fig. 11/1). Do this several times a day. A good time is when you have a shower or a bath. After a while you will find that a yellowish substance seeps out of one or more ducts in your nipples. This is colostrum. The purpose of this exercise is to help the duct systems remain in good order.

You should also prepare your nipples for breast-feeding. From about the 30th week when you shower or bathe wash your nipples with water, dry them carefully and rub a little anhydrous lanolin into them. Then draw out each nipple and roll it gently between your forefinger and thumb a few times. This makes your nipples more flexible and less likely to 'crack' when the baby sucks. Do not believe the myths that you should scrub your nipples or put on methylated spirits to 'harden' them. Nipples should be supple, not hard.

A good way to stimulate your breasts during pregnancy is for your man to fondle your breasts and to play with your nipples with his fingers, or to suck them, when you make love. It helps prepare your breasts, it makes you closer together and it gives you a warm erotic feeling, which is good!

HOW LACTATION OCCURS

Once your baby is born, your breasts begin to produce milk because a hormone, prolactin, is secreted by cells in the pituitary gland just below your brain (see p. 41). During pregnancy the release of prolactin has been prevented by the effects of the high levels of circulating sex hormones – oestrogens and progesterone produced by your placenta. These hormones have prepared your breasts for lactation by their actions on the ducts and alveoli. After the baby is born the level of the sex hormones drops, and messages go to the pituitary cells to start making and releasing prolactin. Prolactin circulates in your blood stream and is taken up by the milk-making cells of the alveoli of the breasts, so the effect of prolactin is to start and to maintain the manufacture of milk deep in your breasts (Fig. 18/5). At first, only the thick colostrum is secreted, but by 24 to 48 hours after birth, milk appears and the amount secreted is regulated by the baby's demand. The process is helped if you want to breast-feed, and if the baby remains with you so that it can be nursed as soon and as often as it wishes, both during the day and at night.

The secretion of milk continues because prolactin continues to be released as your nipple is nuzzled by the baby or when you cuddle your baby. However the secreted milk will remain in the milk glands, distending them, unless the milk-ejection reflex occurs. The reflex forces the milk out of the milk glands to run along the ducts towards the milk reservoirs. This 'let down' of milk is due to contractions of minute muscles which surround the milk glands. The muscles are activated in a complex way, the main component of which is the stimulation of the mother's nipple by a nuzzling baby. A message travels from the stimulated nipple along nerve pathways to the brain, and from there to the pituitary gland. The message tells the pituitary gland to release a muscle contracting substance, called oxytocin, into the blood stream. This is carried in the blood to the tiny muscles

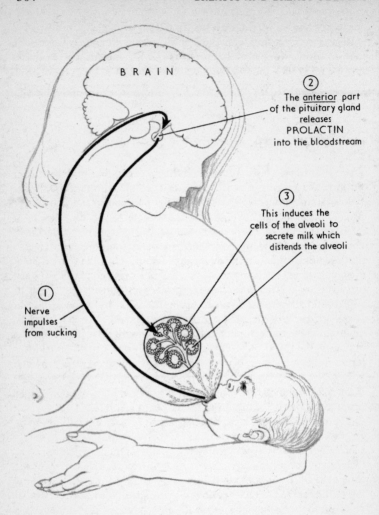

BRAIN

② The <u>anterior</u> part
of the pituitary gland
releases
PROLACTIN
into the bloodstream

③ This induces the
cells of the alveoli to
secrete milk which
distends the alveoli

① Nerve
impulses
from sucking

FIG. 18/5 How milk is secreted

around the milk glands with the result that the muscles contract and
the milk is forced along the milk ducts. (Fig. **18/6**). Milk-ejection, or
'let down' has occurred, and is associated with a gentle tingling in the
breasts and a desire to nurse. The reflex can also be initiated without

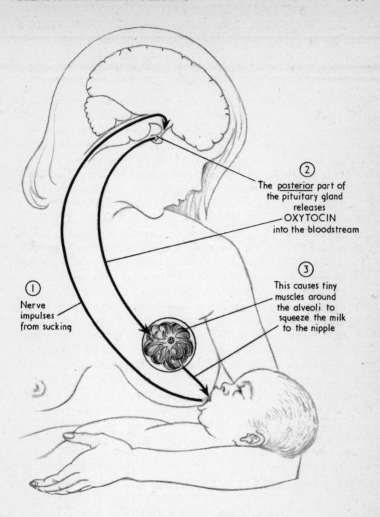

② The posterior part of the pituitary gland releases OXYTOCIN into the bloodstream

① Nerve impulses from sucking

③ This causes tiny muscles around the alveoli to squeeze the milk to the nipple

FIG. 18/6 How milk is 'let-down'

actual stimulation of the nipples. A mother hearing her baby cry, for example, may feel the signs of milk-ejection. But the most potent stimulus to milk-ejection is stimulation of the mother's nipple.

If the milk-ejection reflex does not occur regularly and adequately, the secreted milk distends the milk glands and, by pressure, prevents further milk being made, in addition to causing painful breasts. The consequence is that if a mother says she has 'insufficient milk' it generally means that the milk-ejection reflex is not working properly, although her milk production is normal.

As the pathway of the reflex goes through the brain, the release of the oxytocin needed to cause milk-ejection can be affected by the emotions and by other psychological factors. Dr Niles Newton, a psychologist, and her husband, Dr Michael Newton, an obstetrician, talked with 91 mothers, and asked questions to which the women replied in writing. When the answers were analysed, Dr Newton found that those women who subconsciously, or consciously, showed that they disliked the idea of breast-feeding produced less milk. Continued over a number of days, this would lead inevitably to a hungry, crying baby; to greater maternal anxiety and to the decision to put the baby on the bottle because 'I haven't enough milk and it doesn't agree with the baby'. The converse is also true. If a woman really wants to breast-feed she is far more likely to succeed.

The Newtons found that fear about pain, a mother's anxiety about her ability to breast-feed, disparaging remarks about breast-feeding by friends, and an authoritarian, hurried, attitude by the nursing staff hindered the milk-ejection reflex and made successful breast-feeding less likely to occur. Dr Applebaum who is medical adviser to the La Leche League in the U.S.A., discussing the problem of good milk-ejection, has commented 'a kind sympathetic approach by the nursing staff is important to over-all success in breast-feeding. Too many nurses hand the infant to the mother expecting her to know what to do'. In many surveys in which mothers were asked why they stopped breast-feeding, the most usual answer was 'insufficient milk' or 'the nurse said the milk doesn't agree with my baby'.

To a large extent the mother's anxiety about successful breast-feeding is aggravated by the practice, in many hospitals, of separating the mother from her baby. In many institutions the baby lives for most of the time in a nursery and is only brought to its mother at intervals for feeding. Babies are imitative, so there is generally a good deal of crying in the nursery. This is interpreted as hunger crying by the nursery attendants. To quell the noise and treat the supposed hunger, glucose drinks are given. The wide-holed teat and the sweet drink gives the baby an easy feed, and it begins to like sweet drinks so that it resists and resents having to obtain the less sweet breast milk.

The partly satiated child, when taken to its mother, at time intervals chosen by the nursing staff, not the baby, is not interested in suckling. This in turn reduces the milk supply, because the reflex invoked by stimulating the nipple which causes prolactin release is reduced.

Babies fed 'on demand' gain weight more quickly, after the normal initial weight loss, than babies fed 'by the clock'. Only when the mother and baby live together and are treated by unhurried kindly nurses, and when demand feeding is practised, will the emotional bonds between the two become firm. But all too often hospitals seem to be run for the benefit of authoritarian staff rather than for the benefit of the mother and her baby, which in itself is hardly conducive to the establishment of lactation.

The importance of this infant-mother bonding is that the tactile sensations stimulate the baby's sucking reflex and the mother's milk-ejection reflex. The more the milk-ejection reflex is stimulated in the first four days of life, the more successful is lactation likely to be. This in turn suggests that the reflex is started by more than the actual stimulation of the nipples. The close mother-child contact usual in the developing nations, and lost in recent years in our industrialized, mechanized societies, is a further potent stimulus to successful breast-feeding. The practise of 'rooming-in' of mother and baby and to 'demand feeding' is a return to more rational ways and to a greater chance of successful lactation.

But unless hospitals foster and encourage this return to older practices, breast-feeding will continue to decline. Doris and John Haire points out in their authoritative book *The Nurse's Contribution to Successful Breast-Feeding*, that there is no scientific support for the following practices which are all too common in hospitals in the developed nations:

● Delaying the time of the first feeding for some hours. The fact is an active baby will search for the nipple within minutes of birth, and should do so to practise its sucking reflex. It should then feed 'on demand'.

● Offering the baby glucose water before the first feeding. The scientific fact is that a newborn baby has all the additional fluid it needs in its own body, and needs no extra fluids until breast milk 'comes in' on the 2nd to 4th day. It also does obtain some fluid (colostrum) from the breast.

● Allowing the mother to sleep through the night before her milk comes in, instead of letting her keep her baby beside her and put it on her breast when it needs contact and comfort.

● Insisting that the mother only feeds to a 3-hourly or a 4-hourly schedule 'to bring the milk in and keep it good'.

● Preventing 'demand' feeding, which means that the baby is fed when it gives hunger cries. It may need 6 to 10 feeds a day when on demand feeding.

● Offering the baby water sweetened with glucose after it has fed.

● Demand fed babies rarely need extra water, but if offered it will usually take a small amount.

● Instructing the mother to feed by the clock at intervals of no less than 3-hours when she goes home.

Demand feeding

All this suggests that whenever possible a mother should insist that she demand feed her baby. After all this is what mothers have done since mammals evolved, and it is what the majority of the mothers in the world do today. It was rejected in Western countries about 40 years ago for the routine three-hourly or four-hourly feeding, which was more convenient for hospital routine.

Demand feeding implies that the baby is fed when it is hungry, when it demands food. In 'scheduled feeding' the baby is fed at a time decided by the nursing staff, even if this is inconvenient to the mother, and whether the baby is hungry or not. Babies are even woken up to be fed, and, of course, difficulties arise! It is like waking a man at 11 p.m. four hours after he has eaten a steak, and telling him he has to eat another steak! Some can, many cannot.

For demand feeding to be successful, the baby must 'room-in' with its mother. She is in close contact with it at all times, she cuddles it, she plays with it, she notes its changes in mood, she learns when its cry means hunger. From all these visual, tactile and emotional links, messages are carried to her brain, and the complex system which encourages milk secretion and its flow from the alveoli of the breasts to the collecting ducts is initiated. When the baby is hungry, the mother feeds it, changes it, pets it and then sleeps. A baby enjoys the breast, it nuzzles the nipples, its hands grasp the breast; and as it drinks its toes curl sensuously, its fingers move rhythmically, and in male babies erection of the penis is common. The mother notices these signs of contentment, she is relaxed, and a further flow of milk occurs.

In the first three days after childbirth, however, milk flow is minimal. The baby has sufficient reserves for this period, and is put to the breast merely to encourage the onset of lactation. It should not be put to the breast for too long, or the nipples may become sore; but it can be put for short periods as often as the mother wishes, since it is living beside her.

By the evening of the third day, or the next morning, lactation should have started, the milk should have 'come in', and proper breast-feeding can begin.

You must make sure that your baby is born in a hospital where the nurses want to help you to breast-feed successfully. You should choose a doctor who encourages you in your desire and who can influence the nurses to encourage you. Choose a hospital where the baby is given to you immediately after birth to cuddle and suckle, assuming of course that its birth has been normal; if it has been difficult you would have to take your doctor's advice. Make sure you can cuddle and suckle your baby for short periods every few hours. If you have prepared your nipples properly you need not worry about the baby hurting them.

Ask the nursing staff to let you have your baby beside you all night, unless you feel too tired, even before your milk 'comes in', so that you can cuddle it and give it your nipple to suck. This stimulates milk production. Tell the nurses only to give your baby plain water, not glucose water, after a feed if any extra fluid is needed; and then only after talking to you and your doctor. Demand fed babies do not usually need extra water. Of course, what I have written, applies only to a healthy baby. If your baby is very premature or sick you must take your doctor's advice. But talk it over with him. Do not be shy to ask questions. Doctors, and nurses, are there to help you.

INVERTED NIPPLES

The nipples of the fetus in the womb are normally turned in, or inverted. Usually they evert, or pop-out, in the last weeks of pregnancy, but occasionally they fail to do so. No treatment is required until the woman becomes pregnant. You can tell if your nipples are going to remain inverted by gently squeezing your areola between your forefinger and thumb. If your nipple reacts by starting to come out, it is not permanently inverted, but if it shrinks back, you need treatment. When you see your doctor in early pregnancy if you have inverted nipples ask him, or her, to check the degree of inversion and to tell you about treatment.

One way to treat inverted nipples is to use specially designed breast shields. They are made of plastic. One side is cone shaped, the other relatively flat with a hole in the centre. You put the shields on your breasts so that the hole covers your nipples; and hold them in place by your bra. The shields put a gentle continuous pressure on your nipple area, gradually drawing the nipples through the holes in the shields. You wear the shields from about the 16th week of pregnancy (it varies, depending on how deeply inverted are your nipples). Start wearing the shields for an hour or two at first and increase gradually until by about the 30th week you can wear them comfortably all day. You should not wear them at night. Sometimes the shields cause the escape of colostrum which makes your nipples moist. If this happens use small pads to absorb the liquid as the discharge can make your nipples sore. As well you can coat the nipples with anhydrous lanolin, and take off the shields from time to time to expose your nipples to the air.

There is another, complementary way to help inverted nipples. Direct sucking on the nipple area helps to draw the nipple out. If you and your husband wish he can help by stimulating your nipples with his fingers, and gently sucking the nipple area when you are close together. It is a good, happy and erotically stimulating way to prepare your breasts for successful lactation.

The technique of breast-feeding

The most important factor in successful breast-feeding is to be comfortable. It does not much matter whether the mother breast-feeds her baby when sitting up, on her side, or lying down. If she is most comfortable lying down, the baby lies in the bed beside her and she lies on her side facing it. She then adjusts her position so that the baby can nuzzle her nipple and eventually can take the nipple into its mouth. If the baby stuffs it in too far, it may be unable to breathe, and the mother may need to press her breast down from its nose to give him 'air space'.

If she prefers to feed sitting up, she must get comfortable, and often a chair with arms is preferable to one without. She can put a pillow on the arm of the chair, and then has a convenient prop for her arm as she holds her baby. Once again, the baby may need 'air space' when feeding, and she may need to press her breast away from its nose with her fingers.

It is immaterial which position is adopted for breast-feeding, but it is of great importance to make sure that at least some of the areola is inside the baby's mouth. In the diagram on page 295, it can be seen that the duct from each alveolus expands in the areola to form a sinus, or milk reservoir. These storage areas hold the milk, and when the baby squeezes them with its gums, milk spurts out of the nipple and into the baby's mouth. As the baby relaxes its grip to swallow the milk, more milk comes down from the alveoli to fill the sinuses again. In fact, the 'sucking' action made by the baby is only partly responsible for its obtaining milk; the squeezing effect is far more important. Sucking has another purpose, and this is to keep the areola and nipple well within the baby's mouth, and to draw the milk which spurts all over its mouth and into its throat.

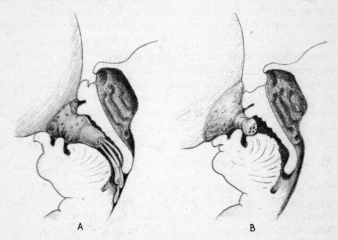

FIG. 18/7 How the nipple should be placed in the baby's mouth
A. Correct – nipple sucked well into mouth; gum chewing on areola
B. Incorrect – nipple being chewed

If the baby only bites onto the nipple, it will get hardly any milk, will become furious and bite harder. This will give the mother a sore nipple. But if the baby takes the nipple and the areola into its mouth, its gums will grip on the areola, leaving the nipple free, and not damaging it (Fig. **18/7**). Should the areola be very large, the mother may have to compress it between her thumb and finger so that the baby can get the nipple well inside its mouth. The mother does not need to hold the baby's head and direct it to the nipple, or to force its mouth open to get the nipple inside; in fact many paediatricians believe that this makes him baffled, bewildered and furious. All she needs to do is to get the baby comfortably nuzzling her nipple. Once the baby wants it, she must make sure the nipple is well inside its mouth, and that it chews on the areola. Nor should she pull the baby off her breast, because it hurts her and annoys the baby. It is easy to detach the baby from the breast, by simply slipping a finger into the corner of its mouth, between its gums, to break the suction.

The schedule of breast-feeding

This has been mentioned already. In the first three days after child-birth, only a thick yellow secretion (called colostrum) is produced, and as the baby has its own reserve stores of food, it is put to the breast for 3 to 5 minutes, between three and six times in the first 24 hours, and then about every 4 hours during the next 2 days, unless it cries when it should be picked up, cuddled and given a breast to suck. The purpose of this is to encourage the milk to 'come in'. Of course, if the baby wakes up and is hungry, the four-hourly routine is replaced by 'demand feeding'.

The milk 'comes in' usually on the 3rd or 4th day, but sometimes later, and either gradually or all at once. By now the baby is hungry and much more wide awake than earlier. It may cry, and the mother who 'rooms-in' with her baby rapidly learns to distinguish the cry of hunger, from the cry of discomfort. The baby is put to the breast, and is given alternate breasts first at alternate feeds. It may get sufficient from one breast, or may need to be put on both at a single feed. Usually, too, the other breast leaks milk when the baby feeds. The baby should never stay on one breast for longer than 12 minutes, as it will have got most of the milk in this time, and if the baby stays on longer the nipple may become sore. If the mother feeds 'on demand', she will generally find it easier than if the baby is fed at fixed times, for the reasons which have already been given. However, with demand feeding, once the milk has 'come in', it is unlikely that the average baby needs to be fed more frequently than every three hours. Fractiousness before this time can be coped with by cuddling, which is probably what the baby wants.

The quantity of milk

It is very difficult to decide from the length of time which the baby spends feeding if it is getting enough milk. As the baby usually gets nearly all the milk available in the first 10 minutes, it may continue to feed because it is comfortable, or because it is getting a little trickle of milk, or because it is asleep. But if the baby is content, it has had enough. Nor can you tell if the baby is satisfied or still hungry by the fact that it cries after a feed. The cry may be due to 'wind', or because the baby is wet, rather than because it is still hungry. Nor can you tell about the quantity, or the quality, of the milk from the fullness of the breasts or the appearance of the milk. In the first week or two the breasts are usually firm, and appear full, although the quantity of milk secreted is not great. After a while, the sequence of production of milk, the 'let down' or passage of milk to the milk sinuses, and the balance between demand and production of milk is established, and the breasts appear less full, although in fact milk production has increased.

The best way of telling if there is sufficient milk is observation of the baby. If it is happy, contented and gaining weight (checked every few days, not after every few feeds), there is enough milk. If the baby is fractious but gaining weight, it is getting enough milk but may be guzzling it down too fast and getting 'wind'. Only if the baby is hungry, crying and not gaining weight, need there be any worry, and even then inadequate milk supply is only one possible reason.

One of the most important ways of being sure that there is sufficient milk is to avoid being worried. The young mother who is full of anxiety about her milk supply, and who fusses constantly that her baby is not getting enough, may well reduce the amount of milk she secretes. Worry is a good way to reduce milk supplies! Modern woman relies too much on scales, and on formulae for feeding. In the developing countries of the world, millions of mothers who have no scales feed their babies 'on demand'; the babies seem to thrive, and to get all the milk they need. Incidentally, it is almost impossible to overfeed a baby.

The quality of breast milk

The quality of the breast milk of a mother who has a normal diet is high. There is no such thing as 'weak milk'. If the baby is fractious, it is because it has to work to feed, or because it is being suckled in the wrong way – not because the milk is weak. Generally speaking, what the mother eats or does will not alter the quality of her milk. She can continue to eat all the foods she is accustomed to eating, and she can drink alcohol, (in moderation, for a drunk mother is hardly a good mother!) tea or coffee. A few substances do cross into the milk and affect the baby. The most annoying drugs are cascara, which no woman needs, and bromides, which can be avoided. A few mothers find that certain foods also affect their baby, although their friends who are breast-feeding find that their babies are not affected by the same foods. It is obviously a peculiarity confined to that mother and her baby, and the simple answer is to avoid that particular food in the future.

Anxiety about the progress of the baby, nervousness and insecurity can reduce the *quantity* of milk secreted, which makes the baby fractious, but this will not alter the *quality*.

Contraception during lactation

Although breast-feeding reduces the chances of conceiving, it is not a certain method. Because of this, many lactating women want to know what additional contraceptive measure they should use. The choice of contraceptives was discussed in Chapter 7, and I stressed that a woman should choose what is right for her. But if she is breast-feeding she is probably wise to avoid the combined oral contraceptives as the milk-supply of some mothers is reduced when taking the Pill, although this is less likely with the new very low-dose Pills. Alternatively, she can use the gestagen-only Pill (see p. 116), which is said to increase the milk-supply rather than the reverse. However, it is not the only choice and you may prefer to have an I.U.D. inserted, or to use a vaginal diaphragm. The choice must be yours after appropriate counselling.

Myths about breast-feeding

A reason given by many mothers – particularly French women – for avoiding breast-feeding is that it will spoil their figures, and cause the breasts to sag. These two statements are untrue. A woman who breast-feeds her baby does not need to stuff herself with food – she has already got a store of fat during pregnancy for this very purpose, which she can burn up. Nor do mothers who feed their babies develop sagging breasts. After a pregnancy the breast is a little more mature and soft, rather than being pointed and firm, but it will not sag, particularly if during the last weeks of pregnancy and during the puerperium the mother wears a well-fitting brassière, day and night.

Another myth is that breast-feeding 'tires out' a mother. Although the care of a new baby does require energy, and consequently the mother should take an increased quantity of milk (for calcium), protein, vegetables and fruit, breast-feeding is probably less tiring that bottle-feeding. In breast-feeding all the mother has to do is put the baby to the breast; if she 'formula feeds', she has to prepare the formula, keep the milk sterile, warm it, feed the baby, clean the bottle, and get the next feed ready. Some women find that they are uncertain how to care for their baby, and worry about the child's progress. These women are apt to feel 'worn out and tired', and blame this on breast-feeding rather than on the disturbed sleep and additional responsibilities which a new baby demands.

Some women find that when they breast-feed their sexual arousal and desire are diminished. It is doubtful if this is due to lactation. A young baby takes up a great deal of time and energy so that less is available for other things, one of which may be your libido. But you can be aroused if your husband helps you by being considerate and spending more time in 'pleasuring' you before sexual intercourse begins. Other women find breast-feeding sexually arousing and pleasurable. If it makes you feel randy do not feel guilty; enjoy the feeling! It is quite normal. And with a helpful man you can enjoy both breast-feeding and sex whether simultaneously or in sequence.

Do not listen to your 'friends' who tell you that breast-feeding is 'taking too much out of you', or the baby 'doesn't seem to be thriving – it's a bit thin!' or 'why don't you put the baby on the bottle – it's so easy'. Ignore them – you know what is best for your baby. You are the expert!

The final myth is a particularly insidious one. This is that a woman who fails to breast-feed her baby has failed as a mother. This is quite untrue. Breast-feeding offers the most suitable milk for the baby, and it brings the mother and her baby into a close, intimate contact; but for psychologists to say that the bottle-fed baby is deprived and will be less stable and happy in later life is just stupid. The mother can show her concern for her baby by caring for it as she feeds it with the bottle, and she can cuddle it between feeds. If she fails to breast-feed or decides not to breast-feed, she is not 'depriving her child' and need not feel guilty. Bottle-fed babies cannot be identified from breast-fed babies in later life.

Do the drugs you take get into your breast milk?

Lactating mothers often express concern that drugs they take, or which are prescribed for them by a doctor may be excreted in breast milk and may affect the baby. Whilst most drugs, including antibiotics, do pass into breast milk the amount is small and will neither benefit nor harm the baby.

Only a few drugs may cause damage to the baby. These include *anti-coagulants* (given to the mother to treat blood clots) which may cause haemorrhages in the baby; *antithyroid drugs* (particularly *thiouracil*) which may depress the infant's thyroid gland; a laxative called *Coloxyl* which may give the baby diarrhoea; *lithium* which may make the baby cold and blue, and *Mysoline* which is sometimes used to treat epilepsy.

If you have been prescribed one of these drugs, stop breast-feeding; if not, you do not need to worry.

Difficulties of breast-feeding

ENGORGEMENT. If the mother determines to follow the plan of 'demand feeding', it may still be necessary to put the baby to the breast at regular intervals in the first three days. By the 3rd or 4th day of the puerperium, the milk 'comes in'. This means that milk production is now in full swing, but that the passage of milk into the ducts and out of the nipple is not yet properly organized. In some women the breasts become heavy, tense and warm. In a few women they are painful. The breasts are said to be 'engorged'. Engorgement is only temporary, lasting for less than 24 hours, and the doctors and nursing staff are fully competent to help the mother.

CRACKED NIPPLES. In normal feeding, the infant grasps the areola of the nipple, and not the nipple itself. The nipple lies free in the baby's mouth. How it should be grasped can be visualized if you suck your thumb, so that the end is freely movable in the mouth. If the nipple is free within the infant's mouth, its gums compress the small reservoirs in the lower part of the nipples and milk squirts out of the openings in the nipples. If the nipple is not far enough in the baby's mouth, the milk does not flow easily, the baby becomes frustrated and sucks harder. This may cause cracked, painful nipples. Cracked and painful nipples can also be caused by letting the baby suck for too long. Normally the baby empties a breast in under 7 minutes, and it is pointless to permit it to suckle on that breast for more than 12 minutes. Cracked nipples can be avoided by preparation during pregnancy and by the proper technique of breast-feeding. As well as this, after a feed you should wash your nipples with water (no soap), dry them carefully and put on anhydrous lanolin. If cracked nipples occur, the baby should be taken off the breast for a couple of days, and the breast emptied by manual expression, the expressed milk being sterilized and fed to the baby in a bottle. An antibiotic ointment may be applied to the breast on a doctor's advice.

INSUFFICIENT MILK PRODUCTION. Fear, anxiety, pain, lack of privacy, and unsympathetic attendants can prevent the milk from passing along the ducts within the breast. In these cases, although milk is secreted, the baby gets very little and cries with hunger. This aggravates the anxiety and a vicious circle is set up. Milk production is best in a mother who is healthy, fairly young, has a good diet and who wants to breast-feed. Milk production is likely to be less if the mother is ill, older and poorly motivated about breast-feeding. Milk production may diminish if the mother starts taking oral contraceptives, but this varies considerably.

Various foods and drugs have been recommended to improve milk production, but none has been proved to be of any value. Drinking excessive water or milk does not improve milk production, nor does the use of iodine drops, special 'lactation foods', or thyroid tablets. The most efficient way of establishing a good milk flow is a knowledge of how milk is produced; a desire to breast-feed; a healthy, hungry baby; and sympathetic, helpful nurses.

MENSTRUATION AND LACTATION. This matter is discussed on p. 260.

MASTITIS. Occasionally infection enters the lactating breast, usually introduced through cracked nipples, during the second or third week of the puerperium. The breasts become engorged, hard, reddened, tender and painful. If this happens and you recognize it early enough you should feed your baby more often so that your breast does not

become engorged with milk, which encourages the infection to
become more severe. As long as you cannot express pus from your
nipples you will not infect the baby. This occurs only rarely. In
addition, your doctor will give you a type of penicillin which is
particularly suitable. It is called flucloxacillin. You take the tablets by
mouth.

But remember an ounce of prevention is worth a pound of cure!
Good antenatal preparation for lactation, proper care of your nipples, demand feeding to avoid engorgement and to establish a strong
'let down' will ensure that your breast is empty after a feed. If you
take these measures you are unlikely to develop mastitis.

Suppressing lactation

As I mentioned a number of women choose not to breast-feed and a
number stop breast-feeding after a few weeks. Unless treatment is
given the breasts rapidly become engorged with milk and are painful
for two or three days, after which pressure in the milk producing
areas, the alveoli, suppresses further lactation. To reduce the pain,
binders and analgesics have been prescribed, and the mother
instructed to limit the amount of fluid she drank. These measures did
help, but not a great deal. For the past 30 years, oestrogen tablets
have been used, as it was found that oestrogen 'fed-back' to suppress
the release of prolactin by the pituitary (p. 303). Recently there has
been some concern that oestrogens used in this way increased the
chance of a woman developing a blood clot in a vein and thrombo-
embolism. This led many doctors to refuse to give oestrogen tablets
and to go back to breast binding.

Today a new drug is available which effectively suppresses lactation and has no dangers. The drug is called bromocriptine. It works
by directly stopping the release of prolactin from the hypothalamus.

Although I believe women should breast-feed, I realise that some
will not, and a very few cannot. For these women, bromocriptine
means that lactation can be stopped without any discomfort. Tablets
of bromocriptine are taken daily for 10 to 14 days.

Chapter 19

The Things that Happen to Women

During life it is inevitable that a woman will have her share of anxiety, of illness, of strain, as well as her share of satisfaction and happiness. But because she is biologically different from man, she may develop conditions unique to woman. Many of these are minor, but require attention. In most instances a woman should consult her doctor, but as doctors are busy men and all too often do not explain adequately to the patient the nature of the condition from which she is suffering, she often remains anxious. This chapter attempts to redress this, and to give a woman the chance of understanding herself better. There is no doubt that fear of the unknown is a potent factor in aggravating disease, and insight into the nature of a disorder is a major step to its cure. For convenience, the conditions which may affect a woman in her reproductive years are considered in as alphabetical an order as is practicable.

ENLARGEMENT OF THE WOMB

The most common cause of enlargement of the womb is pregnancy! But sometimes the womb is enlarged by a muscle tumour, or because of the effects of anxiety.

The muscle tumours are called myomata or 'fibroids'. For some unknown reason, one or more of the muscle fibres which make up the uterus start developing, and quite soon a few small pea-sized tumours appear deep in the muscle wall of the uterus. At this stage no one can detect them, but as the months or years pass – for they grow very slowly – the tumours become the size of a golf ball, a tennis ball or even of a grapefruit. By this time the patient can feel a lump in her abdomen, or if the tumour has grown inwards and distorted the shape of the cavity of the uterus, she may have heavier or irregular menstrual periods. Usually she goes to her doctor, who performs a pelvic examination and can tell from this if there is a single fibroid, or if the womb is misshapen and enlarged by several fibroid tumours. It is unusual for a woman who has children early in life to develop fibroids, and the tumours are more likely to be found in spinsters, or women who have children late in life, which has led to the saying that 'fibroids develop in a disappointed womb'. The tumours are very common, and more than 20 per cent of women have fibroids in their womb. In many cases no treatment is required, as the tumour is not causing any symptoms, but in the few women who have symptoms, treatment is needed. The treatment chosen depends upon the patient's age and her desire to have further children.

If a youngish woman, who is anxious to have children, is found to have fibroids which are causing symptoms, the doctor can often operate to remove the fibroids and leave the uterus. It is a bit like a complicated shelling of peas, and although there is a slight chance that the fibroids may grow again, the chances of pregnancy are good. In an older woman, or a woman who wants no further children, the operation chosen is usually that of hysterectomy, in which the womb is removed.

Another cause of enlargement of the womb is anxiety. The ancient Greeks believed that a woman's emotions were made in her womb. The Greek word for womb is *hysteros* – which is why women were said to be hysterical. Of course, the place in which the emotions occur is the brain, but if the emotions – whether due to anxiety, frustration or unhappiness – operate for a sufficient time, they cause a smooth enlargement of the womb, and heavy periods. All too often, doctors have mistaken this emotionally-stimulated enlargement of the womb for fibroids, and have performed a hysterectomy. This cured the heavy periods, but the disturbed emotions were unaltered, and other disorders (usually unexplained abdominal pain or backache) appeared 3 to 6 months after the operation. Occasionally a surgical operation is needed to cure the condition (which is called myo-hyperplasia), but in most cases what is needed is sympathetic understanding and perhaps some drugs to help temporarily.

ENDOMETRIOSIS

Endometriosis is a strange disorder, which affects spinsters and infertile married women more often than those fertile women who have children early in the reproductive years. The term means that the pieces of the lining of the womb (the endometrium) either form small nests (or cysts) in the muscle of the womb (which will, of course, then become bigger), in the ovaries, or in other parts of the pelvis. These nests of endometrium act like miniature wombs, and at the time of menstruation a tiny amount of bleeding occurs. Since the blood cannot escape, the cyst is stretched and becomes painful. The woman complains of dysmenorrhoea, which increases during menstruation and is worse on the last day. If a cyst has formed in the pelvis behind the womb, as sometimes happens, sexual intercourse can be painful when the husband's penis is moving deeply inside the vagina. Because of dysmenorrhoea, painful sexual intercourse, or failure to become pregnant, the woman attends her doctor. In the past the only treatment was surgery, but today hormone treatment using drugs like those contained in the Pill can cure the condition, and enable the patient to conceive if she so wishes. Some women do need surgery, but often all the gynaecologist has to do is to make a tiny incision below the umbilicus and introduce an instrument, rather like a peri-scope, so that he can see the extent of the disease. This minor operation is done under anaesthesia and is painless. Once the doctor knows how much the endometriosis has involved the genital organs, he can decide if surgery or hormone treatment is best, or if both are needed.

HYSTERECTOMY

One of the most common surgical operations performed on women is removal of the womb, or hysterectomy. In fact, many doctors believe that the operation is done too often for too little reason. An Ameri-can surgeon has written that a woman has about 1,000 dollars-worth of 'expendable parts', a major one being her womb, and by the age of 50 has had most of them removed! This is perhaps extreme, for in many cases a well-performed hysterectomy can cure a patient who was previously miserable. But, even so, the operation is still done too often, for too little reason, and without explaining to the woman its effects. Unfortunately, if the operation is performed for a trivial reason and without proper counselling, a large number of women develop depression which can last for up to 2 years. In careful investigations in England and Australia of women who have had a hysterectomy, the doctors found that over one-third developed depression, and it was sometimes very severe.

Depression after hysterectomy is reduced if a woman, who has been advised to have the operation, is able to talk with her gynaecologist before surgery is performed. It is your right and the doctor's duty to tell you what is wrong with your uterus and why you need the operation. You should not feel that you are wasting the doctor's time, nor that you are asking stupid questions. You should not feel ashamed about asking *any* question and you should expect an answer in clear language that you can understand. Some women believe that they have to have the operation because of some earlier sexual activity, such as masturbation or a previous abortion, or an extramarital affair, and the operation is a punishment. This, of course, is not so. Other women believe, falsely, that without a uterus a woman is no longer a proper woman. This too is untrue.

Hysterectomy does not make a woman sexually mutilated and undesired; it does not shorten or narrow her vagina so that sexual intercourse is impossible, painful or potentially dangerous. Provided that the gynaecologist is skilful, the only after-effects of hysterectomy are that you have no more menstrual periods and pregnancy cannot possibly occur. All the other fears, anxieties and unhappiness connected with the operation occur because a woman has not had the chance to talk, properly and openly, with her doctor.

Myths associated with hysterectomy

'AFTER HYSTERECTOMY I WILL BECOME OLD, UNFEMININE AND UNDESIRABLE'. This is untrue. A woman is sexually desirable because of her character and personality. She is feminine because of the way she has been brought up and because of the female sex hormones which are secreted by her ovaries. It is usual, if a woman is under the age of 45, and often whatever her age, to leave her ovaries in place, so that they can continue to function. And if they need to be removed, oestrogen hormone tablets can be taken to replace those lost. But talk with your doctor.

'AFTER HYSTERECTOMY I WON'T WANT OR ENJOY SEX ANY MORE'. This is untrue. Your enjoyment of sex does not depend on the presence of your uterus, but on the presence of a good, communicating relationship with your man. The operation does not shorten or

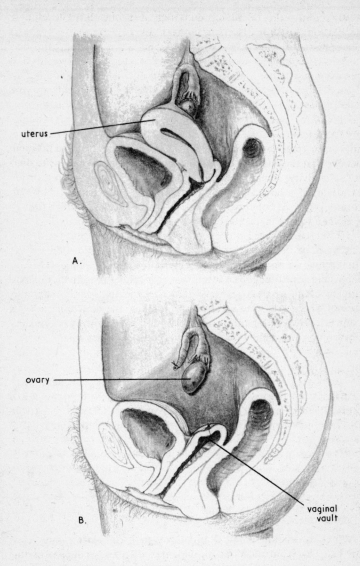

FIG. 19/1 The length of the vagina shown in A is not
shortened by hysterectomy shown in B

narrow your vagina; in fact, if anything it is longer, as you can see (Fig. **19/1**). When the womb is removed the vagina has to be cut and then stitched again at its upper end, and the cervix no longer projects into it. Once the cut has healed properly, which takes between 4 and 6 weeks, you can start enjoying sexual intercourse once again; before that time you can enjoy mutual pleasuring, including digital or oral stimulation of your clitoris (see page 76).

'AFTER HYSTERECTOMY WOMEN BECOME FAT'. This is untrue. Hysterectomy is not followed by obesity, unless the woman takes no exercise after the operation and spends her time eating. If she does this, of course she will get fat.

MENSTRUAL DISORDERS

Because of the complicated control of menstruation which was described in Chapter 4, and because of the impact of the emotions upon the controlling area in the brain, it can be readily understood that from time to time during a woman's life menstrual disorders may occur. These are, in general, of three kinds: the menstrual periods may occur less frequently, or cease altogether; they may occur regularly but be very heavy; or they may become quite irregular in time of onset, in their duration and in the amount of blood lost. These irregularities are more usual before the age of 20 and after the age of 35, but may occur at any time during the reproductive years. Furthermore, many women find that the character of their menstrual period alters during the reproductive years. Often the periods become heavier for a while after childbirth, and as the age of 40 is approached.

The three patterns of menstrual irregularity do need further discussion because many women become very anxious when the periods are not 'normal'.

Less frequent periods or no periods

If the periods occur at longer intervals than usual, and if the interval is at least 14 days more than usual, there may be a problem. The problem is more acute when the periods cease altogether, and the woman has amenorrhoea. Both conditions can be caused by a number of factors, but the most usual one seems to be due to the effect of the emotions, which in turn alter the sequence of hormonal release. If the periods cease altogether, the first thing to do is to make sure that you are not pregnant. And as I have written in Chapter 8, a simple pregnancy test will resolve this. A number of women taking the Pill also develop amenorrhoea. This need be of no concern provided the woman continues to take the Pill as directed. Amenorrhoea also occurs if a girl leaves home to take up a job in a different environment, or if she is under great emotional stress. In the War years, women interned by the Japanese under primitive, unfamiliar conditions, noticed that their periods ceased soon after internment; and today some women find that their menstrual periods cease during bereavement after the death of a loved one. If a woman has less frequent periods occurring over a period of 6 months, or if she has amenorrhoea, she should seek help from a doctor. Infrequent periods are generally of no concern and what a woman needs is to be reassured that she is normal. This can be done once the doctor has made an examination. Treatment using hormones is not indicated, and many women, once they have been reassured, may prefer to have less frequent periods!

If a woman has amenorrhoea, the doctor should exclude pregnancy and find out if the woman is taking the Pill. If she is pregnant she will have to decide whether or not she wants the baby, whilst if she is taking the Pill she need not be concerned that she has no periods, as menstruation has no real function (see p. 45).

However, if the amenorrhoea persists for 9 months or more it is wise for a woman to be seen by a specialist so that he can find out why she is not menstruating. The doctor will do a general and a vaginal examination and will arrange for some blood tests to measure the levels of certain hormones. With this information he can assess whether reassurance or treatment is needed. But I should stress, that provided the amenorrhoea is not due to disease (and usually it is not), and provided the woman does not want to become pregnant, there is no indication for giving hormones to produce a menstrual bleed. It is better to remain without periods.

Heavy regular periods

The pattern of a woman's periods may change so that they become excessively heavy and often last for longer than previously, although their regularity is unchanged. In some women, the problem is aggravated by clots being expelled during menstruation and the woman feels heavy and exhausted.

If the pattern does not revert to normal quickly she should see a doctor. He will examine her generally, making sure she has not become anaemic or has high blood pressure, and also vaginally to be sure that she has not developed a 'fibroid' (see p. 319) or a tumour of her ovary. In many cases he will also recommend that the woman has a diagnostic curettage performed. In this minor operation, the lining of the womb is 'cleaned' off ('scraped' is too strong a verb!) and looked at under the microscope so that the doctor can choose the correct treatment. The operation is performed under an anaesthetic, and the woman need not spend more than a few hours in hospital and certainly does not need to suffer the indignity of having her pubic hair shaved off. Although the operation is loosely called a 'D and C', the proper term, which stresses the fact that it is done *to make a diagnosis*, is a 'diagnostic curettage'.

Not all women with heavy regular periods need a diagnostic curettage, but if a woman is aged 35 or more it is usual to do it, to make quite sure that no cancer of the womb is present.

The choice of treatment should be a matter for discussion with the doctor. Most women will be cured if gestagen hormones are given; and only if these fail need hysterectomy be considered. Unfortunately many doctors – and many women – prefer hysterectomy as a first step. Whilst this may be most successful, it can also lead to many problems unless full discussion has taken place (see p. 321).

Irregular bleeding

If a woman has episodes of bleeding which are irregular in duration, in amount and occur unpredictably, it is inconvenient, disturbing and produces anxiety. She should see her doctor who will examine her and must perform a diagnostic curettage, usually at a time when the woman is not bleeding, so that the most information can be obtained.

With the information obtained from the examination and from the laboratory, the doctor will be better able to discuss the problem with the woman and to advise her. The choices of treatment are to use hormones, or to do a hysterectomy. If the woman wants to have more children, hormones would be used; but in older women or women whose family is complete, both treatments are appropriate. The advantage of hormones is that an operation can be avoided, at least for many women. However, hysterectomy may be the more appropriate treatment. This can only be determined after full discussion between the woman and her gynaecologist, who has spoken with her family doctor, as he knows her family circumstances, which may be important in making a decision.

When this sequence is followed the results of hysterectomy are good; but to repeat what I have written, too many hysterectomies are being performed for too little or for the wrong reasons.

OBESITY

Some women are never satisfied. They are too thin and want to be fatter, or too fat and want to be thinner. Those who are too fat for their height are called obese. The average weight for height is shown in Table 19/1, so you can calculate if you are overweight, or obese. Of course, you may not need to calculate; it may be obvious to your friends and yourself that you are too fat. Obesity is to some extent dependent on a woman's body structure and metabolism. If she comes from an obese family and has obese parents, she is likely to become obese no matter how hard she tries to avoid it. Many women find it infuriating that some of their friends can eat and drink as much as they like and never put on weight, whilst they themselves appear to gain weight merely by looking at food. Looking at food does not put on weight. Eating does, and within the limits established by heredity, fat women are fat because they eat too much and eat the wrong foods. Women who are too fat can lose weight, but it is a slow process and requires great self-control, discipline and persistence.

Because of woman's desire to be something other than she is, and in particular to be thinner, an infinite variety of diets, drugs, regimens, exercises, cures, massages, hydrotherapy and quackery constantly are being recommended. The propagators of these methods have grown rich, a few women have grown thin, but many have not changed; and it is these women who keep the diet-propagators rich, as they in desperation try new methods and adopt other gimmicks. Hardly a week passes without a woman's magazine advising their readers to try this 'six-day tripe diet', or that 'four-day egg and anchovy diet', or the other 'orange, onions and oyster diet'.

It needs to be repeated, a woman can lose weight if she has

self-control, discipline, persistence and only eats the right foods – and they are many.

Table 19/1

Desirable Weight (Kilograms)

Height		Small Frame	Medium Frame	Large Frame
Feet	Inches			
4	8	41.7–44.4	43.6–48.5	47.1–54.0
4	9	42.6–45.8	44.4–49.9	48.0–55.3
4	10	43.5–47.2	45.8–51.3	49.4–56.7
4	11	44.9–48.5	47.2–52.6	50.8–58.0
5	0	46.2–49.9	48.5–54.0	52.2–59.4
5	1	47.6–51.3	49.9–55.3	53.5–60.0
5	2	49.0–52.6	51.3–57.1	54.9–62.6
5	3	50.3–54.0	52.6–59.0	56.7–64.4
5	4	51.7–55.8	54.4–61.2	58.5–66.2
5	5	53.5–57.6	56.2–63.1	60.3–68.0
5	6	54.9–59.4	58.0–64.9	62.1–69.8
5	7	57.1–61.2	59.9–66.7	64.0–71.7
5	8	59.0–63.5	61.7–68.5	65.8–73.9
5	9	60.8–65.3	63.5–70.3	67.6–76.2
5	10	62.6–67.1	65.3–72.1	69.4–78.5

Women (Age 25 and over)

*For girls between 18 and 25, subtract approximately ½ kilogram for each year under 25.

If a woman really wants to lose weight, she has to stick to the diet and obey the rules. Drugs do not cause weight loss, although they may act as a 'prop' to make the hardships of the diet less. One of the most commonly used drugs is amphetamine, which should be avoided because it is an addictive drug. It is far safer to have self-discipline than to use drugs, and the end results are better. Women who use drugs as well as a reducing diet have a much higher chance of putting on weight again later. The woman who sticks to her diet until she has reduced to her desired or 'ideal' weight, without needing drugs, finds it far easier to keep on a diet which will maintain her at that weight. The 'ideal' weight for height and body build is shown in Table 19/1. These weights are of women wearing thin underclothes ('bra' and panties).

Problems may arise when dining out. I know that it might be difficult and impolite to refuse some special, but fattening dish which your hostess has gone to a great deal of trouble to prepare. The solution is to accept a small portion, and to try to eat less, earlier in the day before attending the dinner. If pre-dinner drinks are served, take either soda-water or a single whisky and water. At dinner try to have no more than one glass of wine.

In Table 19/2 you can see the foods you may not eat, the foods which are rationed, and the foods of which you may eat all you wish, within reason, of course! It is doubtful, for example, if you will eat more than 240 g, that is 8 oz, of meat, or more than 4 eggs a day! Table 19/3 gives an example of a diet for one week, but of course you can make up your own if you wish.

Table 19/2

Foods you may not eat
  Fried foods.
  Sugar, jam, marmalade or honey.
  Sweets or chocolates.
  Nuts.
  Butter (beyond the ration of 15 g (½ oz), margarine, fat or oil.
  Bread (except in the ration, see below), cake, biscuits, toast or
    breakfast cereals.
  Macaroni, spaghetti or semolina.
  Rice (except boiled and replacing the potato ration).
  Puddings, ice-cream, dried or tinned fruits.
  Cream.
  Alcohol.

Foods of which you may eat as much as you like (within reason!)

Lean meat, poultry, game, rabbit, liver, kidney, sweetbreads (provided you do not use flour, breadcrumbs or thick sauces).

Fish, steamed, boiled or grilled only.

Eggs.

Vegetables of all kinds – fresh, frozen, dried or tinned (except for baked beans, lima beans, kidney beans, sweet corn, lentils, avocado, sweet potatoes, which are all prohibited).

Salads, tomatoes, cucumbers, beetroot, watercress or parsley (together more than one of these makes a 'combination salad'), but only without oil or mayonnaise, although you can use a lemon and vinegar dressing if you wish.

Fresh fruit, grapefruit, cranberries, strawberries, melon (but only *one* apple, orange, peach or banana if this is chosen to replace the fruits listed).

Soup, clear such as consommé, broth, 'meat extract'.

Salt, pepper, mustard, Worcester sauce for seasoning (but no other sauces).

Saccharin, if desired for sweetening.

Tea, coffee (milk can be added from the ration).

Foods which are rationed

Bread – 3 slices weighing 30 g, or 1 oz, each. Wholemeal bread is preferable to white bread.

Butter – 15 g (½ oz).

Milk   – 300 ml, 10 fluid oz, of whole milk, *or* 600 ml, 20 fluid oz, of skimmed milk or yoghurt.

Potato – boiled, steamed or baked 'in the skin'; but not fried, 'chipped' or roasted. A maximum of 240 g (8 oz) can be eaten.

or Rice   – 120 g (4 oz) can be substituted for the potato.

Table 19/3

A Recommended Diet

(giving approximately 1,600 calories a day)

BREAKFAST   Every day you may choose from grapefruit (a half), strawberries, or a slice of melon; then eat an egg or grilled tomatoes and mushrooms, with one or two slices of bread or toast only; tea or coffee, with milk from the ration.

MONDAY	*Lunch*	Clear soup Egg salad 1 slice of bread Coffee or tea
	Dinner	Steak, tomatoes, celery, green salad, baked potato Apple Coffee or tea
TUESDAY	*Lunch*	Grilled kidneys on toast (1 slice) An apple, an orange or a banana
	Dinner	Boiled chicken, fresh beans, baked potato ½ grapefruit (fresh) Coffee or tea
WEDNESDAY	*Lunch*	Egg and combination salad, 1 potato, boiled or baked in skin
	Dinner	Consommé 2 lamb chops (cut off the fat before grilling), peas, baked potato Coffee or tea
THURSDAY	*Lunch*	Eggs (grilled), mashed potato, spinach or cauliflower Orange, apple or grapefruit
	Dinner	Steak, salad, 1 baked potato Fresh fruit Coffee or tea
FRIDAY	*Lunch*	Poached eggs and spinach 1 slice of bread or toast Coffee or tea

Dinner   Consommé
           Fish, baked potato, courgettes
               (zucchini) or carrots
           Fruit
           Coffee or tea

SATURDAY   *Lunch*   Egg, salad, celery
                     1 slice of wholemeal bread
                     Coffee or tea

           Dinner Boiled chicken and rice, mushrooms,
                         marrow (summer squash)
                     Melon
                     Coffee or tea

SUNDAY   *Lunch*   Sweetbreads or eggs with mushrooms,
                         combination salad
                     1 slice of wholemeal bread
                     Fruit
                     Coffee or tea

           Dinner Vegetable soup
                     Steak, combination salad, baked
                         potato
                     Fruit – orange or apple
                     Coffee or tea

There is no instant method of losing weight. It takes time and discipline. If a woman is 6 kg (14 lb) over-weight, for example, she can calculate that 5 kg of this is due to excess fat and perhaps 1 kg to water retention. Twelve pounds of fat contain about 50,000 calories. The normal, averagely-active woman needs about 2,100 calories a day, and the suggested diet only gives her 1,600 calories a day, so that each day she burns up 500 calories from her stored fat. To lose 50,000 calories will take 100 days. There is no instant cure!! The recommended diet will enable a woman to lose just under 0.4 kg (1 lb) a week, but she will have to accept that in some weeks she will lose less than in others, because at certain times of the month, usually in the week before menstruation, a woman normally retains water. So do not weigh yourself more than once a week.

OVARIES – REMOVAL

The removal of a woman's ovaries by surgery when she is younger than 45 years is followed by very severe 'menopausal symptoms'. These can be very distressing. In the past, unfortunately, many ovaries were removed unnecessarily by surgeons who had not had a proper training in gynaecology. A gynaecologist who has to operate on a young woman because of pelvic disease will use all his skill to preserve her ovaries. This is possible, even if the ovaries are enlarged by cysts. The cysts can be carefully dissected out of the ovaries, leaving enough ovarian tissue to reconstruct an ovary which functions well. Very occasionally a woman younger than 45 years develops ovarian cancer; in this disease it is essential that both ovaries are removed, but treatment with small tablets of oestrogen hormone, given by mouth, will reduce or eliminate menopausal symptoms.

THE 'PREMENSTRUAL SYNDROME' AND 'PELVIC CONGESTION'

In the few days before menstruation many women develop the premenstrual syndrome also called 'premenstrual tension'. This is due to water being retained abnormally in the body under the influence of the female sex hormones. The woman may notice that her breasts become tender and swollen; that she gets 'bags' under her eyes; and that her abdomen feels bloated. Some women develop migraine at this time, whilst others become constipated. Even more annoying, a woman may become irritable with her husband and family (or with her lover), occasionally depressed, sometimes sleepy, and prone to headaches. The syndrome is fairly common, and if severe can be treated by giving tablets which encourage her to get rid of the retained water and consequently to pass more urine, and occasionally by prescribing tranquillizers until menstruation relieves the symptoms.

A new treatment has been announced which may replace tranquillizers and diuretic tablets. Two Dutch gynaecologists have found that a possible cause of the premenstrual syndrome is increased blood levels of the hormone, prolactin (see p. 303). A drug called bromocriptine effectively reduced these high levels and relieved the symptoms of the premenstrual syndrome in almost all of the women they treated. The tablets are taken twice daily from the 10th day of the menstrual cycle.

PELVIC CONGESTION. In 'pelvic congestion' certain symptoms of premenstrual tension persist throughout the menstrual cycle, but are usually more severe in the days before menstruation. The patient complains of feelings of pressure in the pelvis, backache, and vague feelings of being unwell. Often these women have heavier periods. The symptoms are thought to be due to congestion of the pelvic organs with blood, and this in turn is due to emotional stress. Although many women with these symptoms feel that an operation to remove the uterus would help, and many doctors perform a hysterectomy, the results are not good. The best treatment is for the woman to try and resolve her emotional problems, seeking the help of a sympathetic gynaecologist, or a psychiatrist when necessary.

PERIODIC 'BLOATING'. A number of women complain that periodically they develop 'bloating'. When an attack starts, the woman finds her face and hands are puffy, when she wakes up; she may be irritable or depressed, and under some domestic or occupational stress. As the day goes on she finds that her belly becomes distended, and by evening her ankles are swollen. The attack may last only one day or persist for a few days, when constipation seems to be likely, and then disappear only to recur again unexpectedly. Some women find that the 'bloating' is worse in hot weather and, in some, it occurs just before a menstrual period, when it can be confused with the premenstrual syndrome, although usually the weight gain is greater, exceeding 1.5 kg (or 3½ lbs).

The cause is that, for some unknown reason, fluid 'leaks' out of the circulation into the tissues. It is difficult to know how to treat the disorder. First, a woman should know that the irritability and depression are caused by the fluid retention, and should make sure that her sexual partner or her family are aware of this. She needs sympathy not hostility. Second, diuretics help if they are given intermittently, even if the bloating persists. Third, if she is constipated she should not use laxatives but increase her bran intake (see p. 335). Fourth, she should stop smoking, as nicotine seems to aggravate the problem.

IRRITATED COLON. A number of women who have symptoms of 'pelvic congestion' also have a disorder referred to as the 'irritable or irritated colon'. It also is called 'spastic colon'. A woman with this disorder complains of intermittent pain in her abdomen on the left side and low down. As well she finds that her bowels play up. She may have episodes of diarrhoea alternating the constipation and feel 'bloated'. The pain is relieved when she opens her bowels but it returns, particularly after eating.

The condition can be quite disturbing and treatment has been rather unsatisfactory, mainly because it is a psychosomatic disorder. Recent research has shown that patients who have an irritable colon often have a disturbance in the speed with which food moves along their gut, and as well the tension in the affected part of the bowel is increased. The speed of transit of the faeces along the bowel and the tension within the colon can both be regulated by the simple expedient of cutting down sugar and eating coarse bran. If a woman eats wholemeal instead of white bread she needs to eat less bran, and for most women an additional 2 tablespoons of coarse bran eaten daily will relieve the pain and regulate the bowel habits. Because her bowels are not conditioned to 'roughage' she should start by taking 2 teaspoons each day of coarse bran and increase the amount each day until she gets regular soft bulky motions and the pain goes. You can eat the bran alone, like a horse, or mix it with breakfast cereal or yoghurt.

PROLAPSE

If the tissues which support the vagina and uterus are abnormally stretched during childbirth, or if a tear of the perineum is not repaired, the woman may later experience symptoms of prolapse, or what is often called a 'fallen womb'. The prolapse may involve a weakness of the front wall of the vagina – called a *cystocele*; a weakness of the back wall of the vagina, usually associated with damage also to the tissues between the vagina and the rectum – called a *rectocele*; or a weakness of the supports of the womb, which is a *uterine prolapse*.

The weakness of the front vaginal wall – or cystocele – may make a bulge or lump which can be felt just inside the vagina or at its entrance when the patient strains. Unless it is associated with bladder symptoms such as frequency of urination, infection of the urine as shown by laboratory tests, or unless it is very marked, surgery is not required.

The weakness of the back vaginal wall, particularly if there is also an unrepaired tear of the perineum, makes the entrance to the vagina larger, and a lump may be felt there on straining. Once again, unless it causes symptoms, treatment is not really required.

The prolapse of the womb itself only needs treatment if the cervix projects from the vagina, or if the symptoms of 'something falling out' become annoying. The womb normally 'drops' a little down the vagina when the pressure in the abdomen is increased, as in straining to open the bowels, and the cervix may be felt just inside the vaginal entrance. So long as the tissues have good tone and a good blood supply, the minor degree of prolapse does not worry the woman; but after the menopause the blood supply is reduced and the tissues become less flexible, so that the prolapse becomes more obvious and symptoms begin. Prolapse of the womb does not cause backache, despite what is believed.

Once a 'prolapse' causes symptoms, treatment is generally surgical. However today, with better obstetric care, severe prolapse is less common, and the big operations of the past are less often required. Since many patients who have small degrees of prolapse do not need treatment at all, the decision to operate should only be made by an experienced gynaecologist.

'RETROVERSION' OF THE WOMB

Normally the womb lies bent forward at an angle of nearly 90° to that of the vagina, and it is able to rotate about an axis at the level of the cervix (Fig. 19/2). As the bladder fills, it pushes the uterus up and backwards, and if a woman lies on her back her womb may 'tilt backwards'. In 10 per cent of women the womb is normally tilted backwards. The condition is called 'retroversion', and it can occur from time to time in women whose uterus normally lies bent forwards, or anteverted. In the past an amazing variety of gynaecological disorders have been attributed to retroversion of the uterus; these included backache, sterility, vaginal discharge, pelvic pain, headaches, constipation, diminished sexual desire, frequency of urination and 'wind'! The many operations devised to 'correct' the retroversion made the doctors rich, but did little to cure the patient's symptoms which, although temporarily relieved, returned after a while. Retroversion is often called 'twisting' of the womb by doctors

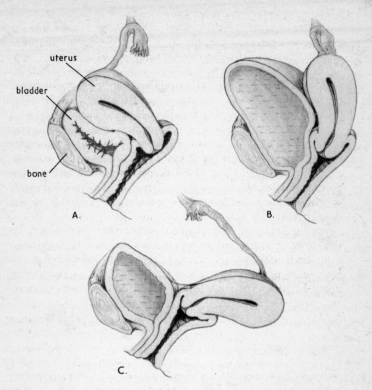

FIG. 19/2 The 'normal' and 'retroverted' uterus, showing
A. how the uterus normally lies in the pelvis; B. how it
may move when the bladder fills and C. a 'retroverted'
uterus

who try to explain the condition to their patients. This is a bad term,
for a twisted womb implies a dangerous condition which needs careful surgery for correction, when all that has happened is that the
uterus has *tilted* backwards, a quite normal event.

It is now known that unless the womb is *fixed* in the retroverted
position by infection or endometriosis, it is of no importance that it is
retroverted, as it causes none of the symptoms attributed to it, and
there is no need for an operation or the use of supporting 'pessaries'
which were once popular.

'TROUBLE WITH THE WATER'

A singularly distressing complaint, which most often occurs after the age of 40, is an 'irritable bladder'. This is not the medical term, and the condition is more properly called 'urgency incontinence', but in fact the patient complains of an 'irritable bladder'. In most cases the woman finds that she gets the urge to empty her bladder at very frequent intervals, and the urge may be stimulated by coughing, jolting in a bus or car, or something of that nature. Once she begins to urinate, she has to go on until her bladder is empty, but because she passes urine so frequently, she only voids a small amount of urine each time. Occasionally an irritable bladder is due to some disorder such as infection, but in most cases it is due to an emotional upset which shows itself in this way. The doctor will have to make tests to decide what is the cause, as only then can he give treatment. This is always medical, and surgery is not needed.

There is another kind of urination trouble which may inconvenience a woman. In this a tiny amount of urine escapes and soils the underclothes whenever the patient strains, coughs or laughs. The woman may be young or old, but has usually given birth to one or more children. The condition is called 'stress incontinence' because the loss of urine occurs after a stress or strain. It can occur whether the bladder is full or apparently empty. The doctor has to differentiate this condition very carefully from urgency incontinence, because the more annoying forms of stress incontinence do require surgical treatment. The lesser forms, when the loss of urine only occurs occasionally, can be treated by the patient doing exercises to strengthen the muscles which support the vagina and the urethra – the short tube connecting the bladder to the outside. The exercises consist of tightening the muscle of the 'tail' without using the abdominal muscles. I describe this as 'trying to make the anus, or back-passage opening, touch the mouth'. A woman can do the exercises in any free moment, and should aim at doing them at least one hundred times a day.

URINARY TRACT INFECTION

The urinary tract starts at the kidney, continues as the tube (the ureter) between the kidney and the bladder, expands as the bladder and then goes on as the tube (the urethra) between the bladder and the outside. Infection of the urinary tract is usually due to the spread of bacteria from the outside up along the urethra to infect the bladder (called 'cystitis'), and then in most cases up the ureter to infect the kidney (called 'pyelonephritis'). Because a woman has a shorter urethra than a man, she is more likely to develop infection of the bladder. Luckily in most cases this is of no importance, as the bladder itself kills the bacteria, so that the urine is sterile, but it appears that about 5 per cent of girls and women harbour active bacteria in their bladders. These bacteria may cause infection at any time, but especially during the first weeks of marriage ('honeymoon cystitis'), and in pregnancy. It is thought that the movement of the penis against the urethra and bladder which occurs in sexual intercourse stimulates the bacteria to grow, and in pregnancy the urine tends to stagnate in the bladder.

The symptoms of urinary tract infection are frequency of urination, and painful urination especially towards the end of voiding. If infection has involved the kidney, backache in the kidney area, fever and chills develop.

If a woman develops these symptoms, she should consult a doctor so that he may have the urine examined for bacteria, and prescribe treatment. Untreated urinary tract infection can lead to kidney damage.

POSTCOITAL CYSTITIS. An unpleasant form of cystitis sometimes begins during a period of frequent sexual intercourse. Usually this clears with treatment but some women have the misfortune to develop cystitis every time they have coitus. This, in turn, prevents any enjoyment because the woman knows it will be followed, within 36 hours, by frequency and pain.

The cause of postcoital cystitis is due to bacteria which live in the urethra being massaged back up into the bladder by the movement of the man's penis in the woman's vagina (If you look at Figs. 1/4 or 19/2 you can see how close the urethra is to the vagina.) Once inside the bladder, bacteria are usually killed by secretions of the cells which line the bladder, but in some women this does not occur. Instead the bacteria thrive, doubling their number every half hour. The result is cystitis.

Doctors have tried many drugs in an attempt to cure this distressing complaint, but with indifferent success. A woman has found an answer which seems to be more successful. It is quite simple. If you suffer from postcoital cystitis, all you have to do is to empty your bladder completely within half-an-hour of sexual intercourse. You will do this more easily if you drink three or four glasses of water immediately after intercourse. Should this simple method not cure you, you should obtain some tablets of the drug, nitrofurantoin, from your doctor, and take one 50 mg tablet each night, in addition to emptying your bladder in the way I have suggested.

VAGINAL DISCHARGE

In several investigations it has been found that the most common reason for a woman to see a doctor is that she has a vaginal discharge. Vaginal discharges are of several kinds, some requiring treatment and others being perfectly normal and of no importance. To understand them it must be remembered that the vagina, like the uterus, is part of the genital tract, and that the tissues which make up the tract are very strongly influenced by the female sex hormones, oestrogen and progesterone. Oestrogen stimulates the tissues to mature, and progesterone further develops them. This is most obvious in pregnancy, but changes occur in the lining tissues of the vagina, the cervix, as well as the uterus during each menstrual cycle. The changes caused by oestrogen make the cells lining the cervix secrete a thin, slightly sticky mucus, and this is most marked midway between the periods. The cells which make up the lining of the vagina are arranged rather like bricks making up a wall. The top cells are thin and large. These top cells are constantly shed into the vagina, rather like leaves falling off a tree; in fact, they are said to 'exfoliate' – which means just that. In the vagina they are acted upon by the helpful bacteria which normally live there, to produce a weak acid. This acid – called lactic acid – prevents dangerous bacteria from growing in the vagina. The vaginal cells and the cervical mucus add to the vaginal discharge. As well, some fluid seeps between the cells of the vaginal wall to join the secretions in the vagina. This seepage is increased during sexual excitement, during anxiety, when sexual frustration occurs, or if the woman is ill or emotionally upset.

It can be seen that the quantity of the normal vaginal secretions can vary very considerably and still be quite normal, just as the quantity of secretions in the mouth (the saliva) varies very considerably. The secretions not only keep the vagina moist, which is desirable, but keep it clean. However, from time to time the increased secretions may stain the woman's panties and cause her concern. Usually, if the discharge is not irritating, it is of little importance and treatment is not required. Indeed, in certain conditions, such as when taking some kinds of oral contraceptive, an increased vaginal discharge may be expected to occur. However, if the amount of the discharge is annoying, the woman should consult her doctor. He will take a swab sample of the discharge and look at it under the microscope before prescribing treatment. This non-irritant vaginal discharge, which may or may not have an odour, is called leukorrhoea – or the 'whites' – but it is bad to give it a name, as it immediately becomes something abnormal in most people's minds, whereas in fact it is quite normal.

Irritating vaginal discharges

If the discharge causes itching and pain in the vagina and around its opening in the vulva, the condition is generally due to some disease and certainly requires investigation. Two main kinds of disorder can cause the trouble. The first, and most common, is when a tiny living organism (called a trichomonad) gets into the vagina. This organism is composed of a single cell, and has a powerful tail (Fig. 19/3). How it gets into the vagina of about one woman in every three is unknown, but there is a lot of evidence that it is transmitted during sexual intercourse. In most women it lives quietly in the velvet-like lining of the vagina, and causes no symptoms; in most men it lives quietly in the urinary tract tube within the penis. But in some women, for some unknown reason, it can cause a severe vaginal and vulval itch. The diagnosis is made after the doctor has taken a specimen from the vagina and looked at it under a microscope, when the organism can be seen wriggling about, its tail thrashing. Treatment is easy and effective. Tablets of metronidazole (Flagyl) are taken three times a day for seven to ten days. Since the sexual partner often harbours the trichomonads without knowing it, treatment should be given to him as well as to the woman.

The second, less common, cause of an itchy vagina is when a fungus gets into the vagina and grows there. This is more common in pregnancy and if the woman has diabetes, as the fungus – called Candida albicans (or monilia) – prefers a sugary, warm atmosphere in which to grow. But fungal infection can occur in other women. The vaginal

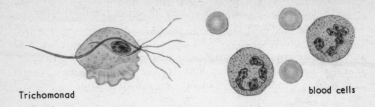

Trichomonad   blood cells

FIG. 19/3 Trichomonads seen under the microscope

discharge can be quite heavy, the itch intolerable, and the woman is in considerable discomfort. Her sexual partner may also be infected and have an itchy penis. Once again, the diagnosis is made by examining a specimen of the discharge under a microscope; branching threads of the fungus will be seen. Two forms of treatment are available. The first is for the woman to paint her vagina with gentian violet three times a week. This is rather messy but effective. It has been replaced by the use of vaginal tablets, called nystatin, which kills the fungus. The woman inserts these tablets, twice daily, high into her vagina for one or two weeks. It is important to continue inserting the tablets if she should start menstruating. If the skin of her vulva is itchy the doctor may give her an ointment, which the man can also use on his penis.

Since the fungus grows best in hot moist conditions she should stop wearing pantihose and change to cotton panties or wear none at all!

Herpes of the vulva

A few women who have monilia also develop small red spots on the labia or around the vaginal entrance. These spots can also appear when monilia is absent. After a day or two the spots turn into big blisters which are exquisitely painful, making the vulva feel like a raw, red hot pad and making it painful to pass urine. This is a condition called herpes genitalis and it is a brute! It is due to a virus called the *Herpes Simplex Type II*, and it can be transmitted by sexual intercourse or can grow on an already irritated area. There is no specific treatment, although many have been suggested; but if you put gentian violet on the ulcers you will obtain some relief and as well you will probably need some form of pain-reliever and an anaesthetic ointment to apply to your vulva. The ulcers heal after about 5 or 6 days but unfortunately the virus remains in the cells deep in the skin even after the ulcers have gone and the disease apparently has been cured, so that the herpes tends to recur.

Of course, other conditions can cause a vaginal discharge, and will be diagnosed after examination by a doctor. One of the most important is a discharge due to gonorrhoea, and this is considered in the next section. Another is the so-called cervical 'erosion'.

Cervical 'erosion'

As noted previously, the lining of the vagina is built up of layers of cells, rather like a wall is built up of bricks, and the same arrangement of cells covers the cervix where it pokes into the upper part of the vagina. However, a sudden change occurs at the edge of the canal leading through the cervix. The cells which line this are a single layer thick. They are large and very active in secreting mucus. During puberty, and again in a first pregnancy, the exact position of the change from the flat wall-like cells of the vaginal part of the cervix to the tall single mucus-secreting cells of the cervical canal moves, and in many women it moves outwards. This means that the tall cells now appear around the entrance to the canal to look like lips (Fig. **19/4**). The same effect can be obtained if you close your mouth and draw in your lips. Your mouth now appears as a slit ringed by pink skin. If you now pout your lips, your mouth is ringed by red lip mucous membrane.

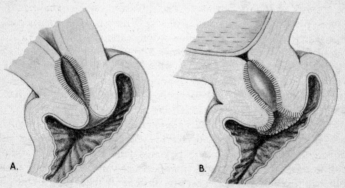

FIG. 19/4 The junction between the lining cells of the cervical canal and those of the cervix move in pregnancy

In the past, the 'pouting' of the cells of the cervical canal was called an 'erosion' or an 'ulcer' because doctors believed it was abnormal. And, of course, it is *not* an ulcer. The treatment of the 'ulcer' was to burn it by applying a cautery stick or by burning it using an electric cautery. It is now known that such treatment is usually unnecessary, and indeed is only needed if at childbirth the mouth of the cervical canal is torn or damaged. However, even in these cases treatment should be withheld for at least six months after childbirth, as the 'pouting' often disappears. Only if it persists beyond this time and leads to a marked vaginal discharge, is cautery needed. The stick cautery is quite useless, and only the electric cautery is of value. The treatment can be given in the doctor's office, but is often best done in hospital under an anaesthetic.

After the cautery of the cervix, the woman will notice that she has a greatly increased quantity of vaginal discharge, often dirty-looking with streaks of blood in the first few days. The discharge is due to the burned area being shed as the cells beneath it make a new lining and push off the old one. The discharge may last for 4 to 6 weeks, but this is normal. At the end of this time, the doctor usually wants to see the patient once again, so that he may inspect the cervix to see how well it has healed.

Vaginal odours

The vagina is self-cleansing, but some women notice that there may be a 'smell'. It is quite normal for the vulva and vagina to have a faint 'odour', just as does the penis, and in general it is quite unnoticeable to other people. However, some women *imagine* that the vaginal odour can be detected by all the passers-by. This is not true, and in fact if a woman bathes each day, the odour will be undetectable. However, the belief of a 'vaginal odour' is encouraged by manufacturers who sell deodorants for 'personal, intimate, feminine freshness', or to give the woman 'day-long protection and a new sense of feminine security'. These sales gimmicks work by making a woman who does not use deodorants feel less feminine and less secure, and appeal to her need for hygiene. In fact, a deodorant works by adding a different smell – usually a perfume – which vanishes in a short time, but inspires the belief that it persists. In general, then, the average girl or woman who bathes each day has no need for vaginal deodorants, but if she wants to spend her money on these unnecessary gimmicks, they are readily, if fairly expensively, available.

Vaginal douching

The use of the vaginal douche for purposes of feminine 'hygiene', to 'remove odour', and immediately after sexual intercourse is a peculiarly American habit, which in recent years has waned in popularity. The idea that the vagina needed washing out was based on false premises, and was connected with the American obsession for personal cleanliness. Whilst it is reasonable and proper to wash the body, including the vulva, daily to remove the accumulated secretions of the sweat glands, the logic of washing out the vagina is less certain. This is because of the vagina's ability to 'cleanse' itself by producing lactic acid. The conclusion must be that there is in general no need for a woman to use vaginal douches, and in fact there is every reason to avoid them.

VENEREAL DISEASES

Venereal diseases are defined as diseases which are transmitted by sexual intercourse. The two traditional venereal diseases have a long history. Gonorrhoea is known to have occurred since ancient times, but syphilis was only introduced in Europe and Asia with the return of Columbus's ships and sailors from the voyage of discovery of America. Except in very rare and special circumstances, the diseases are only spread by sexual intercourse. This means that if a woman develops either syphilis or gonorrhoea, she has caught it from a man who previously caught it from a woman, and so on back in time. Obviously, if promiscuity is reduced, and if men and women fornicate with few partners, or do not have sexual intercourse except with the partner they propose to marry or until after marriage, the spread of the diseases would be limited. Unfortunately, from the viewpoint of control of infection, this ideal situation does not exist, and recently in all countries there has been a rising incidence of the venereal diseases. The causes of this are complex. In part it is due to increasing sexual permissiveness, especially by teenaged women. In part it is due to increased affluence and mobility of people who spend a large amount of time away from their home environment.

Gonorrhoea occurs more frequently than syphilis, and in the

U.S.A. alone it is believed that over 5 million people are infected each year. In a man the disease is diagnosed easily. Within 3 to 5 days of intercourse with an infected woman, or an infected homosexual man, he notices a creamy, purulent discharge from his urethra and finds it hurts him to pass urine. In a woman the same symptoms may occur, when the diagnosis is easy. It is made by taking a specimen of the urethral discharge and looking at it through a microscope after staining the specimen with special dyes. *But over 70 per cent of women who are infected with gonorrhoea have no symptoms*. They act as a 'silent reservoir' for the disease and can transmit gonorrhoea to other men if they are sexually active. The infected man can infect other women. And so it goes on.

Gonorrhoea has more serious consequences for a woman than for a man. The disease may infect the glands at the entrance to her vagina which can swell up forming an abscess. Occasionally, the gonococcus spreads upwards through the uterus to infect the oviducts. This usually occurs during menstruation. Infection of the oviducts is called salpingitis. It is painful, as the oviducts become swollen with pus. And unfortunately if treatment is not given quickly the oviducts may be so damaged that they become kinked and blocked so that the woman can never become pregnant.

Luckily the treatment of gonorrhoea is effective, provided the person seeks help early on in the disease. Penicillin is effective in killing the gonococcus, and its killing power is increased if another drug, called probenecid, is taken at the same time. The usual treatment is for the woman (or the man) to take two tablets of probenecid and to be given an injection of penicillin. She then takes tablets of probenecid 6, 12 and 18 hours later, when she is given a second penicillin injection, and continues to take probenecid every six hours for another two days. A week later, even if she feels well, she must go back for further tests to be made to be sure that she is cured. The tests are repeated each week for two more weeks.

Because of the number of women who have 'silent gonorrhoea', a woman who has three or more sexual partners over a short period of time, would be wise to have smears taken to make sure that none of them has infected her with gonorrhoea. Tiny cottonwool sticks, 'Cotton-buds', are used to take a smear from her urethra and from her cervix. It is a painless procedure.

Syphilis is a more serious condition, and is often hard to detect in a woman. Usually within 14 to 28 days, but sometimes as long as 90 days after sexual intercourse with an infected man, a small sore appears on one of the lips of the vulva (the labia). It is relatively painless, but the labia may become swollen and tender. Usually the sore persists for a few weeks, unless treatment is given, and then disappears. Unfortunately in some infected women the sore, or chancre, may not develop on the labium, but upon the cervix where it is undetected, and only when a faint pink, spotty rash appears on the chest, back and arms does the girl seek medical advice. The rash, if due to syphilis, persists for several weeks, so that a rash which appears and fades over a few days is not due to the disease. However, if a girl develops a pink, spotting rash which lasts for more than 10 days, and if she has had sexual intercourse with more than one man, or even with a man she knows well, it would be wise for her to have a blood test done.

Syphilis carries two dangers to woman unless it is treated. The immediate danger is that when she becomes pregnant, her baby is very likely to develop syphilis whilst still in the womb; the long-term danger is that untreated syphilis causes damage to the nervous system and may lead to madness.

Neither of these two disasters need occur if treatment is obtained early. Syphilis is completely curable if it is treated early in the course of the disease and the infected person follows the directions exactly. Penicillin is given daily by injection for 10–14 days. Following treatment, blood tests for syphilis are made each month for 6 months, and again at 9 and 12 months. If all the tests are negative the person is cured. If the tests become positive a further course of penicillin injections is given.

The sexually transmitted diseases are discussed in greater detail in my book *Sex and V.D.* which you may care to read.

VULVAL ITCHINESS

The skin of the vulval area is particularly sensitive to stimuli, and an itching vulva is a fairly common complaint. If the itch is sufficiently annoying for the woman to seek medical help, she will require proper investigation, as a vulval itch has several causes. Most commonly, it is due to vaginal infection and discharge, or to general diseases such as diabetes or general skin conditions; but in a fairly large number of cases, the itch is an outward sign of an inward frustration, usually of a sexual nature. The itch makes the woman scratch, especially at night; scratching irritates the vulval skin, which causes further itchiness, which causes further scratching, and so on. After careful investigation, the doctor can make a diagnosis and can offer treatment. In this three things need to be known: first, treatment is medical not surgical; secondly, the longer the woman has had the itch before seeking help, the longer it takes to cure; and thirdly, if any cause is found it needs proper treatment, and the patient cannot hope for instant cure. She must be patient and rely upon her doctor.

Chapter 20

An Ounce of Prevention . . .

As most of the diseases which previously killed people in infancy, childhood and adolescence have come under control, the cancers which afflict older people have come under increasing investigation and study. Calculations have been made which show that a woman has a 5 per cent chance of developing cancer of the breast; a 2.7 per cent chance of developing a cancer of the gut; a 2.3 per cent chance of developing cancer of the cervix of the womb; and a 2.0 per cent chance of developing a cancer of the body of the womb. This means that of every 100 females born, 5 will develop cancer of the breast, and 4 will develop cancer of the womb at some time before death. Apart from cancer of the gut, cancer of the genital organs (in which I include the breast) are the most common cancers found in women.

The only sure way to control cancer and to prevent it from killing its host, is to detect it before it has grown very far. Women are luckier than men in this respect, for the breasts and the womb are relatively easily accessible for examination, provided the patient attends for regular periodic check-ups.

The American Cancer Association, in an admirable series of booklets, emphasizes the importance of early detection of cancer, and advises women to consult their doctor immediately if any of the following symptoms or signs appear:

1. Any sore that does not heal quickly, especially about the mouth.
2. Any unusual bleeding or discharge from any natural body opening.
3. Any painless lump, especially in the breasts, lips, tongue or soft tissues.
4. Any persistent indigestion or unexplained weight loss.
5. Any persistent hoarseness or cough or difficulty in swallowing.
6. Any unexplained change in normal bowel habits.

This advice is sensible and timely, and if women followed it, would lead to a reduction in the deaths which occur from cancer. The three signs which may indicate a cancer of the breast or genital tract are: (1) any painless lump in the breast, (2) any unusual bleeding or discharge from the vagina, and (3) a sore or ulcer on the vulva which does not heal quickly. Only by early detection and proper treatment can the fatal outcome of the cancer be prevented. An ounce of prevention is far more valuable than a pound of attempted cure!

CANCER OF THE BREAST

The earliest sign of cancer of the breast is a small, rounded painless lump. Not every lump found in the breast is due to cancer, but every lump is suspect. For this reason, regular self-examination of the breasts is recommended as described in Chapter 18. This self-examination should be supplemented by regular visits to the doctor each year, so that he may also palpate your breasts.

Where facilities exist this annual check may be supplemented by a special X-ray examination of the breasts, called mammography, together with a heat detection test called thermography, if this is available. As the examinations are complicated and expensive, the special tests should be used on women 'at higher risk' for breast cancer. You are 'at higher risk' if anyone in your family has had a breast cancer, especially if this occurred before the age of 40, if you have never been pregnant or have had your first baby after you were 30 years old; if your periods started before the age of 12 or if you menstruated after the age of 50, and if a previous mammogram showed abnormalities. You should also ask for a mammogram if you have very lumpy breasts, as these may prevent your doctor from examining them properly.

The methods are still being evaluated, but the results so far show that mammography and thermography are helpful. Meanwhile every woman should routinely examine her breasts, at monthly intervals, preferably after her menstrual period, during her reproductive years, but equally at monthly intervals after the menopause.

CANCER OF UTERUS: CERVIX AND ENDOMETRIUM

It is unfortunate that by the time cancer of the cervix is visible to the naked eye, it is so far advanced that no matter what treatment is given, one woman in every two will be dead within five years. But if it is detected before it is visible, the disease is 100 per cent curable.

The method used for detection is to take a sample of the cells which cover the cervix. This sample is then fixed in alcohol, and sent to a special cytological laboratory where it is stained with Papanicolaou's stain and examined for 'abnormal cells'. The specimen is called a cervical smear or 'Pap-smear', because Dr. Papanicolaou, who worked in New York, first pointed out that early cancer cells of the cervix were less sticky than normal cells, and were shed (or exfoliated) more readily into the vagina. To take the specimen the doctor inserts a small instrument, called a speculum, into the vagina and looks at the cervix. He then takes a 'scraping' from the cervix using a wooden spatula, similar to that used for depressing the tongue when he wants to look down the throat. He also takes a sample from the upper vagina, and from the canal of the cervix. The whole procedure is quite painless, and the doctor takes the opportunity to do a pelvic examination at the same time to be sure that there is nothing wrong with the uterus or the ovaries.

The pelvic examination and cervical smear should be made twice in the year after the first attendance, and then every one to three years until the woman is 65. The first test is often made when a girl becomes pregnant for the first time, and should certainly be made on every woman who has had sexual intercourse once she reaches the age of 25.

There is evidence that cancer of the cervix is related in some way to sexual intercourse, as the disease is very rare in nuns, and is found most frequently amongst women who have had sexual intercourse in their teens, often with several partners, and have had their first baby before the age of 20. However, by no means every woman with cancer of the cervix has this history. Unfortunately, too, the disease appears to occur more frequently amongst women of the lower socio-economic groups, or more exactly amongst poorer, less educated women. These women are the very ones who do not seek medical care and are reluctant to have routine cervical smears performed.

Any campaign to eliminate cancer of the cervix must include an attempt to get every woman in the area – especially the poor – to have pelvic examinations and cervical smears performed at regular intervals.

The smear is looked at down a microscope by a trained technician and 'abnormal' smears are checked by a qualified doctor. Of every 1,000 smears examined, about 20 will show 'abnormal' cells, and 3 of these will be really worrying. If 'abnormal' cells are found, a further smear is done, and a specimen is taken from the cervix. This specimen may be taken with a tiny punch, after looking at the cervix with a special magnifying instrument called a colposcope. If this instrument is used, the patient does not need an anaesthetic, and the whole procedure can be done without admitting her to hospital. In other cases, the patient does require admission, and a larger piece of the cervix is cut out. This is like coring out an apple, and is called 'conization'. The cervix is stitched and heals easily.

If the pieces of tissue or the 'cone' show very early cancer, treatment is given. Usually if the patient wants to have more children, the cone is sufficient treatment, but if she has completed her family, a hysterectomy is performed. In either case, she will have to continue to attend her doctor after the operation at regular intervals, for further cervical smears. If the tissues show more advanced cancer – and only a very few do – the woman will have to have a much more extensive regimen of radiation therapy or surgery.

Only by regular pelvic examinations and cervical smears will cancer of the cervix be eliminated. Every woman should therefore make sure that she has this simple, painless test done at regular intervals from the time of her first pregnancy or the age of 25, whichever is the earlier, to the age of 65 or later.

The endometrium is the lining of the womb, and cancer can develop in it. It is sometimes called cancer of the body of the womb. Endometrial cancer occurs nearly as frequently as cancer of the cervix, but affects women who are rather older, usually aged between 50 and 60. In recent years an increase in endometrial cancer has been observed. There is some concern that the increase may be due, in part, to the increasing use of oestrogens over long periods to 'keep you young after the menopause' (see p. 363).

Unfortunately 'smear' tests do not readily detect cancer of the body of the womb, and consequently the doctor has to rely on symptoms. Any woman who develops irregular bleeding after the age of 35 should see her doctor. The bleeding is most likely to be due to hormonal changes, but it may be the first sign of cancer of the womb. An even more sinister sign is bleeding which occurs *after* the menopause. However scanty the bleeding is, the woman must see her doctor at once so that he can arrange for a diagnostic curettage if he thinks this is necessary. Luckily cancer of the body of the womb grows very slowly, so that if the woman follows this advice, it is generally curable.

CANCER OF THE VULVA

This is a relatively rare form of cancer found principally in old women and preceded by a vulval itch, usually of long duration. Any elderly woman who has an itchy vulva which persists should seek medical attention. In order to exclude early cancer of the vulval skin, the doctor may need to take tiny pieces of skin. The procedure is done under a local anaesthetic and does not disturb the patient.

CANCER OF THE OVARIES

About 5 per cent of all cancers which develop in women are cancers of the ovaries, and these account for 10 per cent of cancers of the genital tract. In all cases the first sign is enlargement of the ovary, which can be detected on pelvic examination; but 95 per cent of ovarian enlargement is non-cancerous, and only 5 per cent of the enlargements are due to cancer. Cancer is more likely to occur after the age of 40, and particularly likely after the menopause.

Since the growth is silent and slow, the disease is difficult to detect, and the only way is for women aged 40 and over to have periodic pelvic examinations to detect ovarian enlargement. The finding of an enlarged ovary at this age is an indication for surgery, so that the tumour may be removed and examined under the microscope.

Chapter 21

Not the End of Life

At a time which is quite variable and individual for a woman, the remaining egg follicles in the ovary (numbering about 8,000) begin to disappear. This strange and unexplained event occurs some time between the 45th and 55th year of life. The changes are not abrupt, and there is a gradual transition from the normal ovarian activity of the reproductive years, to the relatively inactive ovary of the menopausal years.

The first change in the sequence of events which culminates in the cessation of menstruation, or the menopause, is that the egg follicles in the ovary become increasingly less sensitive to stimulation by the hormones of the pituitary. In addition, there is a change in the quantity of the two pituitary hormones – FSH and LH – which have stimulated the growth of some follicles each month since adolescence. These two changes mean that fewer egg follicles are stimulated, and consequently reduced, but variable, amounts of oestrogen are released during each menstrual cycle. For this reason the lining of the uterus is less satisfactorily stimulated, and the menstrual flow becomes less regular and predictable. The quantity of the blood lost gets less, and the interval between the menstrual periods is usually increased. The co-ordinated control of menstruation, which has been so effective since adolescence, is getting out of gear, as the controlling glands 'unwind' into a quieter phase of life.

As the months pass fewer egg follicles are stimulated and the amount of oestrogen secreted by them diminishes still further, until eventually the menstrual periods cease altogether. The menopause has arrived.

Of course, the sequence may not be so smooth. Some women develop heavy bleeding episodes, as sudden surges of oestrogen occur, followed by long intervals when the menstrual periods are absent. For this is a time of hormonal turbulence, only slightly less than that which occurred at puberty. The whole period of change is more properly called the climacteric, or 'change of life', whilst the ceasing of menstrual periods is called the menopause; but the term menopause is commonly used for both events.

THE CHANGES IN THE BODY

All the changes which occur are due to altered hormone secretion, and result from a fall in oestrogen, an absence of progesterone, and a rise in pituitary hormones. It used to be thought that oestrogen ceased to be produced after the menopause, but now it is known that some continues to be secreted well into old age, but of course the quantity is small.

The main changes which occur in the body of the menopausal woman are due to the diminished secretion of oestrogen. Because oestrogen is most active on the tissues which make up the female genital tract and on the breasts, these are most affected. But because of the continuing but variable amounts of oestrogen secreted, the degree to which they are affected is quite variable.

In the few years before the menopause, the breasts often increase in size as extra fat is deposited; but after the climacteric, this fat is reabsorbed, the gland tissue decreases and the nipples get smaller. These changes take place slowly, but by the age of 65 the breasts are usually flattened and tend to droop. In the same slow manner the uterus, the oviducts and the ovaries become smaller and inactive. The lining wall of the vagina becomes thinner and more easily irritated as the years pass, but this is less likely to occur if sexual intercourse continues to take place. The tissues which surround and support the vagina and the muscles of the floor of the pelvis tend to become flabby, and to lose their elasticity, so that some degree of prolapse may occur. This may be of the front or back wall of the vagina, so that a bulge or lump appears at the vulva when the woman strains; or it may be of the uterus itself, the cervix projecting through the vaginal entrance. The prolapse may look more serious than it really is, because the main lips of the vulva – the labia majora – decrease in size at this time of life. Only a few cases of prolapse give discomfort and need surgery. Most can be left alone. Once again, these changes take place slowly over the years.

MENOPAUSAL SYMPTOMS

More annoying, because they occur earlier and with greater impact, are the 'menopausal symptoms'. Some of these are due to lack of oestrogen, others have not yet been understood completely. In many women the symptoms are minor, and probably no more than one woman in four needs to consult a doctor because of them. Hot flashes, or flushes, may occur, in which a sudden feeling of intense heat sweeps over the body, and a blush spreads over the face and neck. Hot flushes only last a few moments and then go. They tend to recur many times during the day, and are sometimes accompanied by tingling sensations sweeping the body. The hot flushes may be triggered by excitement or emotions, and are the most common menopausal symptoms. They vary in intensity and frequency, but tend to last for months or years, becoming less frequent as time goes by. Almost as common are episodes of sweating, and the onset of irregularities of menstruation. These three symptoms are due to the reduced secretion of oestrogen. Other symptoms which are distressing are depression, insomnia, fatigue, headache and skin changes, but the cause of these is not understood.

PSYCHOLOGICAL CHANGES

Just as the waxing turbulent tides of hormones and the need to adapt to new ways made puberty and adolescence a difficult time, some women find that the waning tides of hormones and the need to adapt to them makes the menopause a difficult time. It is very difficult for doctors to decide if the symptoms of depression, fatigue and insomnia are due to hormonal changes, or to a deep emotional disturbance as the woman looks around and does not like what she sees. Her children are growing up, or have already left the family home; her youthful hopes and desires have dissipated into a routine 'suburban' life; her husband appears to have found other interests, leaving her increasingly alone; her friends have similar problems, and constantly complain about them. She sees these changes, she feels that she has missed something, often a great deal, of what she had imagined life had to offer, and she has to adjust to the strange symptoms of the menopause – or strange to her at any rate. The peculiar irregularity of her periods may subconsciously increase the anxiety that her physical and sexual attractions are waning. She is becoming old, and thinks she is rejected; she has reached the 'end of life'. These vividly felt emotions are, of course, only temporary. Psychiatrists have discovered that many women at the menopause pass through three phases before becoming adjusted to their new life. The first is one in which feelings of anxiety and turmoil are most evident. Usually this period is fairly short and merges into a period which may last months, when irritability, depression and other mood changes are common, and the woman feels rejected by everyone. Nothing is right. In time this phase merges into a phase of readjustment, when all the misery of the previous months seems like a bad dream.

WHAT TO DO AT THE CLIMACTERIC

The first thing for a woman to remember is that the strange feelings which she has are temporary, and that adjustment will come in due course. Women who have interests outside the home find it easier to adjust; but women whose outlook is confined to the house, the backyard, the immediate neighbours and the television set often have problems.

Careful investigations in the U.S.A. and in Britain have shown that about two-thirds of women pass through the 'change of life' without any trouble, or with only a little upset. The remaining one-third need help. Help is available from the family doctor, who knows about the woman and her background. He is particularly well suited to offer sympathetic understanding and the reassurance which is so often needed. He is also able to offer mild sedatives if insomnia is the problem; tranquillizers, if mood changes, irritability and depression are present; or hormones if the hot flushes and sweats are causing the woman concern.

Despite what has been written in many women's magazines, not every woman who seeks medical help at this time needs hormone treatment. If menstruation is still regular and normal in amount, hormones are of little help. Only if the flushes are of such severity or frequency as to cause annoyance are hormones helpful. Oestrogen – which is the hormone usually prescribed – in small doses will control flushings, but it will not rejuvenate the skin, make the hair glisten, put a blush on the cheeks or a sparkle in the eye of the menopausal woman. She can do all these things by her attitude to the 'change of life', and by realizing that it is a *change* and not the end of life.

The dose of oestrogen required to control the number of hot flushes differs, and most doctors try to use the smallest dose needed to regulate them in that particular woman. To help the doctor, the patient is asked to make a 'hot flush count'. She counts the number of hot flushes she gets each day, and the doctor increases or decreases the dose of oestrogen so that she gets no more than five hot flushes a day. This is 'tailoring' the drug to the patient, and is the best way of controlling the symptoms; but sometimes because the patient is impatient or unable to co-operate, the doctor may prescribe 'the Pill' to control hot flushes. This treatment is effective but more expensive, and the woman, of course, will get a return of her periods.

SEXUALITY AFTER THE MENOPAUSE

One of the more insidious myths about a woman's sexuality is that her sexual capacity and sexual desire diminish as she grows older. This is quite untrue; our bodies and minds are capable of sexuality all our lives, from birth to death, but are only capable of reproduction for a part of that time. The idea that only young people enjoy and have the desire for sex is unfair to older women whose sexuality is often enhanced. This is because sexual drive is a learned activity and is not dependent on the sex hormones as some male sexologists believe.

In a U.S. survey of sexuality at and after 'the change of life' it was found that sexual desire and sexual drive were unaltered in 60 per cent of women, 20 per cent had a reduced drive and in 20 per cent sexual desire was increased. Most women enjoy sexual intercourse well into old age, and coitus only ceases because of the death or incapacity of their partner. A few women, who have never really enjoyed sexual intercourse in their youth are not concerned, as they grow older, if coitus becomes less and less frequent. Other women may, for the first time, find a greater sexual fulfilment, either by reaching a new understanding with their partner or with a new partner.

Sexually active older women, with sympathetic partners, report a change in their attitude towards sex. In youth, sex was a rather simplistic, mechanical affair; as the woman grows older she finds that sexual activity has greater variety, a greater subtlety and a greater enjoyment. For many, sex ceases to be mainly genital and expands to include body contact, touching, and hugging, as well as sexual intercourse. Sexuality after the change of life is determined largely by the pattern established in youth: if you have had an active pleasurable sex life when young, you are more likely to have a similarly enjoyable sexual life when you are older.

A woman's sexual potential persists for longer than that of a man, so that any decline is more likely to be due to her partner's failing capacity than her ability to respond. But this can be improved if the partners are willing to try. Studies in the U.S.A. have shown that 7 out of every 10 couples investigated were sexually active after the age of 60, many continuing until their seventies or eighties.

Because women live longer than men and because of the belief that the man should initiate sex, problems do occur. In our society, older women, either single or widowed, have a smaller chance of finding a suitable sexual partner than do older men. This is aggravated by the earlier, erroneous view, that an older woman should not have sexual desires. An older woman, who is single or widowed, should not feel guilty if she has sexual desires. These can be satisfied if she can find a man to whom she can relate.

A woman may feel unable to find a new partner, or does not wish to do so, at least for a while after her husband's death, but still has a powerful sexual drive. She can still enjoy sexuality by masturbating and should feel neither shame nor guilt, nor embarrassment if she does. It is a normal, healthy activity. Studies from the U.S.A. show that older non-married women masturbate twice as frequently as married women of a similar age.

A problem of sexuality in some older women is that intercourse may become painful because the vaginal wall becomes thin and inflamed. This condition is due to a lack of oestrogen, and is easily corrected by the use of tablets of oestrogen placed in the vagina or the use of a vaginal oestrogen cream.

An older woman should not feel embarrassed about showing affection, about cuddling and touching her partner, or about trying different sexual positions. In fact, it may be more than ever necessary for her to encourage her partner to take the initiative in love-making, as some men who have led active sex lives in their youth may have inhibitions about sex as they grow older.

360

POSTMENOPAUSAL BLEEDING

In the years after the menopause, a few women notice that they have a scanty, or more profuse, bloody discharge coming from the vagina. This is an urgent reason for going to consult their doctor. The bleeding may be unimportant, due to the use of oestrogens (which can cause bleeding), or to a vaginal irritation, but in some cases it is caused by cancer of the womb. It is essential to see the doctor as soon as possible after bleeding is discovered. He will examine the woman and almost certainly do a diagnostic curettage and take a cervical smear, so that he may be quite certain that cancer is not present.

GETTING FAT

A woman's weight depends on three things: the disposition to fatness she has inherited from her parents; the amount of food and drink she consumes; and the amount of energy she uses for her activities. She cannot alter her disposition to fatness (and everybody tends to put on a little weight as the years go by), but she can control the other two factors. If she obtains more energy from food and drink than she uses in her daily tasks, the excess will be converted into fat and stored. At the time of the 'change of life' women tend to eat more and to do less, so that their weight increases. Women can avoid excessive weight gain during and after the menopause if they are careful about what they eat, and remember to keep on exercising themselves. This does not mean that the woman needs to do special exercises, although these often help, but that she gardens, goes for walks, plays golf or swims, depending on her inclinations. There is a tendency for women at this time of life to do less housework than formerly, as there is less to do now the family is grown up and helps; to go to more morning tea or coffee parties; to eat cakes more often; and in general to sit around, sometimes thinking, sometimes just sitting. This inertness is a great contributor to the weight gain which occurs at the 'change of life'. It can be avoided if a woman puts her mind to it. Obesity is discussed further in Chapter 19.

'A PILL A DAY KEEPS AGEING AT BAY'

In the past decade, particularly in the U.S.A., there has been considerable discussion about the value of continuing oestrogen tablets long after the need for them for contraception, or to cope with the hot flushes of the climacteric, has passed. Those doctors who believe in oestrogens claim that a daily oestrogen tablet keeps the woman younger and more feminine, prevents the development of heart disease and 'thinning' of the bones, and retards the changes which occur in the tissues of the genital tract. With this belief, they prescribe a daily oestrogen pill until old age. Apart from the expense of such medicines, there is a considerable opinion that they are not necessary, and may be dangerous. Firstly oestrogens continue to be secreted by certain glands in the body after the menopause, and at least one woman in every two is producing sufficient to keep her genital tract tissues supple and well-developed. Secondly, there is no evidence that oestrogen keeps a woman younger or more feminine, that it prevents heart disease, or that it hinders the 'thinning' of the structure of the bones. Third, there is increasing evidence that the use of oestrogen for a long period of time, perhaps more than 12 months, predisposes certain susceptible women to the development of cancer of the uterus. But because so much has been written in women's magazines, this matter needs to be discussed further.

Youth and oestrogen

Women (and men!) have for centuries sought the elixir of youth – a drug which would keep them young for longer. Sensational claims have been made from time to time, that this or that drug delayed the onset of ageing, and more particularly rejuvenated sexual vigour. All of them are fraudulent. In the 1920s it was claimed that 'monkey glands' helped. More recently a secret formula made in Rumania, and known to contain a local anaesthetic, procaine, amongst other ingredients, and an extract of the queen bee, has been claimed to be a potent rejuvenator. None of them have fulfilled their claims, nor can the more sophisticated method of injections of fetal cells developed in Switzerland be said to be effective, at least not when looked at scientifically. The suggestion that oestrogen tablets taken daily will enable a woman to retain her youth is equally fallacious. There is no 'Venus Pill' which will keep a woman eternally youthful. Oestrogen will improve the character of the lining tissues of the uterus and vagina if they are defective, but it will do no more. It will not get rid of wrinkles, eliminate a double chin, a sagging breast or an obese abdomen. It will not restore youth. The real hope for women who are growing old is to adjust to the menopausal years, to keep good physical and mental health, to avoid over-eating and under-exercising, and to cultivate new and challenging interests.

Heart disease and oestrogens

For a while it was thought that oestrogen tablets would delay or reduce heart disease, as it had been found that women under the age of 40, who presumably secreted a good amount of oestrogen, had 20 times less risk of developing heart disease compared with men of the same age. Between the ages of 50 and 60, the difference became far less, and the incidence of heart disease in women was only half that of men. This suggested that oestrogens protected the younger woman, and if oestrogen was given in tablet form after the menopause, the protection would continue. However, most of the evidence from carefully conducted research shows that this is not so, and the most effective way to prevent heart attacks is not for postmenopausal women to take oestrogen tablets, but to avoid overeating, to stop smoking and to keep exercising. A daily swim, or a walk, is a far better preventive of heart disease than an oestrogen pill.

Osteoporosis and oestrogens

Thinning of the bone structure, or osteoporosis, is a strange condition which disables about one woman in every five who is aged more than 65. It occasionally occurs in younger women who have had their ovaries surgically removed before the age of 40. The bones of the back (the vertebrae) are first affected and collapse, so that severe backache and later a decrease in height occur. Because of these findings, it was suggested that the condition was due to a lack of oestrogen, but this failed to explain why men, who have very little oestrogen, did not develop the disease more often. It is unlikely that a lack of oestrogen is the cause, so that a daily oestrogen pill will not prevent the disease, although *large* doses of oestrogen together with calcium improves the lot of the woman who develops osteoporosis. A far better preventive measure is to make sure that the diet contains sufficient calcium, and that the woman takes sufficient exercise.

Oestrogens and uterine cancer

Disturbing reports have come from the U.S.A. which suggests that the routine use of oestrogens, at the time of the change of life, to replace the declining oestrogen from the ovaries, may increase a woman's risk of getting endometrial cancer. If oestrogens are taken for more than one but less than three years the risk is five times that compared with a woman who has taken oestrogens for less than one year. If she takes the 'Venus Pill' for more than three years the risk goes up to ten times the risk if she had taken no oestrogens or had only taken them for short periods.

The lesson seems clear: oestrogens should only be taken for short periods at the menopause and then only to treat hot flushes or a painful vagina.

Oestrogens and statistics

The further myth about oestrogens and ageing is based on false statistics. It is known that 75 years ago the life expectancy of women was only 50 years. This meant that at birth the average woman might expect to live 50 years. Today the life expectancy is 74. This observation suggested that 75 years ago women were born, grew up, had children, reached the menopause and died – 'exploding like sky-rockets without trace' as one writer has said. Today, however, women live longer, and have twenty or more years of life after the menopause without the oestrogen 'support' which had existed earlier. Therefore, it was said, oestrogen tablets were needed to help women 'resist the ageing process' and 'to make the postmenopausal woman's world a better place' – as the pharmaceutical companies who sell oestrogens claim in their advertisement.

Alas, the statistics quoted so often are false. The increase in life expectancy has occurred because the deaths in infancy, childhood and adolescence from infectious diseases have been greatly reduced. In 1900 a woman who reached the age of 25 could expect to live until she was 68. Today she may expect to live until she is 74, so that the difference is not all that great. There are, of course, more older women alive today because there are more people in the world, and because fewer children and girls die before they reach adult life.

Today about 10 per cent of women are aged 65 or over, and in the year 2,000, the same proportion is expected. This is indeed a considerable proportion of the population. Their needs for recreation, for exercise, for social intercourse, for a place in society and in the family will require careful consideration, but to say that in the past women did not live after the menopause is nonsense. Many did, and managed very well without a daily oestrogen tablet!

Oestrogens and the ageing vagina

It is true that if a woman develops a vaginal irritation or finds sexual intercourse painful, the cause may be thinning of the vaginal lining because of deficient oestrogen. This only affects a few post-menopausal women, and is easily corrected by the application into the vagina of a cream containing oestrogen. The use of oestrogen in this way is very sensible and medically correct, whilst its routine use for all women is expensive and ridiculous. It may also be potentially dangerous. There is now some evidence that oestrogens given by mouth or by injection may increase the chance of a woman developing clots in her blood vessels, and as such mishaps are much more common in older women, it is an additional reason for avoiding the routine use of oestrogen tablets.

To be more scientific, some doctors only prescribe oestrogen tablets if a smear taken from the wall of the vagina and examined under a microscope shows a pattern of cells suggesting an oestrogen lack. The approach is more rational, but is still inexact, and it would be better to avoid oestrogens in the postmenopausal years unless there are symptoms which are due to oestrogen deficiency.

GROWING OLD GRACEFULLY

The menopause is only a milestone on a woman's path through life. If she is well adjusted, or becomes well adjusted after receiving medical help, she will pass through the turbulent years, her character unimpaired. She will be ready to meet the excitement and the challenges of the postmenopausal years. Years which can be as full of interest as any other period of life, provided she herself makes sure that they are. She is growing old gracefully. Not ageing, but growing old, for ageing suggests something sinister, the result of unwise or improvident living, and the abuse of the human machine. Growing old begins at the moment of birth, and continues until death. The menopause is but a milestone along the road, and the 'change of life' is not the end of life.

There can be no more appropriate note on which to end a book about 'Everywoman'.

Glossary

Alveoli (pron. Al-*vee*-o-li)
The plural of alveolus, which means a small cavity. The outermost parts of the duct system of the breast, where milk is secreted, are called alveoli.

Amenorrhoea (pron. a-men-or-*e*-a)
The absence of menstruation for an interval twice that (or more) of the patient's usual menstrual cycle.

Amniotic fluid
The fluid in the 'bag of waters' (or the amniotic sac) in which the fetus grows.

Amniocentesis
The procedure of introducing a narrow needle through the abdominal wall into the amniotic sac to obtain a sample of the amniotic fluid.

Analgesic
A pain-relieving drug.

Antenatal period
The period between conception and childbirth. Also called the prenatal period.

Aphrodisiac
A drug or substance which increases sexual desire.

Areola (pron. aree-*o*-la)
The brownish-coloured pigmented area which surrounds the nipple.

Bacillus
A small form of life, made up of a single cell shaped like a tiny rod, often called a germ. Germs may be harmful to man, for example the pneumococcus which causes pneumonia, and the streptococcus which causes sore throats; or they may be helpful, as the lactobacillus which lives in the vagina.

Coitus (pron. *ko*-it-us)
The act of sexual intercourse, or copulation. The verb is 'to copulate'.

Coitus interruptus
Coitus in which the penis is withdrawn from the vagina before male orgasm, and the semen is ejaculated externally to the vagina.

Conception sac
The embryo (or fetus) contained in the fluid-filled amniotic membranes is called the conception sac.

Copulate
To practise sexual intercourse.

Eclampsia
The occurrence of convulsions or fits in a pregnant woman who has other signs of 'toxaemia of pregnancy'.

Ejaculate
To spurt out. Applied in this context to the spurting out of semen at the time of orgasm.

Embryo (pron. *em*-bry-o)
The product of conception (or conceptus) from the day of fertilization of the egg cell (ovum) by the spermatozoon until the beginning of the 7th week. During this short period almost all of the major structures have formed.

'Eye' of the penis
The part of the end of the penis through which the urinary tube passes to reach the outside.

Fetus (pron. *fee*-tus)
The product of conception from the end of the 7th week until birth, at whatever period of the pregnancy this may be, is called a fetus.

FSH
Follicle-stimulating hormone. The substance secreted by the pituitary gland which lies beneath the brain. This hormone stimulates some of the egg follicles of the ovary to manufacture oestrogen.

Gestagen
A synthetic – man-made – substance which acts in the body in a way similar to the natural hormone, progesterone.

Heterosexual
A person whose sexual affections are directed to a person of the other sex.

Homosexual
A noun (i.e. a person is called a homosexual) or an adjective (i.e. a homosexual act) implying that the object of a person's sexual desire is of the same sex. In slang, the male homosexual is called a fairy, a pansy, a queen or a queer, while a female homosexual is referred to as a dike or a butch. Butch is also used as an adjective to describe a female homosexual who displays outward manifestations of masculinity in behaviour or in dress.

Hormone
A substance which is released from special glands into the blood stream and stimulates other glands or tissues into activity.

Lactation
Suckling. The period when the child is nourished from the breast. It also means the secretion or formation of milk.

Lanugo
The downy delicate hair which is found on the body of the fetus. It is replaced after birth by rather thicker hair.

Lesbian
A female homosexual.

LH
Luteinising hormone. The second of the pituitary gonadotrophic, or ovary-stimulating, hormones. It converts the cells of the stimulated egg follicle, from which the egg has been expelled by ovulation, to produce the female sex hormone, progesterone. The cells which produce progesterone become bright yellow (for which the Latin word is '*luteus*'), hence luteinising hormone.

Lochia
The discharge from the uterus which lasts for about 4 weeks after childbirth. For the first few days it is profuse and red, later becoming pale and scanty.

Masturbation
The mechanical stimulation, usually with the hands or fingers, of the penis, the clitoris or other erogenous zones of the body leading to orgasm.

Menarche (pron. men-*ar*-kee)
The time of onset of the first menstrual period.

Menstrual cycle
The interval of time from the start of one menstruation (the 'period') to the next. It includes the time during which bleeding occurs and the interval between bleeding episodes.

Monilia
A fungus infection of the vagina, also called *candidosis*; and *vaginal thrush*.

Oedema (pron. *e-de*ma)
Swelling of the tissues under the skin due to retention of water in these tissues.

Oestrogen (pron. *ee*-strogen)
The female sex hormone manufactured in the ovary, and in pregnancy in the placenta. The word derives from *oestrous*, or heatmaking, because the hormone was found to be necessary to bring animals 'on heat'.

Orgasm
Intense excitement occurring at the climax of sexual intercourse culminating in involuntary jerking movement of the pelvis, a feeling of warmth, well-being and release, and followed by a feeling of relaxation. In the male it is accompanied by the ejaculation, or spurting out, of semen from the penis.

Ovum
The egg cell, which has matured and is ready to be expelled from the ovary, is called the ovum.

Partogram
A graphic display of the progress of labour.

Peer-group
Individuals of approximately the same age and similar social values who form groups.

Penis
The male sexual organ. Normally it lies soft and limp, but during sexual stimulation it becomes erect. Erections may occur spontaneously at night during sleep, after visual stimuli from magazines, from the sight of sexually-desirable girls, or during the preliminaries of love-making. Erection is not under the control of the mind.

Perineum
The area between the thighs which contains the entrance to the vagina and the other female external genitals, which comprise the vulva.

Pica
A longing to eat substances which are not foods, such as clay or coal.

Progesterone (pron. pro-*gest*-erone)
The second main sex hormone produced by the ovaries. The hormone prepares the body, especially the uterus, for pregnancy. Progesterone is also manufactured by the placenta from its earliest days.

Promiscuity
A girl may be considered promiscuous if she has sexual intercourse with several casual acquaintances over a short period of time. Premarital coitus with a single partner is not promiscuity.

Prophylactic treatment
Treatment, usually with drugs, given to prevent the onset or spread of disease.

Psychosomatic disorder
A condition in which a disturbed emotion manifests itself as a disorder of one part of the body or another, and mimics disease of that part.

Puerperium
The period between childbirth and the time when the uterus has returned to its normal size, which is about 6 to 8 weeks.

Regimen
A specific course or plan of diet or drugs to maintain or improve health, or regulate the way of life.

Renal tract
See urinary tract.

Reproductive years, or era
The years during which a woman is ovulating, or able to ovulate, and so is able to have a baby. It is the time when the female sex hormones are regularly and rhythmically produced by the ovaries.

Semen
The fluid ejaculated by the male at orgasm. It consists of spermatozoa, mixed with secretions from the ducts and collecting areas which link the testicles (where the spermatozoa are manufactured) and the penis (from which the semen is ejaculated).

Sexual drive
The desire to have sex. It varies in strength in different people and at different ages of the same person. Probably everyone starts with the same sexual drive but the differences found are due to inhibitions

about sex produced by parental attitudes to sex and those of peer-groups.

Speculum
A small metal instrument, made like a duck's bill which a doctor introduces into a woman's vagina so that he can see her cervix.

'Toxaemia of pregnancy'
A rise of blood pressure occurring in pregnancy, usually associated with the appearance of protein in the urine, is called 'toxaemia of pregnancy'. The term, although convenient, is inexact because no toxin has been found.

Urinary tract
The kidneys, the tubes which connect the kidneys to the bladder (called the ureters), the urinary bladder, and the tube between the bladder and the vulva (called the urethra) form the renal tract. It is also called the urinary tract.

Zona pellucida
The strong translucent outer membrane which surrounds the human egg, rather as the shell surrounds a hen's egg. The zona pellucida only disappears when the fertilized egg reaches the uterine cavity after spending three days in the oviduct.

Further Reading

You may wish to supplement (or confirm!) what you have read in this book with other readings. The following list may help you. Much of the material in *Everywoman* is based on that found in my three textbooks for medical students, doctors and nurses.

Fundamentals of Obstetrics and Gynaecology Vol. 1 Obstetrics (2nd edition 1977) Faber and Faber, London.

Fundamentals of Obstetrics and Gynaecology Vol. 2 Gynaecology (2nd edition 1978) Faber and Faber, London.

Human Reproduction and Society (1974) Faber and Faber, London.

Chapters 3 and 4
Money, J. & Ehrhardt, A. A. (1972). *Man & Woman, Boy & Girl*, Johns Hopkins University Press, Baltimore.

Chapters 4 and 5
Brecher, E. (1969). *The Sex Researchers*, Little, Brown and Co., Boston.
Hite, S. (1976). *The Hite Report: a nationwide study of female sexuality*, Collier-Macmillan, London.
Masters, W. & Johson, V. (1966). *The Human Sexual Response*, Little, Brown & Co. Boston.

Chapter 7
Llewellyn-Jones, D. (1975). *People Populating*, Faber and Faber, London.

Chapters 8–17
Kitzinger, Sheila (1970). *The Experience of Childbirth*, Pelican, London.

Leboyer, F. (1975). *Birth Without Violence*, Wildwood House, London.

Pearce, Caroline (1976). Newsletter, Nursing Mothers of Australia Journal, 12 April.

Chapter 18
Jolly, H (1976). *The Book of Child Care*, Allen & Unwin, London.
Phillip, V. (1976). *Successful Breast Feeding,* Nursing Mothers Association, Australia.

Chapter 19
Boston Health Collective, (2nd edition 1976). *Our Bodies, Ourselves*, Simon & Schuster, New York.

INDEX